Hematopathology

Editor

YURI FEDORIW

SURGICAL PATHOLOGY CLINICS

www.surgpath.theclinics.com

Consulting Editor

JASON L. HORNICK

March 2016 • Volume 9 • Number 1

ELSEVIER

1600 John F. Kennedy Boulevard • Suite 1800 • Philadelphia, Pennsylvania, 19103-2899

http://www.theclinics.com

SURGICAL PATHOLOGY CLINICS Volume 9, Number 1
March 2016 ISSN 1875-9181, ISBN-13: 978-0-323-41667-2

Editor: Lauren Boyle
Developmental Editor: Donald Mumford

Surgical Pathology Clinics (ISSN 1875-9181) is published quarterly by Elsevier Inc., 360 Park Avenue South, New York, NY 10010. Months of issue are March, June, September, and December. Business and Editorial Office: Elsevier Inc., 1600 John F. Kennedy Blvd., Ste. 1800, Philadelphia, PA 19103-2899. Accounting and Circulation Offices: Elsevier Inc., 3251 Riverport Lane, Maryland Heights, MO 63043. Periodicals postage paid at New York, NY and at additional mailing offices. Subscription prices are $200.00 per year (US individuals), $263.00 per year (US institutions), $100.00 per year (US students/residents), $250.00 per year (Canadian individuals), $300.00 per year (Canadian Institutions), $250.00 per year (foreign individuals), $300.00 per year (foreign institutions), and $120.00 per year (international & Canadian students/residents). Foreign air speed delivery is included in all *Clinics'* subscription prices. All prices are subject to change without notice. **POSTMASTER:** Send address changes to *Surgical Pathology Clinics*, Elsevier, 3251 Riverport Lane, Maryland Heights, MO 63043. **Customer Service: 1-800-654-2452 (US). From outside the United States, call 1-314-447-8871. Fax: 1-314-447-8029. E-mail: JournalsCustomerServiceusa@elsevier.com (for print support) and JournalsOnlineSupport-usa@elsevier.com (for online support).**

Reprints. For copies of 100 or more, of articles in this publication, please contact the Commercial Reprints Department, Elsevier Inc., 360 Park Avenue South, New York, NY 10010-1710. Tel. 212-633-3874; Fax: 212-633-3820; E-mail: reprints@elsevier.com.

Surgical Pathology Clinics of North America is covered in *MEDLINE/PubMed (Index Medicus)*.

Contributors

CONSULTING EDITOR

JASON L. HORNICK, MD, PhD
Director of Surgical Pathology, Director,
Immunohistochemistry Laboratory, Brigham
and Women's Hospital, Associate Professor of
Pathology, Harvard Medical School, Boston,
Massachusetts

EDITOR

YURI FEDORIW, MD
Associate Professor of Pathology and
Laboratory Medicine, Director of
Hematopathology, University of North
Carolina, Chapel Hill, North Carolina

AUTHORS

NATHANAEL G. BAILEY, MD
Assistant Professor, Division of
Hematopathology, Department of Pathology,
University of Michigan, Ann Arbor, Michigan

AMIR BEHDAD, MD
Division of Hematopathology, Assistant
Professor, Department of Pathology,
Northwestern Memorial Hospital,
Northwestern University, Feinberg School of
Medicine, Chicago, Illinois

CHRISTINE E. BOOKHOUT, MD
Resident, Department of Pathology and
Laboratory Medicine, University of North
Carolina, Chapel Hill, North Carolina

DAVID R. CZUCHLEWSKI, MD
Associate Professor, Department of Pathology,
University of New Mexico, Albuquerque,
New Mexico

AHMET DOGAN, MD, PhD
Chief, Hematopathology Service, Department
of Pathology and Laboratory Medicine,
Memorial Sloan Kettering Cancer Center,
New York, New York

YURI FEDORIW, MD
Associate Professor of Pathology and
Laboratory Medicine, Director of
Hematopathology, University of North
Carolina, Chapel Hill, North Carolina

CHARLES M. HARMON, MD
Department of Pathology, University of
Michigan Hospitals and Health Systems, Ann
Arbor, Michigan

ROBERT P. HASSERJIAN, MD
Associate Professor, Department of
Pathology, Massachusetts General Hospital,
Harvard Medical School, Boston,
Massachusetts

ERIC D. HSI, MD
Chair, Department of Laboratory Medicine,
Robert J. Tomsich Pathology and Laboratory
Medicine Institute, Cleveland Clinic, Cleveland,
Ohio

K. DAVID LI, MD
Assistant Professor, Hematopathology,
Department of Pathology, University of Utah/
ARUP Laboratories, Salt Lake City, Utah

LAWRENCE K. LOW, MD, PhD
Clinical Instructor, Department of Pathology,
City of Hope National Medical Center, Duarte,
California

STEPHANIE P. MATHEWS, MD
Assistant Professor, Division of
Hematopathology, Department of Pathology
and Laboratory Medicine, University of North
Carolina School of Medicine, Chapel Hill, North
Carolina

NATHAN D. MONTGOMERY, MD, PhD
Hematopathology Fellow, Division of
Hematopathology, Department of
Pathology and Laboratory Medicine,
University of North Carolina School of
Medicine, Chapel Hill, North Carolina

VALENTINA NARDI, MD
Instructor; Assistant Pathologist, Department
of Pathology, Massachusetts General Hospital,
Harvard Medical School, Boston,
Massachusetts

HORATIU OLTEANU, MD, PhD
Associate Professor, Department of Pathology,
Medical College of Wisconsin, Milwaukee,
Wisconsin

SARAH L. ONDREJKA, DO
Associate Staff, Department of Laboratory
Medicine, Robert J. Tomsich Pathology and
Laboratory Medicine Institute, Cleveland
Clinic, Cleveland, Ohio

LoANN C. PETERSON, MD
Professor, Department of Pathology,
Northwestern University Feinberg School of
Medicine, Chicago, Illinois

KAAREN K. REICHARD, MD
Associate Professor of Pathology, Chair,
Division of Hematopathology, Department of
Laboratory Medicine and Pathology, Mayo
Clinic, Rochester, Minnesota

MARIAN A. ROLLINS-RAVAL, MD, MPH
Assistant Professor, Department of
Pathology and Laboratory Medicine,
University of North Carolina, Chapel Hill,
North Carolina

MOHAMED E. SALAMA, MD
Professor, Hematopathology, Department
of Pathology, University of Utah/ARUP
Laboratories, Salt Lake City, Utah

LAUREN B. SMITH, MD
Department of Pathology, University of
Michigan Hospitals and Health Systems, Ann
Arbor, Michigan

JOO Y. SONG, MD
Assistant Professor, Department of Pathology,
City of Hope National Medical Center, Duarte,
California

ADAM J. WOOD, DO
Division of Hematopathology, Department of
Laboratory Medicine and Pathology, Mayo
Clinic, Rochester, Minnesota

MINA L. XU, MD
Department of Pathology and Laboratory
Medicine, Yale University School of Medicine,
New Haven, Connecticut

Contents

> As the cost of health care continues to rise and reimbursement rates decrease, there
> is a growing demand and need to cut overall costs, enhance quality of services, and
> maintain as a top priority the needs and safety of the patient. In this article, we pro-
> vide an introduction to test utilization and outline a general approach to creating an
> efficient, cost-effective test utilization strategy. We also present and discuss 2 test
> utilization algorithms that are evidence-based and may be of clinical utility as we
> move toward the future of doing the necessary tests at the right time.

> B-cell non-Hodgkin lymphomas with plasmacytic differentiation are a diverse group
> of entities with extremely variable morphologic features. Diagnostic challenges can
> arise in differentiating lymphoplasmacytic lymphoma from marginal zone lymphoma
> and other low-grade B-cell lymphomas. In addition, plasmablastic lymphomas can
> be difficult to distinguish from diffuse large B-cell lymphoma or other high-grade
> lymphomas. Judicious use of immunohistochemical studies and molecular testing
> can assist in appropriate classification.

> Follicular lymphoma is a far more heterogeneous entity than originally appreciated.
> Clinical and biological variants are increasingly more granularly defined, expanding
> the spectrum of disease. Some variants associate with age, whereas others with
> anatomic site. Identification of these biologically distinct diseases has real prog-
> nostic and predictive value for patients today and likely will be more relevant in
> the future. Understanding of follicular lymphoma precursors has also made their
> identification both scientifically and clinically relevant. This review summarizes the
> features and understanding of follicular lymphoma, variants, and precursor lesions.

> High-grade B-cell lymphomas (HGBCLs) are a heterogeneous group of neoplasms
> that include subsets of diffuse large B-cell lymphoma, Burkitt lymphoma, and
> lymphomas with features intermediate between diffuse large B-cell lymphoma and
> Burkitt lymphoma. Morphologically indistinguishable HGBCLs may demonstrate
> variable clinical courses and responses to therapy. The morphologic evaluation and
> classification of these neoplasms must be followed by further genetic and immuno-
> phenotypic work-up. These additional diagnostic modalities lead to a comprehensive

Immunoglobulin G4–related lymphadenopathy (IgG4-RLAD) occurs in the setting of extranodal IgG4-related disease (IgG4-RD), an immune-mediated process described in many organ systems characterized by lymphoplasmacytic infiltrates with abundant IgG4-positive plasma cells and fibrosis. Although the morphologic features in the lymph node sometimes resemble those seen at the extranodal sites, 5 microscopic patterns have been described, most of which resemble reactive lymphoid hyperplasia. This morphologic variability leads to unique diagnostic challenges and a broad differential diagnosis. As IgG4-RD may be exquisitely responsive to steroids or other immunotherapy, histologic recognition and inclusion of IgG4-RLAD in the differential diagnosis is vital.

Nodal-based peripheral T-cell lymphomas are heterogeneous malignancies with overlapping morphology and clinical features. However, the current World Health Organization classification scheme separates these tumors into prognostically relevant categories. Since its publication, efforts to uncover the gene expression profiles and molecular alterations have subdivided these categories further, and distinct subgroups are emerging with specific profiles that reflect the cell of origin for these tumors and their microenvironment. Identification of the perturbed biologic pathways may prove useful in selecting patients for specific therapies and associating biomarkers with survival and relapse.

Cytogenetic analysis of acute myeloid leukemia (AML) and myelodysplastic syndrome (MDS) is essential for disease diagnosis, classification, prognostic stratification, and treatment guidance. Molecular genetic analysis of *CEBPA*, *NPM1*, and *FLT3* is already standard of care in patients with AML, and mutations in several additional genes are assuming increasing importance. Mutational analysis of certain genes, such as *SF3B1*, is also becoming an important tool to distinguish subsets of MDS that have different biologic behaviors. It is still uncertain how to optimally combine karyotype with mutation data in diagnosis and risk-stratification of AML and MDS, particularly in cases with multiple mutations and/or several mutationally distinct subclones.

The forthcoming update of the World Health Organization (WHO) classification of hematopoietic neoplasms will feature "Myeloid Neoplasms with Germline Predisposition" as a new provisional diagnostic entity. This designation will be applied to some cases of acute myeloid leukemia and myelodysplastic syndrome arising in the setting of constitutional mutations that render patients susceptible to the development of myeloid malignancies. For the diagnostic pathologist, recognizing these cases and confirming the diagnosis will demand a sophisticated grasp of clinical genetics and molecular techniques. This article presents a concise review of this new provisional WHO entity, including strategies for clinical practice.

K. David Li and Mohamed E. Salama

This article highlights the most common morphologic features identified in the bone marrow after chemotherapy for hematologic malignancies, growth-stimulating agents, and specific targeted therapies. The key is to be aware of these changes while reviewing post-therapeutic bone marrow biopsies and to not mistake reactive patterns for neoplastic processes. In addition, given the development and prevalent use of targeted therapy, such as tyrosine kinase inhibitors and immune modulators, knowledge of drug-specific morphologic changes is required for proper bone marrow interpretation and diagnosis.

SURGICAL PATHOLOGY CLINICS

Preface

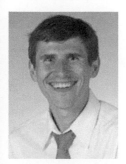

Yuri Fedoriw, MD
Editor

The practice of pathology, and ultimately the care of patients, is becoming more dependent on specialized techniques. While in-house testing for the vast array of available diagnostic, prognostic, and predictive markers is not possible at every institution or practice, awareness of their applicability and impact on patient care is the responsibility of both the pathologist and the treating clinician. This is particularly true in an era when patients are increasingly knowledgeable about genomic and proteomic analyses and these studies are easily accessible. This issue of *Surgical Pathology Clinics* aims to address select areas of hematopathology, highlight concepts that shape our practice, and underscore the expanding role of the pathologist as a consultant. Some reviews that follow discuss approaches to common diagnostic challenges, including evaluation of low-grade lymphomas, transformation, and lymphoproliferations rich in IgG$_4$-positive plasma cells. Others describe how evolving insights into disease pathogenesis are being rapidly applied to the care of patients with both myeloid and lymphoid diseases. Also included is a review on laboratory test utilization and management principles related specifically to hematopathology. Importantly, as the costs associated with testing increase in the face of diminishing reimbursement, constant re-evaluation of the diagnostic process is necessary. The presented concepts are widely applicable in diagnostic practice, and the authors hope that the reviews prove enlightening and serve as a useful resource.

Yuri Fedoriw, MD
University of North Carolina School of Medicine
Department of Pathology and Laboratory Medicine
NC Cancer Hospital C3162-D
101 Manning Drive
Chapel Hill, NC 27599, USA

E-mail address:
yuri.fedoriw@unchealth.unc.edu

Surgical Pathology 9 (2016) xi
http://dx.doi.org/10.1016/j.path.2016.01.001
1875-9181/16/$ – see front matter © 2016 Published by Elsevier Inc.

Laboratory Test Utilization Management
General Principles and Applications in Hematopathology

Kaaren K. Reichard, MD*, Adam J. Wood, DO

KEYWORDS

- Test utilization • Clinical value • Guidelines • Algorithms • Infrastructure • Multidisciplinary
- Intervention • Strategy

ABSTRACT

As the cost of health care continues to rise and reimbursement rates decrease, there is a growing demand and need to cut overall costs, enhance quality of services, and maintain as a top priority the needs and safety of the patient. In this article, we provide an introduction to test utilization and outline a general approach to creating an efficient, cost-effective test utilization strategy. We also present and discuss 2 test utilization algorithms that are evidence-based and may be of clinical utility as we move toward the future of doing the necessary tests at the right time.

Key Features

- Test utilization is a strategy for performing appropriate laboratory and pathology testing with the goal of providing high-quality, cost-effective patient care.
- Test utilization is important for good patient care and good medical practice, and there is an economic demand for it.
- Test utilization is a complex issue: a good approach is likely multifaceted with a multidisciplinary effort.
- Pathologists should assume a leadership role in test utilization given their training experience in laboratory testing, and administrative and managerial skills.

OVERVIEW

The explosive growth of medical knowledge, imaging and technologies, access to medical care, and laboratory tests has led to a vast array of diverse information for medical practitioners to know and manage. As a result, practitioners may have difficulty efficiently navigating the enormous assortment of testing options thereby leading to medical testing overuse, misuse, and/or underuse.[1,2] Adding further to any potential confusion about which test(s) is/are the right one(s) to order, is that laboratories often set up tests without much help or guidance provided to the ordering individual as to which tests provide what information regarding a certain disease process. From a laboratory perspective, an opportunity therefore exists to collaborate with our clinical colleagues and share our collective expertise with regard to which tests might not be necessary and which tests might be necessary.[3]

There are 2 fundamental components that underlie a laboratory test utilization management

Disclosure: The authors do not have any commercial or financial conflicts of interest as well as any funding sources.

Division of Hematopathology, Department of Laboratory Medicine and Pathology, Mayo Clinic, 200 First Street Southwest, Rochester, MN 55905, USA

* Corresponding author. Division of Hematopathology, Department of Laboratory Medicine and Pathology, Mayo Clinic, 200 First Street Southwest, Hilton 8-00C, Rochester, MN 55905.

E-mail address: reichard.kaaren@mayo.edu

Surgical Pathology 9 (2016) 1–10
http://dx.doi.org/10.1016/j.path.2015.10.002

program: founding principles and an implementation strategy. A high-level overview of test utilization principles and strategies for implementation comprises the first half of this article. The second half provides 2 evidence-based, data-driven examples of test utilization practice in the discipline of hematopathology.

TEST UTILIZATION MANAGEMENT PRINCIPLES

Test utilization management principles are key and vital components of the current and future success of the practice of medicine. Three basic principles supporting a test utilization approach include good patient care, sound medical practice, and economic demand. Importantly, these principles resonate not only with 1 or 2 medical specialties but rather with and influence all clinical medicine disciplines (Box 1).

Good patient care is an essential tenet of an optimal test utilization practice. The needs of each individual patient come first, and as good stewards of health care, all those involved in health care delivery aim to "above all, do no harm." From the perspective of the laboratory, we aim to do the right test, at the right time, for the right patient and obtain the right result.[4] By embracing and adhering to this principle, one reduces unnecessary testing and saves time. Additionally, potential pitfalls of equivocal or false-positive results that could result in unnecessary additional tests or incorrect patient management are avoided.

There are many factors that constitute sound medical practice, including physician and other health care worker competency, practicing with standard-of-care principles and knowledge, working honestly and with integrity, and respecting all individuals involved in medical care. The test utilization component of good medical practice comes from the perspective of practicing competently and using diagnostic testing modalities correctly and judiciously. Laboratory professionals take pride in knowing the value they provide by performing and accurately reporting the right tests for each individual patient. It has been stated that more than 50% of medical decisions are made based on laboratory results; thus, it is imperative

that the right tests are being performed and that the unnecessary tests are not.[5,6]

With the continued economic challenges in health care, decreasing reimbursements, and limited resources, a test utilization strategy, as part of overall patient care management, is not just a reality but a necessity. Every year the annual cost of health care in the United States continues to increase. This is due, in part, to the increased cost of laboratory testing in general, but unnecessary, overused, and duplicative testing are also significant contributing factors.[1,6–9] Thus, there is a growing economic need for reforming current test ordering/utilization practices and embracing a test utilization management plan. As overall reimbursement rates continue to drop and the fee-for-service payment model shifts to a bundled payment model, any testing that is performed will be a cost to the laboratory. Therefore, bundled tests with increased operating costs may not be financially sustainable. As such, these options will force the laboratory to move to a cost-cutting/saving test utilization model so as to perform as efficiently and effectively as possible.[4] A targeted testing approach for each patient/disease entity will result in decreased, out-of-pocket expenses for the patient whose testing charges are not covered by a health insurance company, and decreased costs and improved efficiency for the laboratory.

STRATEGY FOR TEST UTILIZATION MANAGEMENT IMPLEMENTATION

A test utilization management system has value for patients, physicians, and health care overall, but implementation can be challenging and time-consuming. A successful strategy includes a multi-pronged approach, including support from the institution, identification and inclusion of the key stakeholders (eg, institutional leadership, clinicians, health care workers, managers, laboratorians, and pathologists), a careful and methodical approach, a data-driven process, and a recurring review process to ensure continued current medical applicability and appropriate updating.[1,3,9,10] Box 2 outlines key components that could underlie one approach toward developing a test utilization implementation strategy.

To begin the work toward successful implementation of a laboratory test utilization management program, it is critical that there is full support by institutional leadership and an adequate organizational infrastructure. Senior administration and institutional/hospital leaders provide the highest level of oversight for the strategic planning and

Box 1
Three key factors that support the importance of test utilization
1. Good patient care
2. Sound medical practice
3. Economic demand

<table>
<tr><td>

Box 2
One approach to developing a test utilization implementation strategy

1. Ensure institutional leadership support and presence of adequate infrastructure

2. Define the problem with the current standard of practice and establish the need to address it

3. Decide on a type of intervention that will address the problem defined above (see **Box 3**)

4. Establish the clinical indications, overall value, and application of a diagnostic test for a certain disease

5. Review the current clinical practice guidelines

6. Formulate a data-driven, evidence-based strategy

7. Consider your stakeholders, especially your clinical colleagues, and share the proposed strategy with them

8. Launch your test utilization strategy

9. Audit laboratory and clinical personnel

10. Reevaluate your strategy on an annual basis

</td><td>

Box 3
A nonexhaustive list of the different types of interventions that can be used in test utilization strategies

- Restrict ordering to clinicians with certain credentials
- Changes to computerized provider order entry:
  - Using pop-ups
  - Removing tests from quick-pick screens
  - Removing research-only test
- Banning of certain tests:
  - Obsolete tests
  - Referral tests that are also offered in-house
- Send and hold specimens
- Add prerequisites/requirements that must be fulfilled before an order can be placed
- Requiring laboratory approval for specified tests
- Selective review process
- Test send-out review
- Test formularies
- Test guidelines
- Analytical algorithms
- Hard stops and gatekeeper functions
- Restrict the frequency of specified tests
- Real-time test-selection support
- Educational activities
- Utilization audits and report cards
- Required genetic counseling before approving test

Data from Refs.[3,11,15,82]

</td></tr>
</table>

operational logistics of an institution.[11] With the backing of the institution, laboratorians then work with clinical colleagues and key health care personnel to effect the right outcome.[1,12–14] Pathologists, who have administrative leadership experience, laboratory management responsibilities, and knowledge regarding laboratory testing, are uniquely positioned to be leaders in this process.[1,15,16]

Next steps include identifying an area of the practice that would benefit from laboratory test utilization implementation. This identification process also includes taking into consideration the clinical, financial, and operational impacts.[1,13] Once a problem area is identified and agreed on as requiring intervention, a type of intervention that will address the problem is delineated (**Box 3**).

The development of a laboratory test utilization guideline or algorithm as an intervention occurs as a multistep process. The clinical indications, overall value, and application of a diagnostic test for a certain disease are established.[9] Subsequently, the laboratory team performs a retrospective review and correlation of in-house test results with the patient clinical status.[17] Simultaneously, other team members review the current literature

regarding the diagnostic test and disease in question, including national and international guidelines (for example, the National Comprehensive Cancer Network guidelines), recommendations, published best practices, and peer-reviewed journals.[10] After identifying appropriate tests, supported by current standard of practice guidelines, a data-driven, evidence-based guideline or analytical algorithm can be formulated.[13]

At the appropriate point(s) in this process, all stakeholders should be included. For example, clinical colleagues and geneticists who are part of the disease-oriented group(s) relevant to the test utilization strategy are critical collaborators.

Laboratory personnel, management, and specialists in information technology should also be consulted to ensure that the proposed strategy is a feasible one from the laboratory and operational standpoints. At times, it may be necessary to actively engage your stakeholders and this can be done using various educational tools that may include recorded videos, Grand Round presentations, and publications.[9]

Once an algorithm/implemented guideline is in place, it is necessary that it be audited on a routine, at least annual, basis. Auditing a test utilization guideline or algorithm supports sustained success of the strategy, helps to ensure compliance, confirms that a standardized approach is working, and is a critical step in efficient test utilization. Key concepts during an audit include assessment that the testing being performed remains relevant, that there are/are not new technologies or tests that should be considered and finally, that the diagnostic approach to the disease entity is unchanged. The data from auditing highlight comparative differences/similarities between practicing individuals, provide information on how a test(s) is being used, indicate whether the intended outcome was achieved, and help to identify problem areas that need updating, modifying, or reeducation.[3,4,9,13]

Beyond just the scope of one's local clinical and laboratory practice, implementation of efficient and successful test utilization strategies demonstrates our broader value to health care organizations and insurance companies as the economic environment continues to change. Ongoing comparison of disease workup under the previous model of care with a new test utilization strategy highlights standardization, decreased unnecessary testing, and improved targeted diagnostics. Thus, we prove evidence of added value while still putting the needs of the patient first and creating a sustainable and operational laboratory.

THE PRACTICE OF HEMATOPATHOLOGY AND TEST UTILIZATION

The discipline of hematopathology increasingly embraces the concept of utilization management as evidenced by a growing number of peer-reviewed publications, educational seminars and workshops, and presentations at pathology national meetings on this topic. As a direct result of these efforts, data-driven, effective, test utilization algorithms have been proposed and exist in some practices.[18–26] Algorithms incorporate important clinical parameters, comparative studies of testing modalities, practice data, published literature, and national and international guidelines (where applicable). They may vary slightly between individual pathology practices based on case mix, clinical trial enrollment, and practice expertise. However, in general, algorithms hold true to the principles of the right test(s) at the right time for the right diagnosis.

In this section, we present 2 examples of test utilization approaches for hematologic conditions: (1) the initial workup and diagnosis of myelodysplastic syndromes and (2) bone marrow testing in the staging for involvement by lymphoma diagnosed in an extramedullary site. A key point to remember with the consideration of implementation of an algorithm into routine clinical practice is that these approaches are meant for most patient cases (80%). They are by no means meant to be exclusive or "one size fits all." Outlier cases are well known to pathologists and in no way should deter testing that may be necessary in the evaluation of such a case. In general, our approach has been the "80/20 rule" wherein 80% of cases can be successfully managed with the algorithm. A second key point, as mentioned previously, is that medicine and technologies continually evolve and therefore algorithms need to be reviewed and updated on a regular basis or whenever a transformative event occurs. Algorithms, as a whole, provide an excellent framework within which to begin the assessment of a case and ensure that best practices are followed.

ALGORITHMIC APPROACH TO THE INITIAL WORKUP AND DIAGNOSIS OF MYELODYSPLASTIC SYNDROME

Myelodysplastic syndromes (MDSs) are a heterogeneous group of clonal stem cell myeloid disorders with a predilection for evolution into acute myeloid leukemia.[27–33] Pathologically, MDS is diagnosed by morphologic dysplasia in a bone marrow specimen in the setting of persistent cytopenias and adequate exclusion of non-neoplastic mimickers of dysplasia (eg, nutritional deficiency, toxin/drug exposure). On occasion (fewer than 5%–10% of all cases), bone marrows performed for unexplained persistent cytopenias show no diagnostic dysplastic features; however, a clonal MDS-associated abnormality (eg, chromosomal analysis, fluorescence in situ hybridization [FISH], and molecular mutations [Next Generation sequencing]) may be detected. These cases represent situations of clonal hematopoiesis of uncertain significance or clonal hematopoiesis of indeterminate potential.[27,34–36] Flow cytometry is another useful technique in the evaluation of myeloid disorders, but its role currently as a diagnostic tool in MDS remains supportive.[37–40]

Although morphology plays the key diagnostic role in MDS at the present time, prognostication in MDS is influenced by multiple factors. These factors include, but are not limited to, blast count in the peripheral blood and bone marrow, presence of Auer rods, degree of cytopenias, and number and type of chromosomal abnormalities.[33,41–43] Recent data indicate that certain molecular alterations also may now play a prognostic role in MDS.[35,44–46]

Given that morphology drives the diagnosis of MDS and that a variety of tools (clinical features, morphology, complete blood cell count values, chromosomal and molecular genetic findings) drive MDS prognosis, a data-driven, test utilization strategy for the initial workup of MDS can be proposed (**Fig. 1**). As mentioned previously, such a strategy is not intended to be dogmatic, nor does it preclude one from deviating in exceptional circumstances, but is meant to assist in the efficient and appropriate workup of a particular disease entity. A robust algorithm is evidence-based and integrates and incorporates findings from practice data, peer-reviewed published literature, clinician expertise, national guidelines (eg, National Comprehensive Cancer Network) and international recommendations (eg, international prognostic scoring system for MDS).[41–43,47,48]

Typically a bone marrow examination to assess for MDS is initiated by a clinician based on his or her clinical suspicion. This initial evaluation includes morphologic review and chromosomal analysis. Bone marrow morphologic requirements should include a peripheral blood smear in addition to complete blood cell count data, particulate, Wright-Giemsa–stained aspirate smears, and an adequate, hematoxylin-eosin–stained, bone marrow core biopsy. If morphologic review renders a firm diagnosis of MDS, the chromosomal study provides additional prognostic and therapeutic (eg, lenalidomide treatment for deletion 5q)

information.[41–43,45,49–52] If the chromosomal study yields 20 adequate metaphase spreads and there is a resultant resolved karyotype, then FISH studies for the commonly recurring genetic abnormalities (−5/5q, −7/7q, +8, del20q, del17p, −13/13q) are not generally needed.[53–56] If the chromosomal study yields fewer than 20 adequate metaphases and/or the karyotype is unresolved, additional FISH testing should be considered for possible prognostic assessment. These general practice principles are based on the findings of the chromosomal study and apply not only to cases of morphologic MDS but also to cases in which the morphology is either equivocal or not diagnostic of MDS. The finding of MDS-associated abnormalities in those latter instances is of uncertain significance in the absence of unequivocal features of MDS.[27,57]

The recent and rapid discovery of recurring molecular mutations in MDS is yet another tool that is set to transform our diagnostic and prognostic approach to MDS.[35,45,46,58–61] However, it is still too early in this process to be able to carefully and methodically assess the test utilization principles for this technology at this point (see **Box 1**). An MDS algorithm is a good example of the critical value that an annual review and reassessment of the test utilization guideline has so as to determine what the evolving/current best practices and/or new technologies are and whether the guideline/algorithm needs updating. Given all the advances and innovation that continue to occur in medicine, our approach to MDS for best medical practice will undoubtedly evolve.[45,58]

ALGORITHMIC APPROACH TO THE EVALUATION OF BONE MARROW SPECIMENS PERFORMED FOR STAGING OF LYMPHOMA

Bone marrow biopsies are routinely performed to stage concurrently diagnosed Hodgkin and non-Hodgkin lymphoma in an extramedullary tissue

Fig. 1. Algorithmic approach to test utilization in MDSs. MDS FISH does not increase the detection of MDS if chromosome analysis is successful and 20 metaphases are analyzed. Thus, MDS FISH studies should be ordered at the discretion of the cytogeneticist if <20 metaphases are identified, if there is an unresolved karyotype, or if only 1 abnormal metaphase is identified. [a] Consider Next Generation Sequencing testing for select gene mutations, as clinically warranted.

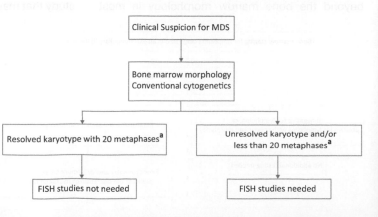

biopsy. Staging for lymphoma in the bone marrow may be important for prognostication and therapeutic options.[62,63] Similar to other tissues biopsied to assess for a hematologic neoplasm, there is an extensive suite of ancillary studies that are at a pathologist's disposal to further clarify and classify a disease process. These testing modalities include morphology/step section levels, immunohistochemistry, flow cytometry, molecular testing, chromosomal analysis, and FISH testing. Each of these testing modalities has well-recognized value in the diagnosis and prognosis of lymphoma in tissues. However, in the context of evaluating bone marrows performed to stage diagnosed lymphoma, the utility of and value added from performing these testing modalities should be clarified.

Multiple, peer-reviewed articles have systematically reported on the utility of the available testing modalities in the evaluation of a bone marrow performed for the purpose of staging lymphoma (morphology/step section levels, immunohistochemistry, flow cytometry, molecular testing, chromosomal analysis, and FISH testing).[64,65] The utility of these various testing modalities in the bone marrow staging of lymphoma is controversial; however, most would agree that the highest impact modality is morphologic review of an adequate and generous biopsy specimen (Fig. 2). The patterns of bone marrow involvement by Hodgkin and non-Hodgkin lymphoma are well-recognized and documented.[64,66] With this knowledge, pathologists readily determine the presence or absence of morphologic involvement of the bone marrow by lymphoma.

Flow cytometric immunophenotyping is a useful ancillary tool in the diagnosis and classification of B-cell and T-cell lymphomas. In bone marrow specimens obtained for the purpose of staging extramedullary diagnosed lymphoma, the role for flow cytometry has also been investigated. Although its role is controversial among several peer-reviewed published articles,[67–72] in general, flow cytometry does not add significant additional information beyond the bone marrow morphology in most cases (80%).[68,70,73] The concordance rate beyond bone marrow morphology and flow cytometry exceeds 80% in most studies. Hanson and colleagues[73] concluded that flow cytometric evaluation is not cost-effective in the setting of an adequate morphologic evaluation. In the study by Wolach and colleagues,[70] positive flow cytometry (FC) in the setting of negative bone marrow (BM) histology at diffuse large B-cell lymphoma (DLBCL) diagnosis did not significantly affect overall survival (OS) or progression free survival (PFS). Iancu and colleagues[68] found that 3-color flow cytometric immunophenotyping adds little information to the evaluation of staging BM specimens of follicular lymphoma (FL) patients. Concordance between the 2 methods was detected in 411 (85%) cases (27% BMB+/FC+; 58% BMB−/FC−), whereas discordance was present in 75 (15%) (P<.001): 58 cases (12%) were BMB+/FC− and 17 (3%) were BMB−/FC+ in the study by Merli and colleagues.[69] Given the incidence of monoclonal B lymphocytosis and occasional cases of subtle bone marrow involvement by marginal zone lymphoma and intrasinusoidal lymphoma, it is not surprising that discrepancies exist.[74] It is therefore of utmost importance to determine in which very specific scenarios would flow cytometry contribute valuable information in the setting of a morphologically normal bone marrow.

Immunohistochemistry (IHC) is another useful tool in the hematopathology armamentarium for disease classification. However, its role in the setting of an adequate bone marrow morphology specimen in staging lymphoma is not clear. It is doubtful that in most cases IHC would make a meaningful contribution to the interpretation of a staging lymphoma bone marrow in otherwise straightforward concordant involvement or lack of involvement (see Fig. 2). Exceptions could be investigated as necessary on a case-by-case basis (eg, assessment for intrasinusoidal involvement by marginal zone lymphoma).

Conventional karyotyping is an optional ancillary study that may be performed in the setting of bone

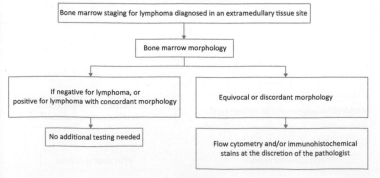

Fig. 2. Guideline for bone marrow testing performed for staging for lymphoma diagnosed in an extramedullary tissue site.

marrow staging for lymphoma. However, a routine cytogenetic study is costly, time-consuming, and labor intensive. Two, large, recent, independent retrospective studies have shown that routine cytogenetic studies in staging of extramedullary diagnosed lymphoma in the bone marrow provides no additional diagnostic information beyond the histomorphologic findings.[25,75]

FISH plays an important role in the prognostication and occasional diagnosis of non-Hodgkin lymphomas.[76–78] FISH studies, as a general rule, when needed for the latter purposes, should be performed on the primary diagnostic specimen. In the setting of a staging bone marrow for extramedullary diagnosed lymphoma, FISH is of doubtful utility whether there is morphologic evidence of marrow involvement by lymphoma or not. Although it could be argued that detection of a low-level abnormality could indicate occult bone marrow involvement by lymphoma, the true significance of such a finding in the absence of morphologic confirmation is unclear and could potentially be spurious.[79] Conversely, morphologic bone marrow involvement by lymphoma does not require confirmation by a FISH study.

Clonal immunoglobulin heavy chain gene (IgH) rearrangements may support the presence of a clonal B-cell population in the appropriate clinical, morphologic, and immunophenotypic setting. In bone marrows performed to stage extramedullary lymphoma, assessment for a clonal IgH gene rearrangement does not routinely contribute additional meaningful information. In the setting of morphologic bone marrow involvement by lymphoma, IgH gene rearrangement studies provide no additional diagnostic information. Conversely, in cases lacking morphologic bone marrow involvement by lymphoma, apparent IgH clonality detection could lead to a significant misinterpretation or misdiagnosis of bone marrow involvement by lymphoma. It is known that IgH clones may occur in reactive conditions and when there is a limited B-cell repertoire.[80] Detection of a clone in a morphologically negative bone marrow may have a prognostic role in follicular lymphoma,[81] but should be confirmed in larger studies.

SUMMARY

Efficient, cost-effective test utilization is a key component of sound medical practice, judicious management of health care resources, decreasing health care costs, ensuring patient safety, and improving the quality of health care services.[1,9] Pathologists and laboratorians must be engaged in this process along with clinical colleagues and all health care contributors. Utilization

management also allows the laboratory to demonstrate value to insurance companies, provides justification for a sustainable and data-driven operation for patient care, and is an important parameter of evidence-based medicine. Pathologists are uniquely positioned to be at the forefront of test utilization and lead the efforts during this needed time of change. The field of hematopathology has been a leader in incorporating ancillary testing into the diagnostic classification of disease. As ancillary testing continues to evolve and transform our practice, hematopathology is a key area in which efficient test utilization can be and must be applied.

ACKNOWLEDGMENTS

We gratefully acknowledge the work and significant contributions of Dr Curtis A. Hanson and Dr Paul J. Kurtin to the field of test utilization, application of utilization management to the field of hematopathology, and assistance with this work.

REFERENCES

1. Kim JY, Dzik WH, Dighe AS, et al. Utilization management in a large urban academic medical center: a 10-year experience. Am J Clin Pathol 2011;135(1):108–18.
2. Procop GW, Keating C, Stagno P, et al. Reducing duplicate testing: a comparison of two clinical decision support tools. Am J Clin Pathol 2015;143(5):623–6.
3. Hanson CA. Helping clinicians maneuver through the diagnostics maze. Critical Values 2012;5(2):16–9.
4. Futrell K. Test order optimization: The laboratory's formula for being a partner in a value-based or outcome-based ACO reimbursement environment. Adv for Admin of the Lab 2015;24(5):16–8.
5. Dickerson JA, Cole B, Conta JH, et al. Improving the value of costly genetic reference laboratory testing with active utilization management. Arch Pathol Lab Med 2014;138(1):110–3.
6. Alexander CB. Reducing healthcare costs through appropriate test utilization. Critical Values 2012;2012:6–8.
7. Robinson A. Rationale for cost-effective laboratory medicine. Clin Microbiol Rev 1994;7(2):185–99.
8. Sisko A, Truffer C, Smith S, et al. Health spending projections through 2018: recession effects add uncertainty to the outlook. Health Aff 2009;28(2):w346–57.
9. Hanson C, Plumhoff E. Test utilization and the clinical laboratory. Mayo Medical Laboratories Communique 2012;37(3):1–4.

10. Wilson ML. Decreasing inappropriate laboratory test utilization: controlling costs and improving quality of care. Am J Clin Pathol 2015;143(5):614–6.

11. Malone B. The future of lab utilization management. Are lab formularies the answer? Clinical Laboratory News 2012;38(1).

12. Check W. Powering down on excessive test use. CAP Today 2014;2014.

13. Titus K. Lab teams up to curb unneeded testing. CAP Today 2012;2012.

14. Warren JS. Laboratory test utilization program: structure and impact in a large academic medical center. Am J Clin Pathol 2013;139(3):289–97.

15. Lewandrowski KB, Dighe A. Clinical pathologists needed to implement utilization management programs. Critical Values 2012;5:25–7.

16. Zhao JJ, Liberman A. Pathologists' roles in clinical utilization management. A financing model for managed care. Am J Clin Pathol 2000;113(3):336–42.

17. Titus K. With molecular PMN testing, think positive. CAP Today 2015;2015.

18. Seegmiller AC, Kim AS, Mosse CA, et al. Optimizing personalized bone marrow testing using an evidence-based, interdisciplinary team approach. Am J Clin Pathol 2013;140(5):643–50.

19. Reichard KK, Chen D, Pardanani A, et al. Morphologically occult systemic mastocytosis in bone marrow: clinicopathologic features and an algorithmic approach to diagnosis. Am J Clin Pathol 2015;144(3):493–502.

20. Healey R, Naugler C, de Koning L, et al. A classification tree approach for improving the utilization of flow cytometry testing of blood specimens for B-cell non-Hodgkin lymphoproliferative disorders. Leuk Lymphoma 2015;56(9):2619–24.

21. He R, Wiktor AE, Hanson CA, et al. Conventional karyotyping and fluorescence in situ hybridization: an effective utilization strategy in diagnostic adult acute myeloid leukemia. Am J Clin Pathol 2015;143(6):873–8.

22. Oberley MJ, Fitzgerald S, Yang DT, et al. Value-based flow testing of chronic lymphoproliferative disorders: a quality improvement project to develop an algorithm to streamline testing and reduce costs. Am J Clin Pathol 2014;142(3):411–8.

23. Jevremovic D, Dronca RS, Morice WG, et al. CD5+ B-cell lymphoproliferative disorders: beyond chronic lymphocytic leukemia and mantle cell lymphoma. Leuk Res 2010;34(9):1235–8.

24. He R. Myeloproliferative neoplasm: morphology, molecular updates and cost-effective test utilization. Mayo Medical Laboratories Hot Topic Video and Transcript, 2015. Available at: http://www.mayo medicallaboratories.com/articles/hot-topic/2015/07-15-myeloproliferative-neoplasm/index.html. Accessed September 12, 2015.

25. Kurtin PJ. Bone marrow genetic studies for malignant lymphoma staging: optimizing laboratory testing for hematologic disorders series. Mayo Medical Laboratories Hot Topic Video and Transcript, 2013. Available at: http://www.mayomedicallaboratories. com/articles/hot-topic/2013/01-15-malignant-lymphoma-staging/index.html. Accessed September 12, 2015.

26. Malignant lymphoma, guideline for bone marrow staging studies. Mayo Medical Laboratories Diagnostic Testing Algorithms—Hematology, 2015. Available at: http://www.mayomedicallaboratories. com/it-mmfiles/Malignant_Lymphoma__Guideline_for_ Bone_Marrow_Staging_Studies.pdf. Accessed September 28, 2015.

27. Swerdlow SH, International Agency for Research on Cancer, World Health Organization. WHO classification of tumours of haematopoietic and lymphoid tissues, 4th edition World Health Organization classification of tumours. Lyon (France): International Agency for Research on Cancer; 2008. p. 439.

28. Bueso-Ramos CE, Kanagal-Shamanna R, Routbort MJ, et al. Therapy-related myeloid neoplasms. Am J Clin Pathol 2015;144(2):207–18.

29. Steensma DP. Myelodysplastic syndromes: diagnosis and treatment. Mayo Clin Proc 2015;90(7):969–83.

30. Vardiman J, Reichard K. Acute myeloid leukemia with myelodysplasia-related changes. Am J Clin Pathol 2015;144(1):29–43.

31. Vardiman J. The classification of MDS: from FAB to WHO and beyond. Leuk Res 2012;36(12):1453–8.

32. Tefferi A, Vardiman JW. Myelodysplastic syndromes. N Engl J Med 2009;361(19):1872–85.

33. Garcia-Manero G. Myelodysplastic syndromes: 2015 update on diagnosis, risk-stratification and management. Am J Hematol 2015;90(9):831–41.

34. Steensma DP, Bejar R, Jaiswal S, et al. Clonal hematopoiesis of indeterminate potential and its distinction from myelodysplastic syndromes. Blood 2015; 126(1):9–16.

35. Bejar R. Myelodysplastic syndromes diagnosis: what is the role of molecular testing? Curr Hematol Malig Rep 2015;10(3):282–91.

36. Genovese G, Kähler AK, Handsaker RE, et al. Clonal hematopoiesis and blood-cancer risk inferred from blood DNA sequence. N Engl J Med 2014;371(26):2477–87.

37. Porwit A. Is there a role for flow cytometry in the evaluation of patients with myelodysplastic syndromes? Curr Hematol Malig Rep 2015;10(3):309–17.

38. Porwit A, van de Loosdrecht AA, Bettelheim P, et al. Revisiting guidelines for integration of flow cytometry results in the WHO classification of myelodysplastic syndromes—proposal from the International/European LeukemiaNet Working Group for Flow Cytometry in MDS. Leukemia 2014;28(9):1793–8.

39. Westers TM, Ireland R, Kern W, et al. Standardization of flow cytometry in myelodysplastic syndromes: a report from an international consortium and the European LeukemiaNet Working Group. Leukemia 2012;26(7):1730–41.

40. Porwit A. Role of flow cytometry in diagnostics of myelodysplastic syndromes–beyond the WHO 2008 classification. Semin Diagn Pathol 2011; 28(4):273–82.

41. Della Porta MG, Tuechler H, Malcovati L, et al. Validation of WHO classification-based Prognostic Scoring System (WPSS) for myelodysplastic syndromes and comparison with the revised International Prognostic Scoring System (IPSS-R). A study of the International Working Group for Prognosis in Myelodysplasia (IWG-PM). Leukemia 2015;29(7):1502–13.

42. Greenberg PL, Tuechler H, Schanz J, et al. Revised international prognostic scoring system for myelodysplastic syndromes. Blood 2012;120(12): 2454–65.

43. Jonas BA, Greenberg PL. MDS prognostic scoring systems—past, present, and future. Best Pract Res Clin Haematol 2015;28(1):3–13.

44. Nazha A, Sekeres MA, Gore SD, et al. Molecular testing in myelodysplastic syndromes for the practicing oncologist: will the progress fulfill the promise? Oncologist 2015;20(9):1069–76.

45. Lee EJ, Podoltsev N, Gore SD, et al. The evolving field of prognostication and risk stratification in MDS: recent developments and future directions. Blood Rev 2015. [Epub ahead of print].

46. Bejar R. Clinical and genetic predictors of prognosis in myelodysplastic syndromes. Haematologica 2014;99(6):956–64.

47. Greenberg PL, Stone RM, Bejar R, et al. Myelodysplastic syndromes, version 2.2015. J Natl Compr Canc Netw 2015;13(3):261–72.

48. Greenberg PL, Attar E, Bennett JM, et al. Myelodysplastic syndromes: clinical practice guidelines in oncology. J Natl Compr Canc Netw 2013;11(7): 838–74.

49. Greenberg P, Cox C, LeBeau MM, et al. International scoring system for evaluating prognosis in myelodysplastic syndromes. Blood 1997;89(6):2079–88.

50. List A, Dewald G, Bennett J, et al. Lenalidomide in the myelodysplastic syndrome with chromosome 5q deletion. N Engl J Med 2006;355(14):1456–65.

51. Raza A, Reeves JA, Feldman EJ, et al. Phase 2 study of lenalidomide in transfusion-dependent, low-risk, and intermediate-1 risk myelodysplastic syndromes with karyotypes other than deletion 5q. Blood 2008;111(1):86–93.

52. Sekeres MA, Swern AS, Fenaux P, et al. Validation of the IPSS-R in lenalidomide-treated, lower-risk myelodysplastic syndrome patients with del(5q). Blood Cancer J 2014;4:e242.

53. Pitchford CW, Hettinga AC, Reichard KK. Fluorescence in situ hybridization testing for -5/5q, -7/7q, +8, and del(20q) in primary myelodysplastic syndrome correlates with conventional cytogenetics in the setting of an adequate study. Am J Clin Pathol 2010;133(2):260–4.

54. Douet-Guilbert N, Herry A, Le Bris MJ, et al. Interphase FISH does not improve the detection of DEL(5q) and DEL(20q) in myelodysplastic syndromes. Anticancer Res 2011;31(3):1007–10.

55. Romeo M, Chauffaille Mde L, Silva MR, et al. Comparison of cytogenetics with FISH in 40 myelodysplastic syndrome patients. Leuk Res 2002;26(11): 993–6.

56. Seegmiller AC, Wasserman A, Kim AS, et al. Limited utility of fluorescence in situ hybridization for common abnormalities of myelodysplastic syndrome at first presentation and follow-up of myeloid neoplasms. Leuk Lymphoma 2014;55(3):601–5.

57. Steensma DP, Dewald GW, Hodnefield JM, et al. Clonal cytogenetic abnormalities in bone marrow specimens without clear morphologic evidence of dysplasia: a form fruste of myelodysplasia? Leuk Res 2003;27(3):235–42.

58. Bacher U, Kohlmann A, Haferlach T. Mutational profiling in patients with MDS: ready for every-day use in the clinic? Best Pract Res Clin Haematol 2015;28(1):32–42.

59. Lindsley RC, Ebert BL. Molecular pathophysiology of myelodysplastic syndromes. Annu Rev Pathol 2013;8:21–47.

60. Bejar R, Ebert BL. The genetic basis of myelodysplastic syndromes. Hematol Oncol Clin North Am 2010;24(2):295–315.

61. Visconte V, Tiu RV, Rogers HJ. Pathogenesis of myelodysplastic syndromes: an overview of molecular and non-molecular aspects of the disease. Blood Res 2014;49(4):216–27.

62. Ansell SM. Non-Hodgkin lymphoma: diagnosis and treatment. Mayo Clin Proc 2015;90(8):1152–63.

63. Mauz-Korholz C, Metzger ML, Kelly KM, et al. Pediatric Hodgkin lymphoma. J Clin Oncol 2015;33(27): 2975–85.

64. Zhang QY, Foucar K. Bone marrow involvement by Hodgkin and non-Hodgkin lymphomas. Hematol Oncol Clin North Am 2009;23(4):873–902.

65. Talaulikar D, Dahlstrom JE. Staging bone marrow in diffuse large B-cell lymphoma: the role of ancillary investigations. Pathology 2009;41(3):214–22.

66. Arber DA, George TI. Bone marrow biopsy involvement by non-Hodgkin's lymphoma: frequency of lymphoma types, patterns, blood involvement, and discordance with other sites in 450 specimens. Am J Surg Pathol 2005;29(12):1549–57.

67. Kim B, Lee ST, Kim HJ, et al. Bone marrow flow cytometry in staging of patients with B-cell non-Hodgkin lymphoma. Ann Lab Med 2015;35(2): 187–93.

68. Iancu D, Hao S, Lin P, et al. Follicular lymphoma in staging bone marrow specimens: correlation of histologic findings with the results of flow cytometry immunophenotypic analysis. Arch Pathol Lab Med 2007;131(2):282–7.

69. Merli M, Arcaini L, Boveri E, et al. Assessment of bone marrow involvement in non-Hodgkin's lymphomas: comparison between histology and flow cytometry. Eur J Haematol 2010;85(5):405–15.

70. Wolach O, Fraser A, Luchiansky M, et al. Can flow cytometry of bone marrow aspirate predict outcome of patients with diffuse large B cell lymphoma? A retrospective single centre study. Hematol Oncol 2015;33(1):42–7.

71. Talaulikar D, Dahlstrom JE, Shadbolt B, et al. Occult bone marrow involvement in patients with diffuse large B-cell lymphoma: results of a pilot study. Pathology 2007;39(6):580–5.

72. Schmidt B, Kremer M, Götze K, et al. Bone marrow involvement in follicular lymphoma: comparison of histology and flow cytometry as staging procedures. Leuk Lymphoma 2006;47(9):1857–62.

73. Hanson CA, Kurtin PJ, Katzmann JA, et al. Immunophenotypic analysis of peripheral blood and bone marrow in the staging of B-cell malignant lymphoma. Blood 1999;94(11):3889–96.

74. Tierens AM, Holte H, Warsame A, et al. Low levels of monoclonal small B cells in the bone marrow of patients with diffuse large B-cell lymphoma of activated B-cell type but not of germinal center B-cell type. Haematologica 2010;95(8):1334–41.

75. Nardi V, Pulluqi O, Abramson JS, et al. Routine conventional karyotyping of lymphoma staging bone marrow samples does not contribute clinically relevant information. Am J Hematol 2015;90(6):529–33.

76. Ochs RC, Bagg A. Molecular genetic characterization of lymphoma: application to cytology diagnosis. Diagn Cytopathol 2012;40(6):542–55.

77. Ondrejka SL, Hsi ED. Pathology of B-cell lymphomas: diagnosis and biomarker discovery. Cancer Treat Res 2015;165:27–50.

78. Xing X, Feldman AL. Anaplastic large cell lymphomas: ALK positive, ALK negative, and primary cutaneous. Adv Anat Pathol 2015;22(1):29–49.

79. Huh HJ, Min HC, Cho HI, et al. Investigation of bone marrow involvement in malignant lymphoma using fluorescence in situ hybridization: possible utility in the detection of micrometastasis. Cancer Genet Cytogenet 2008;186(1):1–5.

80. Shin S, Kim AH, Park J, et al. Analysis of immunoglobulin and T cell receptor gene rearrangement in the bone marrow of lymphoid neoplasia using BIOMED-2 multiplex polymerase chain reaction. Int J Med Sci 2013;10(11):1510–7.

81. Berget E, Helgeland L, Liseth K, et al. Prognostic value of bone marrow involvement by clonal immunoglobulin gene rearrangements in follicular lymphoma. J Clin Pathol 2014;67(12):1072–7.

82. Solomon DH, Hashimoto H, Daltroy L, et al. Techniques to improve physicians' use of diagnostic tests: a new conceptual framework. JAMA 1998;280(23):2020–7.

B-cell Non-Hodgkin Lymphomas with Plasmacytic Differentiation

Charles M. Harmon, MD[a], Lauren B. Smith, MD[b],*

KEYWORDS

- Lymphoplasmacytic • MALT • Nodal marginal zone • Splenic • Plasmablastic • Plasmacytic
- Lymphoma

Key points

- Significant overlap exists between low-grade B-cell lymphomas with plasmacytic differentiation.
- Testing for *MYD88* (L265P) can be a useful adjunct in differentiating lymphoplasmacytic lymphoma (LPL) from other small B-cell lymphomas with plasmacytic differentiation when morphologic and immunophenotypic findings are equivocal.
- Cases of immunoblastic morphology raise a broad differential diagnosis, including immunoblastic diffuse large B-cell lymphoma (I-DLBCL), plasmablastic lymphoma, ALK-positive large B-cell lymphoma (ALK+ LBCL), and the solid variant of primary effusion lymphoma (PEL).
- Clinicopathologic correlation may be necessary to distinguish plasmablastic lymphoma (PBL) from anaplastic plasmacytoma because the morphologic features and immunophenotype can be similar.

ABSTRACT

B-cell non-Hodgkin lymphomas with plasmacytic differentiation are a diverse group of entities with extremely variable morphologic features. Diagnostic challenges can arise in differentiating lymphoplasmacytic lymphoma from marginal zone lymphoma and other low-grade B-cell lymphomas. In addition, plasmablastic lymphomas can be difficult to distinguish from diffuse large B-cell lymphoma or other high-grade lymphomas. Judicious use of immunohistochemical studies and molecular testing can assist in appropriate classification.

LYMPHOPLASMACYTIC LYMPHOMA

OVERVIEW

LPL is a B-cell lymphoma composed of a spectrum of small B lymphocytes, plasmacytoid lymphocytes, and plasma cells.[1] According to the 2008 World Health Organization (WHO) classification scheme, LPL is a diagnosis of exclusion because its definition is that of a lymphoma "which does not fulfill the criteria for any of the other small B-cell lymphoid neoplasms."[1] Mutations in the *MYD88* gene, however, that result in an amino acid change (L265P), have recently been identified in approximately 90% of cases of LPL.[2–8] Although most patients with LPL have an immunoglobulin M (IgM) paraprotein, some patients may have a non-IgM paraprotein, whereas others may not have any detectable paraprotein. Although the terms, *LPL* and *Waldenström macroglobulinemia (WM)* are sometimes used interchangeably, WM is a clinicopathologic entity that is defined as LPL with an IgM paraprotein and bone marrow (BM) involvement.[1] Thus, although all cases of WM are also LPL, a minority of cases of LPL do not satisfy criteria for a diagnosis of WM.

LPL is a disease of older adults, with a median age at diagnosis of 63 years in African Americans

The authors have no relevant personal financial relationships or financial conflicts of interest to disclose.
[a] Department of Pathology, University of Michigan Hospitals and Health Systems, 1301 Catherine Street, Ann Arbor, MI 48109, USA; [b] Department of Pathology, University of Michigan Hospitals and Health Systems, 5320 Medical Science I, 1301 Catherine Street, Ann Arbor, MI 48109-5602, USA
* Corresponding author.
E-mail address: lbsmith@med.umich.edu

Surgical Pathology 9 (2016) 11–28
http://dx.doi.org/10.1016/j.path.2015.09.007
1875-9181/16/$ – see front matter © 2016 Elsevier Inc. All rights reserved.

surgpath.theclinics.com

and of 73 years in white patients.[9] There is a male predominance, and the disease is more common in whites than in blacks.[10] Although the most common presenting symptom is fatigue related to anemia, the presence of an IgM paraprotein may also result in peripheral neuropathy, hemolytic anemia, coagulopathy, cryoglobulinemia, and hyperviscosity.[10]

GROSS AND MICROSCOPIC FEATURES

LPL most commonly involves the BM with less frequent involvement of lymph nodes and spleen.[1] Rarely, LPL presents as a primarily node-based lymphoma. BM involvement by LPL manifests histologically as an interstitial infiltrate sometimes mixed with nodular and paratrabecular aggregates.[11] Less commonly, LPL involves the BM in a diffuse pattern. The infiltrate of LPL morphologically consists of a mixture of small lymphocytes, plasmacytoid lymphocytes, and plasma cells (Fig. 1). Although nonspecific, the presence of intermixed mast cells and hemosiderin is characteristic of LPL.[12]

Lymph node involvement by LPL is most commonly characterized by a lymphoplasmacytic infiltrate within the paracortex and in the parasinusoidal regions with patent sinuses and relative sparing of the lymph node architecture. Proliferation centers, which are a characteristic feature of nodal involvement by chronic lymphocytic leukemia/small lymphocytic leukemia (CLL/SLL), are not seen in LPL.[1] Prominent monocytoid features

and follicular colonization are also typically absent in LPL and are more commonly seen in marginal zone lymphoma (MZL).[12] As in the BM, intermixed mast cells and hemosiderin are often present (Box 1).

In contrast to other small B-cell lymphomas, the immunophenotypic profile of LPL is not distinctive and displays significant overlap with other B-cell lymphoproliferative disorders.

The small B-lymphocytes of LPL express pan-B-cell markers, including CD19, CD20, CD22, CD79a, and PAX5. LPL is usually negative for CD10, CD5, and CD23. Dim or partial expression of CD5 and/or CD23 may be seen, however, in LPL, with occasional coexpression of these markers.[13,14] The plasma cells of LPL almost always express CD45, CD19, CD38, and CD138. Although the plasma cell component usually demonstrates cytoplasmic immunoglobulin light chain restriction, polytypic expression of light chains is seen in a small minority of cases.[13] In contrast to non-neoplastic plasma cells, plasma cell myeloma (PCM), and MZL with plasmacytic differentiation, a portion of the plasma cells in LPL may aberrantly coexpress PAX5 with CD138.[13,15]

DIAGNOSIS AND DIFFERENTIAL DIAGNOSIS

As discussed previously, the diagnosis of LPL requires exclusion of other small B-cell lymphomas with plasmacytic differentiation, including MZL, follicular lymphoma (FL), and CLL/SLL. Less commonly, mantle cell lymphoma (MCL) may

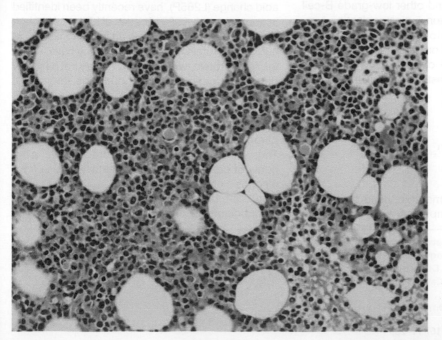

Fig. 1. BM biopsy showing an infiltrate of small lymphocytes and plasma cells, including occasional Dutcher bodies, in a case of LPL (hematoxylin-eosin, original magnification ×400).

also show plasmacytic differentiation. CLL/SLL, FL, and MCL can usually be readily distinguished from LPL based on distinct immunophenotypic and morphologic differences. In contrast to CLL/SLL, LPL is usually negative for CD5 and CD23. In the event of CD5/CD23 coexpression in LPL, CLL/SLL may be excluded based on bright surface immunoglobulin light chain expression and bright expression of CD20.[13] Proliferation centers, a characteristic feature of CLL/SLL involving lymph nodes, are absent in LPL. FL can be differentiated from LPL by its expression of CD10, whereas MCL can be distinguished based on its expression of CD5 and cyclin D1. MZL usually represents the most problematic differential diagnosis because its immunophenotypic and morphologic features show significant overlap with those of LPL. In the BM, a paratrabecular pattern of involvement favors a diagnosis of LPL.[16] Increased numbers of mast cells, although not entirely specific, are also seen more commonly in LPL than in MZL.[16] In the lymph node, MZL may demonstrate prominent monocytoid features and follicular colonization, whereas these characteristics are unusual in LPL.[12]

Although PCM in BM and plasmacytoma in tissue may be considered in the differential diagnosis, these can usually be differentiated from LPL by the predominance of plasma cells without small lymphocytes or plasmacytoid lymphocytes and a B-cell clone by flow cytometry. In contrast to the immunophenotype of the plasma cell component of LPL, PCM is nearly always CD19− and does not coexpress CD138 and PAX5.[15] An IgM paraprotein, if present, makes PCM unlikely because less than 1% of PCMs produce IgM.[17] An exception is PCM with t(11;14)(q13;q32) involving the *IGH* and *CCND1* genes, which may have a prominent lymphoplasmacytic morphologic appearance and produce a IgM paraprotein.[18] Immunohistochemical staining for cyclin

D1 can be useful in this differential diagnosis because PCM with t(11;14)(q13;q32) displays nuclear expression of cyclin D1, whereas LPL does not.[18] In addition, lytic bone lesions are a specific feature of PCM in this context because such lesions are not typically seen in LPL.[19]

Although not entirely specific, the *MYD88* (L265P) mutation is present in approximately 90% of cases of LPL.[2–8] In contrast, *MYD88* (L265P) is present in only 2% to 3% of CLL/SLL, approximately 7% of extranodal MZL, and 4% to 15% of splenic MZL (SMZL).[2,3,8,20] Although cases of nodal MZL (NMZL) with *MYD88* (L265P) have been reported, this seems to be rare.[2,20,21] *MYD88* (L265P) is absent in PCM (including IgM PCM).[2,20] Thus, polymerase chain reaction–based assays for *MYD88* (L265P) can be a useful adjunct in distinguishing LPL from its mimics when morphologic, immunophenotypic, and/or clinical findings are equivocal (**Boxes 2 and 3**).

PROGNOSIS

LPL usually follows an indolent clinical course with a median overall survival (OS) of 8 years.[22] Factors associated with a worse prognosis include age greater than 65 years, hemoglobin less than or equal to 11.5 g/dL, platelet count less than or equal to 100,000/μL, β_2-microglobulin greater than 3 mg/L, and monoclonal IgM greater than 7 g/dL.[23] Median survival time ranges from 43.5 months to 142.5 months based on these factors.[23] The absence of *MYD88* (L265P) is associated with an adverse prognosis.[24] Although the presence of del(6q) is associated with adverse characteristics, such as increased levels of paraprotein and β_2-microglobulin, it has not been shown to have an impact on OS.[25–27] The treatment of LPL ranges from observation for those patients who are asymptomatic and without cytopenias to combination chemotherapy in the setting of bulky disease, profound cytopenias, or constitutional symptoms.[10] Plasmapheresis is effective in the treatment of hyperviscosity due to an IgM paraprotein.

EXTRANODAL MARGINAL ZONE LYMPHOMA OF MUCOSA-ASSOCIATED LYMPHOID TISSUE

OVERVIEW

MZL encompasses several diagnostic entities that share in common a resemblance to the normal B cells of the marginal zone. The WHO classification recognizes 3 distinct subtypes of MZL based on the primary site of involvement: extranodal, nodal, and splenic.[28–30] Depending on the subtype, there is substantial variation in the clinical and pathologic features of MZL.

Extranodal MZL of mucosa-associated lymphoid tissue (MALT) lymphoma, as the name implies, arises at extranodal sites, such as the gastrointestinal (GI) tract, salivary glands, lungs, skin, thyroid, and orbit. Regardless of the site, there is an association with conditions that cause chronic inflammation, whether infectious or autoimmune. In the stomach, MALT lymphoma is strongly associated with gastritis caused by *Helicobacter pylori*.[31] MALT lymphomas arising in the salivary glands and thyroid are associated with Sjögren syndrome and lymphocytic (Hashimoto) thyroiditis, respectively. Although less firmly established than *H pylori* gastritis, infections caused by *Chlamydophila psittaci*, *Borrelia burgdorferi*, *Campylobacter jejuni*, and *Achromobacter xylosoxidans* have been described as possible risk factors for the development of MALT lymphoma of the ocular adnexa, skin, small intestine, and lung, respectively.[32–36]

GROSS AND MICROSCOPIC FEATURES

The GI tract is the most common site of involvement by MALT lymphoma, with the stomach the most commonly involved segment within the GI tract.[37] Histologic features of MALT lymphoma resemble acquired, benign MALT. An infiltrate of predominantly small lymphocytes surrounds reactive follicles in a marginal zone distribution. These neoplastic lymphocytes may colonize or overrun the germinal centers of the reactive follicles. The lymphomatous infiltrate is often composed of a heterogeneous mixture of centrocyte-like cells, with small to medium-sized irregular nuclei, inconspicuous nucleoli, and moderately abundant pale cytoplasm; monocytoid cells with greater amounts of pale cytoplasm; and scattered larger cells that resemble immunoblasts or centroblasts. In addition, plasmacytic differentiation can be seen in approximately 30% of cases.[38] The degree of plasmacytic differentiation present in MALT lymphoma is highly variable, ranging from minimal to plasmacytoma-like (**Fig. 2**).[39] Lymphoepithelial lesions (LELs), defined as infiltration of the epithelium by 3 or more lymphoid cells with accompanying structural disruption and distortion, are also a characteristic feature of MALT lymphoma.[40] MALT lymphoma secondarily involves lymph nodes in a marginal zone distribution with extension of the lymphomatous infiltrate into the interfollicular areas. As in extranodal sites, the infiltrate is typically polymorphous with a mixture of centrocyte-like cells, monocytoid cells, and large transformed cells (**Box 4**).

The neoplastic lymphocytes of MALT lymphoma express CD20, CD79a, CD21, and CD35.[28] MALT lymphoma displays a nonspecific immunophenotype, however, because it lacks expression of CD5, CD10, and CD23. Aberrant expression of CD43 is present in approximately half of cases.[41] Because of the lack of a positive defining marker, the diagnosis of MALT lymphoma has rested largely on the observation of characteristic histopathologic features and the lack of markers associated with other small B-cell lymphomas. Expression of immunoglobulin superfamily receptor translocation-associated 1 (IRTA1), however, a protein expressed by a subpopulation of normal B cells of the tonsil and Peyer patch, has been demonstrated in 93% of MALT lymphomas and 73% of NMZLs by immunohistochemical staining.[42] In contrast, all cases of CLL/SLL, LPL, SMZL, FL, and MCL were reportedly negative for IRTA1 when positivity was defined as IRTA1 expression in at least 30% of neoplastic cells.[42] Expression of myeloid cell nuclear differentiation antigen (MNDA) has also been recently described in 61% to 95% of MALT lymphomas, 67% to 75% of NMZLs, and 24% to 100% of SMZLs.[43,44] This marker may have diagnostic utility in excluding FL because it is expressed in only 4% to 5% of grade 1 to 2 FLs. The usefulness of MNDA may be limited, however, in differentiating MZLs from other small B-cell lymphomas because expression of MNDA is also frequently seen in LPL (25%–83% of cases), MCL (6%–82% of cases), and CLL/SLL (13%–65% of cases).[43,44]

Several different chromosomal translocations associated with MALT lymphoma have been

Fig. 2. Extranodal MZL of MALT with extensive plasmacytic differentiation, including numerous Russell bodies (hematoxylin-eosin, original magnification ×400).

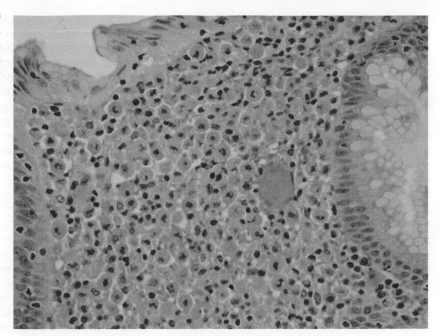

described: t(11;18)(q21;q21) involving *BIRC3* at 11q21 and *MALT1* at 18q21; t(14;18)(q32;q21) involving *IGH* at 14q32 and *MALT1*; t(1:14) (p22;q32) involving *BCL10* at 1p22 and *IGH*; and t(3;14)(p13;q32) involving *FOXP1* at 3p13 and *IGH*.[45,46] These translocations are not present, however, in all cases and the frequency at which each occurs varies widely depending on anatomic site.[45] The common pathophysiologic mechanism of the t(11;18)(q21;q21), t(14:18)(q32;q21), and t(1;14)(p22;q32) translocations is activation of nuclear factor (NF)-κB, thereby promoting B-cell survival.[47] The exact function of the t(3;14)(p13;q32) translocation is as yet unknown.[46]

Box 4
Key features of mucosa-associated lymphoid tissue lymphoma

- Associated with chronic inflammation (infectious or autoimmune)

- Infiltrate of small lymphocytes that surround, colonize, and/or overrun reactive germinal centers

- Monocytoid appearance may be prominent

- Larger transformed cells may be intermixed

- LELs often present

- Plasmacytic differentiation in 30% of cases

- Immunophenotype: CD20⁺, CD79a⁺, CD21⁺, CD35⁺, CD43±, CD5⁻, CD10⁻, CD23⁻

DIAGNOSIS AND DIFFERENTIAL DIAGNOSIS

The differential diagnosis of MALT lymphoma includes reactive MALT and other small B-cell lymphomas. Prominent LELs, sheets of monocytoid B-cells, and Dutcher bodies in accompanying plasma cells favor a diagnosis of MALT lymphoma over reactive lesions. If plasmacytic differentiation is present, demonstration of light-chain restriction indicates a neoplastic process. Absence of light chain restriction in plasma cells does not, however, exclude lymphoma because intermixed reactive plasma cells that are not clonally related to the neoplastic lymphocytes may be seen in MALT lymphoma. The presence of aberrant CD43 expression, seen in approximately half of MALT lymphomas, is indicative of a neoplasm.[41] Assessment of B-cell clonality by polymerase chain reaction–based assays for immunoglobulin heavy chain (IgH) gene rearrangement should be done with great caution because this technique can show a monoclonal population in approximately 13% of biopsies with *H pylori* gastritis in the absence of MALT lymphoma.[48]

MALT lymphoma can usually be differentiated from CLL/SLL by the absence of CD5 and CD23 expression; FL by lack of CD10 and BCL6 expression; and MCL by the absence of CD5 and cyclin D1 expression. CD5, however, is expressed in some cases of otherwise typical MALT lymphoma.[49] When colonization of reactive follicles is prominent, MALT lymphoma may mimic the morphologic features of FL. MALT lymphoma cells that have colonized the germinal centers are negative, however, for CD10 and BCL6, thus aiding in this distinction. As discussed previously, absence of the *MYD88* (L265P) mutation favors a diagnosis of MALT lymphoma over LPL.

Although scattered large cells are usually present in MALT lymphoma, a diagnosis of large cell transformation should not be made unless solid or sheet-like aggregates of large cells are present.[28] When MALT lymphoma colonizes germinal centers, however, the neoplastic cells can assume the appearance of large centroblasts under the influence of the follicular environment.[41] Care should be taken not to interpret these changes as transformation to a diffuse large B-cell lymphoma (DLBCL). Demonstration that the aggregates of large cells are confined to colonized germinal centers by immunohistochemical staining for CD21 or CD23 can aid in this distinction (**Boxes 5** and **6**).

PROGNOSIS

The prognosis of MALT lymphoma is favorable, with a 5-year OS of approximately 70% to 80%.[50,51] The treatment of MALT lymphoma depends on the site of involvement (gastric vs nongastric) and the stage of disease. Gastric MALT lymphoma is usually effectively treated by antibiotic therapy to eradicate *H pylori*, thereby eliminating the *H pylori*–specific intratumoral T cells that provide CD40/CD40L-mediated signaling and T_H2-type cytokines that promote the growth and differentiation of MALT lymphoma cells.[46] The presence of t(11;18)(q21;q21) in gastric MALT lymphoma, however, has been shown to predict resistance to *H pylori* eradication therapy.[52] In contrast, the treatment of nongastric MALT lymphomas depends on the stage of disease. Stage I–II MALT lymphoma is treated by locoregional radiotherapy, whereas stage III–IV disease is often treated with rituximab with or without chemotherapy. Because of the suspected etiologic link with infection by *Chlamydophila psittaci*, antibiotic therapy has also been used to treat MALT lymphoma of the ocular adnexa.[33] Although the success of such an approach has not been as dramatic as that seen in gastric MALT lymphoma, the overall response rate of antibiotic therapy is approximately 45% in cases of MALT lymphoma affecting the ocular adnexa.[53]

NODAL MARGINAL ZONE LYMPHOMA

OVERVIEW

NMZL is defined in the WHO classification as a primary nodal B-cell neoplasm that displays morphologic features similar to those seen in lymph nodes that are secondarily involved by MALT lymphoma or SMZL.[30] To exclude SMZL and MALT lymphoma, patients should not have evidence of extranodal disease other than involvement of the BM and peripheral blood.

NMZL is rare, accounting for 1% to 2% of non-Hodgkin lymphoma, and the median age at diagnosis ranges from 50 to 63 years, depending on the study.[54–56] Some studies have reported an association between NMZL and hepatitis C infection, whereas others have not found such a link.[57]

GROSS AND MICROSCOPIC FEATURES

The peripheral lymph nodes are involved in nearly all cases, whereas abdominal and/or thoracic lymph nodes are involved in approximately 20% to 50% of patients.[55] The reported frequency of BM involvement varies widely, from 19% to 62%, depending on the study.[55,56,58,59] By definition, the spleen and other extranodal sites are uninvolved.

A majority of cases of NMZL display a diffuse architectural pattern in which sheets of neoplastic cells efface the lymph node architecture, often with a minor component of vague nodularity.[60] Other patterns of lymph node involvement include a nodular/follicular pattern, in which follicular colonization of neoplastic cells forms discrete nodules with intervening uninvolved interfollicular areas; an interfollicular pattern that is characterized by involvement of the interfollicular areas by the lymphomatous infiltrate with sparing of interspersed reactive follicles; and a perifollicular pattern, in which the neoplastic cells surround uninvolved secondary follicles in an annular distribution (**Fig. 3**).[58,60] A majority of NMZLs are characterized by cellular polymorphism with a

---

Box 5
Differential diagnosis of mucosa-associated lymphoid tissue lymphoma

- Reactive MALT: typically lacks prominent LELs, sheets of monocytoid B-cells, Dutcher bodies, and aberrant CD43 expression

- CLL/SLL: CD5$^+$, CD23$^+$, CD20 dim, surface light chain dim

- FL: CD10$^+$, BCL6$^+$

- MCL: CD5$^+$, cyclin D1$^+$

- LPL: absence of prominent follicular colonization. Lack of monocytoid features. *MYD88* (L265P) positive

---

Box 6
Pitfalls of mucosa-associated lymphoid tissue lymphoma

- IGH gene rearrangement studies may show a clonal population in biopsies of *H pylori* gastritis in the absence of lymphoma
- Follicular colonization by MALT lymphoma with numerous centroblast-like cells may mimic DLBCL and be mistaken for transformation

---

mixture of centrocyte-like cells, monocytoid cells, and intermixed large transformed cells. Although an increased number of intermixed large cells (>20%) can frequently be seen in NMZL, the proportion of large cells does not seem to significantly affect outcome.[54,58] Plasmacytic differentiation is a frequent finding in NMZL, reported in 22% to 47% of cases (**Box 7**).[57]

Like other small B-cell lymphomas, the neoplastic cells of NMZL express CD19, CD20, PAX5, and CD79a. Most cases of NMZL express BCL2, but CD10, BCL6, and cyclin D1 are negative. Although CD5 and CD23 are usually negative, expression of these markers has been reported in a minority of cases.[59] The reported frequency of CD43 expression in NMZL varies widely, from 5% to 75% of cases.[57] As discussed previously, IRTA1 and MNDA are expressed in 73% and 67% to 75% of NMZLs, respectively.[42–44]

Although cytogenetic abnormalities that are specific to NMZL have not been identified, gains of 1q, 2p, 3p, 3q, 6p, and 6q as well as losses of 1q and 6q have been frequently reported in NZML.[57] Other reported cytogenetic abnormalities seen in NMZL include trisomies 3, 7, 12, and 18.[30,57] The recurrent translocations that have been reported, however, in MALT lymphoma are not seen in NMZL.

DIAGNOSIS AND DIFFERENTIAL DIAGNOSIS

NMZL can usually be differentiated from CLL/SLL, MCL, and FL based on differences in immunophenotype. CLL/SLL can be excluded based on the lack of CD5 and CD23 expression in most cases of NMZL. Similarly NMZL can be distinguished from MCL based on the absence of CD5 and cyclin D1 expression. In some cases, NMZL with prominent germinal center colonization by the neoplastic cells can closely mimic FL. Further complicating this distinction is expression of BCL2 by NMZL cells that have colonized germinal centers. In contrast to FL, however, NMZL cells colonizing germinal centers are negative for CD10 and BCL6.[60] As discussed previously, recently described immunohistochemical stains for MNDA and IRTA1 may prove useful in excluding FL.[42–44]

LPL involving the lymph node may be difficult to differentiate from NMZL with plasmacytic

Fig. 3. MZL showing a residual germinal center and a perifollicular infiltrate of monocytoid B cells and plasma cells (hematoxylin-eosin, original magnification ×200).

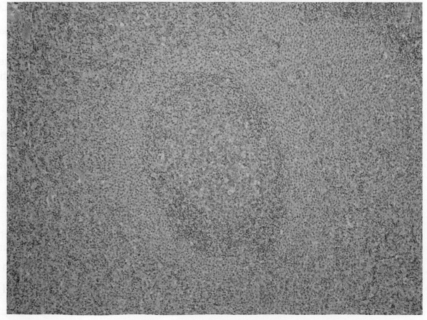

> **Box 7**
> **Key features of nodal marginal zone lymphoma**
>
> - Primary nodal B-cell neoplasm that displays morphologic features similar to lymph nodes secondarily involved by MALT lymphoma or SMZL
> - Most common architectural pattern is effacement of lymph node architecture by diffuse sheets of neoplastic cells
> - Nodular, interfollicular, and perifollicular patterns are less common
> - Polymorphic infiltrate of centrocyte-like cells, monocytoid cells, and large transformed cells
> - Plasmacytic differentiation in 22% to 47% of cases
> - Immunophenotype: CD19[+], CD20[+], CD79a[+], CD43[±], PAX5[+], BCL-2[+], CD5[−], CD10[−], CD23[−], BCL6[−], cyclin D1[−]

differentiation. Features that favor NMZL over LPL include prominent monocytoid features and follicular colonization, whereas numerous mast cells are more commonly seen in LPL.[12] Testing for the *MYD88* (L265P) mutation can be helpful in this distinction because this mutation is present in approximately 90% of LPL but is uncommon in NMZL.[2,8,20,21]

Because MALT lymphoma and SMZL can secondarily involve lymph nodes in a pattern that is similar to NMZL, correlation with clinical and radiographic findings is necessary when considering a diagnosis of NMZL because involvement of extranodal sites other than BM must be excluded.

Monocytoid B-cell hyperplasia can be seen in a variety of reactive conditions, especially in *Toxoplasma* lymphadenitis. Monocytoid B-cell hyperplasia in the setting of toxoplasmosis, however, is usually accompanied by florid follicular hyperplasia with clusters of epithelioid histiocytes that encroach on germinal centers, features not seen in NMZL. Immunohistochemical staining for BCL2 can be helpful because monocytoid B-cells seen in reactive conditions are BCL2 negative, whereas neoplastic monocytoid B-cells of NMZL are usually positive for BCL2 (**Boxes 8 and 9**).[61]

PROGNOSIS

The prognosis reported in most studies is less favorable than MALT lymphoma or SMZL, with a 5-year OS ranging from 55% to 89%.[62] Unfortunately, there is currently no consensus as to the optimal treatment of NMZL.[57] Patients with localized (stage I–II) disease are often treated with surgery with or without radiotherapy. Advanced-stage disease that is asymptomatic may be observed, whereas symptomatic advanced disease may be treated with rituximab,

cyclophosphamide, doxorubicin, vincristine, and prednisone (R-CHOP) or other similar regimens.[62]

SPLENIC MARGINAL ZONE LYMPHOMA

OVERVIEW

SMZL is a disease of older adults, with a median age at diagnosis of 68 years.[63] The disease is rare, accounting for only 1% to 2% of all non-Hodgkin lymphomas.[64] As the name implies, the spleen is invariably involved by SMZL, and patients tend to present with splenomegaly. A vast majority of SMZLs involve the BM. Although splenic hilar lymph nodes are involved in a majority of cases, peripheral lymphadenopathy is uncommon.[64] Peripheral blood involvement is detected in 64% to 84% of cases.[64]

GROSS AND MICROSCOPIC FEATURES

The spleen is often markedly enlarged with a median weight of 1750 g.[63] The gross appearance of the spleen is characterized by a micronodular appearance with dramatic expansion of the white

> **Box 8**
> **Differential diagnosis of nodal marginal zone lymphoma**
>
> - LPL: lack of prominent monocytoid features and follicular colonization. Numerous mast cells. *MYD88* (L265P) positive
> - FL: BCL6[+], CD10[+]
> - CLL/SLL: ± proliferation centers, CD5[+], CD23[+], CD20 dim, surface light chain dim
> - MCL: CD5[+], cyclin D1[+]
> - Reactive monocytoid B-cell hyperplasia lacks BCL2 expression

- NMZL with prominent follicular colonization may closely mimic FL

- MALT lymphoma and SMZL secondarily involving lymph nodes may be morphologically indistinguishable from NMZL

pulp. Histologically, these nodules are composed of a central zone of small lymphocytes that are surrounded by an outer zone of medium-sized lymphocytes with more abundant pale cytoplasm (marginal zone cells) (**Fig. 4**). Residual germinal centers may be present at the center of these nodules. The red pulp may be secondarily involved by a diffuse infiltrate of neoplastic cells with frequent infiltration of the sinuses. As is the case with other types of MZL, plasmacytic differentiation may be present, reported in 20% to 70% of cases.[39] SMZL usually involves the BM in a nodular interstitial pattern. Although not entirely specific for SMZL, a prominent intrasinusoidal lymphomatous infiltrate in the BM is characteristic. The splenic hilar lymph nodes are often involved by SMZL in a nodular pattern that surrounds and replaces the germinal centers. The two distinct zones seen in the spleen, however, are usually absent with more intermixing of small cells with marginal zone lymphocytes (**Box 10**).

Similar to other types of MZL, tumor cells of SMZL are CD20+, CD79a+, CD5−, CD10−,

CD23−, BCL2+, and BCL6−.[64] In contrast to NMZL and MALT lymphoma, expression of CD43 is not present in SMZL. Although expression of CD103 is usually absent, it can be seen occasionally. SMZL is negative, however, for annexin A1 and cyclin D1.[65,66] The tumor cells of SMZL usually express both surface IgM and IgD.

The most common chromosomal abnormalities in SMZL are allelic loss of 7q31–32 in up to 40% of cases and gain of 3/3q in approximately 20% of cases.[67,68] Activating mutations of *NOTCH2*, a gene encoding a protein required in marginal zone B-cell development, have been identified in 6.5% to 25% of cases of SMZL.[69–71] More recently, mutations of *KLF2*, which impair its ability to suppress NF-κB activation, have been reported in 42% of SMZL.[72] Because initial reported data suggest that *NOTCH2* and *KLF2* mutations are rare or absent in other small B-cell lymphomas, identification of these mutations has potential diagnostic utility.

DIAGNOSIS AND DIFFERENTIAL DIAGNOSIS

Other small B-cell lymphomas, in particular MCL and FL, can involve the spleen with a prominent expansion of the white pulp that results in a micronodular/miliary pattern that resembles the changes seen in SMZL. SMZL, however, can usually be readily distinguished from FL and MCL by its lack of expression of CD10/BCL6 and CD5/cyclin D1, respectively.

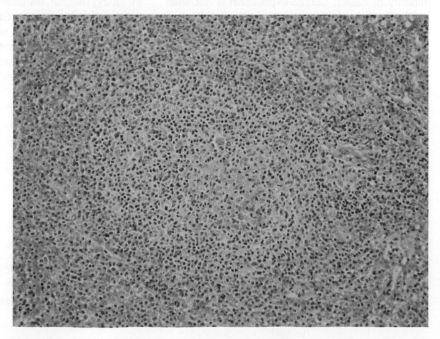

Fig. 4. Nodular infiltrates of small lymphocytes and plasma cells in the white pulp of the spleen (hematoxylin-eosin, original magnification ×200).

Box 10
Key features of splenic marginal zone lymphoma

- Spleen is always involved with frequent involvement of the BM
- Nodules composed of a central zone of small lymphocytes surrounded by an outer zone of medium-sized lymphocytes with abundant pale cytoplasm
- Nodular and intrasinusoidal pattern of involvement of the BM
- Immunophenotype: CD20[+], CD79a[+], BCL2[+], CD103[±], CD5[−], CD10[−], CD23[−], BCL6[−], annexin A1[−], cyclin D1[−]
- Mutations of *KLF2* and *NOTCH2* in approximately 40% and approximately 25% of cases, respectively

---

Because SMZL can display significant plasma-cytic differentiation and an IgM paraprotein, LPL may also be considered in the differential diagnosis. In addition, LPL displays a similar immunophenotype to SMZL because both are CD5[−]/CD10[−]. Serum hyperviscosity, if present, favors a diagnosis of LPL as this is uncommon in SMZL.[39] Testing for the *MYD88* (L265P) mutation may be helpful as this mutation is found in approximately 90% of cases of LPL but only uncommonly found in SMZL.[8]

In BM biopsies performed for patients with splenomegaly, hairy cell leukemia (HCL), and HCL-variant (HCL-v) may be considered in the differential diagnosis of SMZL. In contrast to the nodular pattern of BM involvement seen in SMZL, HCL and HCL-v usually involve the BM in an interstitial or sinusoidal distribution manner.[73,74] Although SMZL is usually positive for CD11c with occasional expression of CD25 and/or CD103 in a minority of cases, CD123 expression is not seen in SMZL. This is in contrast to HCL, which expresses CD123 in addition to strong coexpression of CD11c, CD25, and CD103 in nearly all cases. Furthermore, SMZL is negative for annexin A1, whereas nearly all cases of HCL are positive for this marker.[65] There is a greater degree of immunophenotypic overlap between SMZL and HCL-v because each can be positive for CD11c and

CD103 but negative for CD123.[75] Immunohistochemical staining for annexin A1 does not distinguish between SMZL and HCL-v because both are negative. SMZL and HCL-v are readily distinguished, however, based on splenic morphology because HCL-v is characterized by diffuse red pulp infiltration with blood lake formation whereas SMZL predominantly expands the white pulp in the pattern described previously with a lesser degree of red pulp involvement (**Boxes 11 and 12**).

PROGNOSIS

SMZL is an indolent disease with a 5-year relative survival rate of approximately 80%.[76,77] Parameters that predict a worse prognosis include hemoglobin less than 12 g/dL, lactate dehydrogenase greater than normal, and albumin less than 3.5 g/dL.[78] The presence of *NOTCH2* mutations in SMZL is also associated with adverse outcomes, including relapse, transformation, and death.[69]

Not all patients with SMZL require immediate treatment, and those who are asymptomatic without marked splenomegaly or cytopenias are often observed. In patients who require treatment, rituximab with or without splenectomy may be considered.[79] In certain circumstances, rituximab may be combined with various chemotherapeutic regimens.[80] There is currently a lack of

---

Box 11
Differential diagnosis of splenic marginal zone lymphoma

- FL: CD10[+], BCL6[+]
- MCL: CD5[+], cyclin D1[+]
- LPL: serum hyperviscosity, frequent mast cells, *MYD88* (L265P) positive
- HCL: interstitial pattern of BM involvement, diffuse red pulp pattern of splenic involvement with blood lake formation, CD123[+], annexin A1[+]
- HCL-v: interstitial pattern of BM involvement, diffuse red pulp pattern of splenic involvement with blood lake formation

---

Box 12
Pitfalls of splenic marginal zone lymphoma

- SMZL and HCL-v may have significant immunophenotypic overlap in BM biopsy specimens because both may be positive for CD11c and CD103 but negative for CD123 and annexin A1

---

prospective randomized clinical trials, however, comparing the efficacy of these different approaches. An epidemiologic link between hepatitis C infection and SMZL has been reported, and small studies have reported regression of SMZL on treatment with interferon and/or ribavirin for concurrent hepatitis C.[81–83]

PLASMABLASTIC LYMPHOMA

OVERVIEW

PBL is a high-grade neoplasm composed of large cells with prominent nucleoli that resemble B immunoblasts with the immunophenotype of plasma cells.[84] Although a majority of cases occur in the setting of HIV infection, PBL can also occur in HIV-negative individuals, most frequently in the setting of immunosuppression for organ transplantation or in elderly patients.[85] Approximately 75% of cases occur in male patients.[85] PBL is rare, comprising only 2% of HIV-related non-Hodgkin lymphomas.[86] Although pediatric cases have been reported in the literature, a majority of cases occur in adults with a median age of 50 years.[84]

GROSS AND MICROSCOPIC FEATURES

The most common site of involvement is the oral cavity/jaw followed by the GI tract and lymph nodes.[85] Less common sites include skin, bone, and the genitourinary tract. Microscopically, cases of PBL display a diffuse infiltrate composed of large cells with abundant cytoplasm, vesicular chromatin, and prominent, often central, nucleoli that resemble immunoblasts (**Fig. 5**). Many cases of PBL are composed of cells with cytologic characteristics of plasmacytic differentiation, including eccentric nuclei and perinuclear hofs. Frequent mitoses, apoptotic figures, and intermixed tingible body macrophages are also typically present. Cases presenting in the oral cavity of an HIV-positive patient most often have an immunoblastic appearance, whereas PBL involving other extranodal sites and lymph nodes often displays more obvious plasmacytic differentiation (**Fig. 6, Box 13**).[84]

PBL is usually positive for markers associated with plasmacytic differentiation, including CD138, CD38, and IRF4/MUM1.[87] PBL is negative for markers of B-cell differentiation, including CD19, CD20, and PAX5.[85,87] CD79a expression,

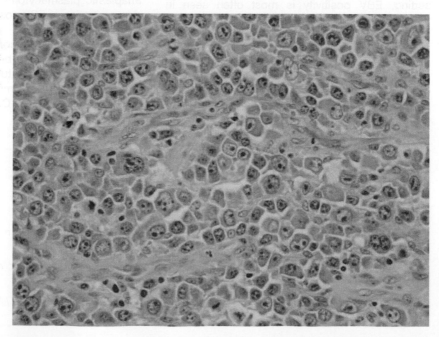

Fig. 5. PBL with pleomorphic cells, many with central nucleoli and abundant eosinophilic cytoplasm (hematoxylin-eosin, original magnification ×400).

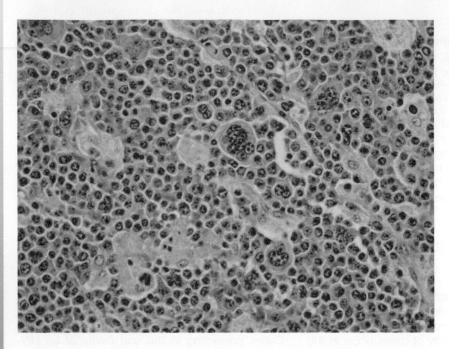

Fig. *6.* PBL with numerous plasma cells and pleomorphic, large multinucleated cells (hematoxylin-eosin, original magnification ×400).

however, is common. Expression of CD30 and EMA is frequently seen in PBL, but CD45 is typically negative or only weakly positive.[84] Approximately 50% of cases harbor rearrangements involving the *MYC* gene, and a similar percentage of cases are positive for MYC by immunohistochemical staining.[85,88,89] Although Epstein Barr virus-encoded RNA (EBER) is positive in a majority of cases, EBV positivity varies based on the clinical setting. EBV positivity is most often seen in the setting of AIDS-related PBL (75% of cases) and PBL in transplant recipients (67% of cases) but is also seen in a smaller proportion of cases of PBL in immunocompetent patients (50%).[90] Immunohistochemical staining for HHV-8 is negative in PBL.[90]

DIAGNOSIS AND DIFFERENTIAL DIAGNOSIS

PBL can be difficult to distinguish from anaplastic (plasmablastic) plasmacytoma because the morphologic and immunophenotypic features of these entities are extremely similar.[87,91] Clinical features, however, such as osteolytic lesions, hypercalcemia, diffuse BM involvement, and the presence of an M protein, support a diagnosis of anaplastic plasmacytoma. HIV infection and the demonstration of EBV positivity in the tumor favor PBL.[91]

ALK[+] LBCL may be considered in the differential diagnosis of PBL because it also demonstrates morphologic features of immunoblast-like cells (**Fig. 7**) and an immunophenotype that is similar to PBL (CD38[+], CD138[+], CD20[-], PAX5[-],

---

Box 13
Key features of plasmablastic lymphoma

- Associated with HIV infection or other causes of immunosuppression

- Oral cavity/jaw is most common site

- Diffuse infiltrate of large cells with abundant cytoplasm, vesicular chromatin, and prominent, often central, nucleoli resembling immunoblasts

- Cytologic characteristics of plasmacytic differentiation, including eccentric nuclei and perinuclear hofs

- Immunophenotype: CD38[+], CD138[+], IRF4/MUM1[+], CD79a[±], CD45[±], EBER[+], MYC[±], CD19[-], CD20[-], PAX5[-], HHV-8[-]

Fig. 7. ALK⁺ LBCL with large atypical cells, many with abundant cytoplasm (hematoxylin-eosin, original magnification ×400).

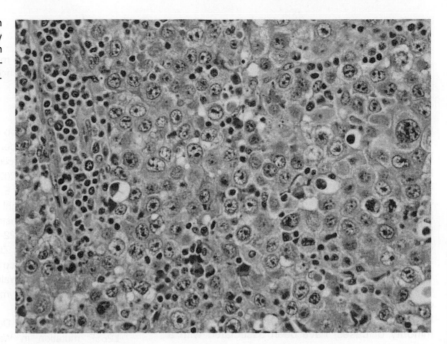

and CD45⁻).[92,93] As the name implies, ALK⁺ LBCL is strongly positive for ALK protein in a granular cytoplasmic staining pattern and thus can be readily distinguished from PBL, which is negative for ALK. ALK expression in ALK⁺ LBCL is most often due to t(2;17)(p23;q23) which results in a clathrin-ALK fusion protein.[94] Although *MYC* rearrangements are absent in ALK⁺ LBCL, immunohistochemical staining for MYC is often positive, possibly due to activation of STAT3.[93]

Given the immunoblastic cytologic features that are typical of PBL, I-DLBCL may be considered in the differential diagnosis. Immunophenotypic differences can aid, however, in this distinction because I-DLBCL expresses CD20 and PAX5 but is negative for CD138.[85,95] In addition, EBV infection is not seen in Immunoblastic DLBCL (I-DLBCL). As in PBL, however, translocations involving *MYC* are

frequently seen in I-DLBCL. Not surprisingly, most cases of I-DLBCL are also positive on immunohistochemical staining for MYC.[95]

PEL can rarely present as a solid tumor mass, referred to as extracavitary PEL. Because extracavitary PEL can display immunoblastic and/or plasmablastic morphology, it should be considered in the differential diagnosis of PBL. Furthermore, PEL demonstrates an immunophenotype that is similar to PBL with frequent expression of plasma cell–related antigens (CD38⁺, CD138⁺, and IRF4⁺/MUM1⁺) and absence of pan–B-cell markers (CD19⁻, CD20⁻, CD79a⁻, and PAX5⁻).[96–98] Other similarities to PBL include a strong association with HIV infection and frequent EBV positivity of the tumor cells. PEL is universally associated with human herpesvirus 8 (HHV-8) infection, whereas PBL is negative for HHV-8 (**Boxes 14** and **15**).

Box 14
Differential diagnosis of plasmablastic lymphoma

- Anaplastic plasmacytoma: osteolytic lesions, hypercalcemia, diffuse BM involvement, M-protein, absence of EBV positivity, absence of HIV infection

- ALK⁺ LBCL: expression of ALK (usually in a granular cytoplasmic staining pattern)

- I-DLBCL: CD20⁺, PAX5⁺, CD138⁻, EBER⁻

- PEL: HHV-8⁺

> **Box 15**
> **Pitfalls of plasmablastic lymphoma**
> - It may be difficult to distinguish PBL from anaplastic plasmacytoma based on morphology and immu-nophenotype. EBV positivity and HIV infection favor PBL, whereas the presence of osteolytic lesions, hypercalcemia, and/or an M-protein favor plasmacytoma

PROGNOSIS

PBL follows an aggressive clinical course with a poor prognosis. HIV-positive patients have been reported to have a median OS time of 14 months and a 5-year OS rate of 31%.[99] Some studies have suggested that HIV-negative patients with PBL have a worse median OS time (9 months) and OS rate (10% at 2 years) than patients who are HIV-positive.[100] A recent meta-analysis, however, incorporating data from 277 reported cases of PBL, found no significant difference in survival of HIV-positive and HIV-negative PBL patients.[90] EBV positivity and CD45 expression (present in a minority of cases) have been associated with a better outcome, whereas *MYC* rearrangement or amplification is associated with a worse outcome.[90] A proliferation rate greater than 80%, as assessed by immunohistochemical staining for Ki-67, has also been shown to be associated with worse OS.[101]

Although there is currently no firmly established standard of care in regard to therapy for PBL, treatment typically includes the use of intensive chemotherapy regimens, such as etoposide, pred-nisone, vincristine, cyclophosphamide, and doxo-rubicin (EPOCH).[85] Small studies have shown possible improvement in OS in both HIV-positive and HIV-negative patients who are treated with autologous stem cell transplantation in first remission.[102,103]

REFERENCES

1. Swerdlow SH, Berger F, Pileri SA, et al. Lympho-plasmacytic lymphoma. In: Swerdlow SH, Campo E, Harris NL, et al, editors. WHO classifica-tion of tumours of haematopoietic and lymphoid tis-sues. 4th edition. Lyon (France): IARC; 2008. p. 194–5.
2. Treon SP, Xu L, Yang G, et al. MYD88 L265P so-matic mutation in Waldenstrom's macroglobuli-nemia. N Engl J Med 2012;367:826–33.
3. Gachard N, Parrens M, Soubeyran I, et al. IGHV gene features and MYD88 L265P mutation sepa-rate the three marginal zone lymphoma entities and Waldenstrom macroglobulinemia/lymphoplas-macytic lymphomas. Leukemia 2013;27:183–9.
4. Xu L, Hunter ZR, Yang G, et al. MYD88 L265P in Waldenstrom macroglobulinemia, immunoglobulin

M monoclonal gammopathy, and other B-cell lym-phoproliferative disorders using conventional and quantitative allele-specific polymerase chain reac-tion. Blood 2013;121:2051–8.
5. Jimenez C, Sebastian E, Chillon MC, et al. MYD88 L265P is a marker highly characteristic of, but not restricted to, Waldenstrom's macroglobulinemia. Leukemia 2013;27:1722–8.
6. Varettoni M, Arcaini L, Zibellini S, et al. Prevalence and clinical significance of the MYD88 (L265P) so-matic mutation in Waldenstrom's macroglobuli-nemia and related lymphoid neoplasms. Blood 2013;121:2522–8.
7. Poulain S, Roumier C, Decambron A, et al. MYD88 L265P mutation in Waldenstrom macroglobuli-nemia. Blood 2013;121:4504–11.
8. Insuasti-Beltran G, Gale JM, Wilson CS, et al. Sig-nificance of MYD88 L265P mutation status in the subclassification of low-grade B-Cell lymphoma/leukemia. Arch Pathol Lab Med 2015;139:1035–41.
9. Ailawadhi S, Kardosh A, Yang D, et al. Outcome disparities among ethnic subgroups of Walden-strom's macroglobulinemia: a population-based study. Oncology 2014;86:253–62.
10. Gertz MA. Waldenstrom macroglobulinemia: 2015 update on diagnosis, risk stratification, and man-agement. Am J Hematol 2015;90:346–54.
11. Arber DA, George TI. Bone marrow biopsy involve-ment by non-Hodgkin's lymphoma: frequency of lymphoma types, patterns, blood involvement, and discordance with other sites in 450 specimens. Am J Surg Pathol 2005;29:1549–57.
12. Lin P, Molina TJ, Cook JR, et al. Lymphoplasma-cytic lymphoma and other non-marginal zone lym-phomas with plasmacytic differentiation. Am J Clin Pathol 2011;136:195–210.
13. Morice WG, Chen D, Kurtin PJ, et al. Novel immuno-phenotypic features of marrow lymphoplasmacytic lymphoma and correlation with Waldenstrom's macroglobulinemia. Mod Pathol 2009;22:807–16.
14. Konoplev S, Medeiros LJ, Bueso-Ramos CE, et al. Immunophenotypic profile of lymphoplasmacytic lymphoma/Waldenstrom macroglobulinemia. Am J Clin Pathol 2005;124:414–20.
15. Roberts MJ, Chadburn A, Ma S, et al. Nuclear pro-tein dysregulation in lymphoplasmacytic lym-phoma/waldenstrom macroglobulinemia. Am J Clin Pathol 2013;139:210–9.

16. Bassarova A, Troen G, Spetalen S, et al. Lympho-plasmacytic lymphoma and marginal zone lymphoma in the bone marrow: paratrabecular involvement as an important distinguishing feature. Am J Clin Pathol 2015;143:797–806.

17. Kyle RA, Gertz MA, Witzig TE, et al. Review of 1027 patients with newly diagnosed multiple myeloma. Mayo Clin Proc 2003;78:21–33.

18. King RL, Howard MT, Hodnefield JM, et al. IgM multiple myeloma: pathologic evaluation of a rare entity. Am J Clin Pathol 2013;140:519–24.

19. Schuster SR, Rajkumar SV, Dispenzieri A, et al. IgM multiple myeloma: disease definition, prognosis, and differentiation from Waldenstrom's macroglobulinemia. Am J Hematol 2010;85:853–5.

20. Martinez-Lopez A, Curiel-Olmo S, Mollejo M, et al. MYD88 (L265P) Somatic Mutation in Marginal Zone B-cell Lymphoma. Am J Surg Pathol 2015;39:644–51.

21. Hamadeh F, MacNamara SP, Aguilera NS, et al. MYD88 L265P mutation analysis helps define nodal lymphoplasmacytic lymphoma. Mod Pathol 2015;28:564–74.

22. Castillo JJ, Olszewski AJ, Kanan S, et al. Overall survival and competing risks of death in patients with Waldenstrom macroglobulinaemia: an analysis of the surveillance, epidemiology and end results database. Br J Haematol 2015;169:81–9.

23. Morel P, Duhamel A, Gobbi P, et al. International prognostic scoring system for Waldenstrom macroglobulinemia. Blood 2009;113:4163–70.

24. Treon SP, Cao Y, Xu L, et al. Somatic mutations in MYD88 and CXCR4 are determinants of clinical presentation and overall survival in Waldenstrom macroglobulinemia. Blood 2014;123:2791–6.

25. Nguyen-Khac F, Lambert J, Chapiro E, et al. Chromosomal aberrations and their prognostic value in a series of 174 untreated patients with Waldenstrom's macroglobulinemia. Haematologica 2013;98:649–54.

26. Ocio EM, Schop RF, Gonzalez B, et al. 6q deletion in Waldenstrom macroglobulinemia is associated with features of adverse prognosis. Br J Haematol 2007;136:80–6.

27. Chang H, Qi C, Trieu Y, et al. Prognostic relevance of 6q deletion in Waldenstrom's macroglobulinemia: a multicenter study. Clin Lymphoma Myeloma 2009;9:36–8.

28. Isaacson PG, Chott A, Nakamura S, et al. Extranodal marginal zone lymphoma of mucosa-associated lymphoid tissue (MALT lymphoma). In: Swerdlow SH, Campo E, Harris NL, et al, editors. WHO classification of tumours of haematopoietic and lymphoid tissues. 4th edition. Lyon (France): IARC; 2008. p. 214–7.

29. Isaacson PG, Piris MA, Berger F, et al. Splenic marginal zone lymphoma. In: Swerdlow SH, Campo E, Harris NL, et al, editors. WHO classification of tumours of haematopoietic and lymphoid tissues. 4th edition. Lyon (France): IARC; 2008. p. 185–7.

30. Campo E, Pileri SA, Jaffe ES, et al. Nodal marginal zone lymphoma. In: Swerdlow SH, Campo E, Harris NL, et al, editors. WHO classification of tumours of haematopoietic and lymphoid tissues. 4th edition. Lyon (France): IARC; 2008. p. 218–9.

31. Bhandari A, Crowe SE. Helicobacter pylori in gastric malignancies. Curr Gastroenterol Rep 2012;14:489–96.

32. Thieblemont C, Bertoni F, Copie-Bergman C, et al. Chronic inflammation and extra-nodal marginal-zone lymphomas of MALT-type. Semin Cancer Biol 2014;24:33–42.

33. Ferreri AJ, Guidoboni M, Ponzoni M, et al. Evidence for an association between Chlamydia psittaci and ocular adnexal lymphomas. J Natl Cancer Inst 2004;96:586–94.

34. Lecuit M, Abachin E, Martin A, et al. Immunoproliferative small intestinal disease associated with Campylobacter jejuni. N Engl J Med 2004;350:239–48.

35. Adam P, Czapiewski P, Colak S, et al. Prevalence of Achromobacter xylosoxidans in pulmonary mucosa-associated lymphoid tissue lymphoma in different regions of Europe. Br J Haematol 2014;164:804–10.

36. Ferreri AJ, Govi S, Ponzoni M. Marginal zone lymphomas and infectious agents. Semin Cancer Biol 2013;23:431–40.

37. Thieblemont C, Bastion Y, Berger F, et al. Mucosa-associated lymphoid tissue gastrointestinal and nongastrointestinal lymphoma behavior: analysis of 108 patients. J Clin Oncol 1997;15:1624–30.

38. Wohrer S, Troch M, Streubel B, et al. Pathology and clinical course of MALT lymphoma with plasmacytic differentiation. Ann Oncol 2007;18:2020–4.

39. Molina TJ, Lin P, Swerdlow SH, et al. Marginal zone lymphomas with plasmacytic differentiation and related disorders. Am J Clin Pathol 2011;136:211–25.

40. Papadaki L, Wotherspoon AC, Isaacson PG. The lymphoepithelial lesion of gastric low-grade B-cell lymphoma of mucosa-associated lymphoid tissue (MALT): an ultrastructural study. Histopathology 1992;21:415–21.

41. Isaacson PG, Du MQ. Gastrointestinal lymphoma: where morphology meets molecular biology. J Pathol 2005;205:255–74.

42. Falini B, Agostinelli C, Bigerna B, et al. IRTA1 is selectively expressed in nodal and extranodal marginal zone lymphomas. Histopathology 2012;61:930–41.

43. Kanellis G, Roncador G, Arribas A, et al. Identification of MNDA as a new marker for nodal marginal zone lymphoma. Leukemia 2009;23:1847–57.

44. Metcalf RA, Monabati A, Vyas M, et al. Myeloid cell nuclear differentiation antigen is expressed in a subset of marginal zone lymphomas and is useful in the differential diagnosis with follicular lymphoma. Hum Pathol 2014;45:1730–6.

45. Remstein ED, Dogan A, Einerson RR, et al. The incidence and anatomic site specificity of chromosomal translocations in primary extranodal marginal zone B-cell lymphoma of mucosa-associated lymphoid tissue (MALT lymphoma) in North America. Am J Surg Pathol 2006;30:1546–53.

46. Zucca E, Bertoni F, Vannata B, et al. Emerging role of infectious etiologies in the pathogenesis of marginal zone B-cell lymphomas. Clin Cancer Res 2014;20:5207–16.

47. Sagaert X, De Wolf-Peeters C, Noels H, et al. The pathogenesis of MALT lymphomas: where do we stand? Leukemia 2007;21:389–96.

48. Hsi ED, Greenson JK, Singleton TP, et al. Detection of immunoglobulin heavy chain gene rearrangement by polymerase chain reaction in chronic active gastritis associated with Helicobacter pylori. Hum Pathol 1996;27:290–6.

49. Jaso J, Chen L, Li S, et al. CD5-positive mucosa-associated lymphoid tissue (MALT) lymphoma: a clinicopathologic study of 14 cases. Hum Pathol 2012;43:1436–43.

50. A clinical evaluation of the International Lymphoma Study Group classification of non-Hodgkin's lymphoma. The Non-Hodgkin's Lymphoma Classification Project. Blood 1997;89:3909–18.

51. Nathwani BN, Anderson JR, Armitage JO, et al. Marginal zone B-cell lymphoma: A clinical comparison of nodal and mucosa-associated lymphoid tissue types. Non-Hodgkin's Lymphoma Classification Project. J Clin Oncol 1999;17:2486–92.

52. Liu H, Ruskon-Fourmestraux A, Lavergne-Slove A, et al. Resistance of t(11;18) positive gastric mucosa-associated lymphoid tissue lymphoma to Helicobacter pylori eradication therapy. Lancet 2001;357:39–40.

53. Kiesewetter B, Raderer M. Antibiotic therapy in nongastrointestinal MALT lymphoma: a review of the literature. Blood 2013;122:1350–7.

54. Traverse-Glehen A, Bertoni F, Thieblemont C, et al. Nodal marginal zone B-cell lymphoma: a diagnostic and therapeutic dilemma. Oncology (Williston Park) 2012;26:92–9, 103–4.

55. Arcaini L, Paulli M, Burcheri S, et al. Primary nodal marginal zone B-cell lymphoma: clinical features and prognostic assessment of a rare disease. Br J Haematol 2007;136:301–4.

56. Oh SY, Ryoo BY, Kim WS, et al. Nodal marginal zone B-cell lymphoma: Analysis of 36 cases. Clinical presentation and treatment outcomes of nodal marginal zone B-cell lymphoma. Ann Hematol 2006;85:781–6.

57. van den Brand M, van Krieken JH. Recognizing nodal marginal zone lymphoma: recent advances and pitfalls. A systematic review. Haematologica 2013;98:1003–13.

58. Traverse-Glehen A, Felman P, Callet-Bauchu E, et al. A clinicopathological study of nodal marginal zone B-cell lymphoma. A report on 21 cases. Histopathology 2006;48:162–73.

59. Camacho FI, Algara P, Mollejo M, et al. Nodal marginal zone lymphoma: a heterogeneous tumor: a comprehensive analysis of a series of 27 cases. Am J Surg Pathol 2003;27:762–71.

60. Salama ME, Lossos IS, Warnke RA, et al. Immunoarchitectural patterns in nodal marginal zone B-cell lymphoma: a study of 51 cases. Am J Clin Pathol 2009;132:39–49.

61. Camacho FI, Garcia JF, Sanchez-Verde L, et al. Unique phenotypic profile of monocytoid B cells: differences in comparison with the phenotypic profile observed in marginal zone B cells and so-called monocytoid B cell lymphoma. Am J Pathol 2001;158:1363–9.

62. Angelopoulou MK, Kalpadakis C, Pangalis GA, et al. Nodal marginal zone lymphoma. Leuk Lymphoma 2014;55:1240–50.

63. Franco V, Florena AM, Iannitto E. Splenic marginal zone lymphoma. Blood 2003;101:2464–72.

64. Mollejo M, Camacho FI, Algara P, et al. Nodal and splenic marginal zone B cell lymphomas. Hematol Oncol 2005;23:108–18.

65. Sherman MJ, Hanson CA, Hoyer JD. An assessment of the usefulness of immunohistochemical stains in the diagnosis of hairy cell leukemia. Am J Clin Pathol 2011;136:390–9.

66. Savilo E, Campo E, Mollejo M, et al. Absence of cyclin D1 protein expression in splenic marginal zone lymphoma. Mod Pathol 1998;11:601–6.

67. Mateo M, Mollejo M, Villuendas R, et al. 7q31-32 allelic loss is a frequent finding in splenic marginal zone lymphoma. Am J Pathol 1999;154:1583–9.

68. Sole F, Salido M, Espinet B, et al. Splenic marginal zone B-cell lymphomas: two cytogenetic subtypes, one with gain of 3q and the other with loss of 7q. Haematologica 2001;86:71–7.

69. Kiel MJ, Velusamy T, Betz BL, et al. Whole-genome sequencing identifies recurrent somatic NOTCH2 mutations in splenic marginal zone lymphoma. J Exp Med 2012;209:1553–65.

70. Rossi D, Trifonov V, Fangazio M, et al. The coding genome of splenic marginal zone lymphoma: activation of NOTCH2 and other pathways regulating marginal zone development. J Exp Med 2012;209:1537–51.

71. Martinez N, Almaraz C, Vaque JP, et al. Whole-exome sequencing in splenic marginal zone

lymphoma reveals mutations in genes involved in marginal zone differentiation. Leukemia 2014;28: 1334–40.

72. Clipson A, Wang M, de Leval L, et al. KLF2 mutation is the most frequent somatic change in splenic marginal zone lymphoma and identifies a subset with distinct genotype. Leukemia 2015;29: 1177–85.

73. Foucar K, Falini B, Catovsky D, et al. Hairy cell leukemia. In: Swerdlow SH, Campo E, Harris NL, et al, editors. WHO classification of tumours of haematopoietic and lymphoid tissues. 4th edition. Lyon (France): IARC; 2008. p. 188–90.

74. Piris M, Foucar K, Mollejo M, et al. Splenic B-cell lymphoma/leukemia, unclassifiable. In: Swerdlow SH, Campo E, Harris NL, et al, editors. WHO classification of tumours of haematopoietic and lymphoid tissues. 4th edition. Lyon (France): IARC; 2008. p. 191–3.

75. Behdad A, Bailey NG. Diagnosis of splenic B-cell lymphomas in the bone marrow: a review of histopathologic, immunophenotypic, and genetic findings. Arch Pathol Lab Med 2014;138:1295–301.

76. Liu L, Wang H, Chen Y, et al. Splenic marginal zone lymphoma: a population-based study on the 2001-2008 incidence and survival in the United States. Leuk Lymphoma 2013;54:1380–6.

77. Olszewski AJ, Castillo JJ. Survival of patients with marginal zone lymphoma: analysis of the surveillance, epidemiology, and end results database. Cancer 2013;119:629–38.

78. Arcaini L, Lazzarino M, Colombo N, et al. Splenic marginal zone lymphoma: a prognostic model for clinical use. Blood 2006;107:4643–9.

79. Else M, Marin-Niebla A, de la Cruz F, et al. Rituximab, used alone or in combination, is superior to other treatment modalities in splenic marginal zone lymphoma. Br J Haematol 2012;159:322–8.

80. Matutes E. Splenic marginal zone lymphoma: disease features and management. Expert Rev Hematol 2013;6:735–45.

81. Chuang SS, Liao YL, Chang ST, et al. Hepatitis C virus infection is significantly associated with malignant lymphoma in Taiwan, particularly with nodal and splenic marginal zone lymphomas. J Clin Pathol 2010;63:595–8.

82. Hermine O, Lefrere F, Bronowicki JP, et al. Regression of splenic lymphoma with villous lymphocytes after treatment of hepatitis C virus infection. N Engl J Med 2002;347:89–94.

83. Saadoun D, Suarez F, Lefrere F, et al. Splenic lymphoma with villous lymphocytes, associated with type II cryoglobulinemia and HCV infection: a new entity? Blood 2005;105:74–6.

84. Stein J, Harris NL, Campo E. Plasmablastic lymphoma. In: Swerdlow SH, Campo E, Harris NL, et al, editors. WHO classification of tumours of haematopoietic and lymphoid tissues. 4th edition. Lyon (France): IARC; 2008. p. 256–7.

85. Castillo JJ, Bibas M, Miranda RN. The biology and treatment of plasmablastic lymphoma. Blood 2015; 125:2323–30.

86. Carbone A. AIDS-related non-Hodgkin's lymphomas: from pathology and molecular pathogenesis to treatment. Hum Pathol 2002;33:392–404.

87. Vega F, Chang CC, Medeiros LJ, et al. Plasmablastic lymphomas and plasmablastic plasma cell myelomas have nearly identical immunophenotypic profiles. Mod Pathol 2005;18:806–15.

88. Valera A, Balague O, Colomo L, et al. IG/MYC rearrangements are the main cytogenetic alteration in plasmablastic lymphomas. Am J Surg Pathol 2010;34:1686–94.

89. Castillo JJ, Furman M, Beltran BE, et al. Human immunodeficiency virus-associated plasmablastic lymphoma: poor prognosis in the era of highly active antiretroviral therapy. Cancer 2012;118: 5270–7.

90. Morscio J, Dierickx D, Nijs J, et al. Clinicopathologic comparison of plasmablastic lymphoma in HIV-positive, immunocompetent, and posttransplant patients: single-center series of 25 cases and meta-analysis of 277 reported cases. Am J Surg Pathol 2014;38:875–86.

91. Lorsbach RB, Hsi ED, Dogan A, et al. Plasma cell myeloma and related neoplasms. Am J Clin Pathol 2011;136:168–82.

92. Delsol G, Campo E, Gascoyne RD. ALK-positive large B-cell lymphoma. In: Swerdlow SH, Campo E, Harris NL, et al, editors. WHO classification of tumours of haematopoietic and lymphoid tissues. 4th ed. Lyon (France): IARC; 2008. p. 254–5.

93. Valera A, Colomo L, Martinez A, et al. ALK-positive large B-cell lymphomas express a terminal B-cell differentiation program and activated STAT3 but lack MYC rearrangements. Mod Pathol 2013;26: 1329–37.

94. Morgan EA, Nascimento AF. Anaplastic lymphoma kinase-positive large B-cell lymphoma: an underrecognized aggressive lymphoma. Adv Hematol 2012;2012:529572.

95. Horn H, Staiger AM, Vohringer M, et al. Diffuse large B-cell lymphomas of immunoblastic type are a major reservoir for MYC-IGH translocations. Am J Surg Pathol 2015;39:61–6.

96. Chadburn A, Hyjek E, Mathew S, et al. KSHV-positive solid lymphomas represent an extra-cavitary variant of primary effusion lymphoma. Am J Surg Pathol 2004;28:1401–16.

97. Carbone A, Gloghini A, Cozzi MR, et al. Expression of MUM1/IRF4 selectively clusters with primary effusion lymphoma among lymphomatous effusions: implications for disease histogenesis and pathogenesis. Br J Haematol 2000;111:247–57.

98. Said J, Cesarman E. Primary effusion lymphoma. In: Swerdlow SH, Campo E, Harris NL, et al, editors. WHO classification of tumours of haematopoietic and lymphoid tissues. 4th edition. Lyon (France): IARC; 2008. p. 260–1.

99. Castillo JJ, Winer ES, Stachurski D, et al. Prognostic factors in chemotherapy-treated patients with HIV-associated Plasmablastic lymphoma. Oncologist 2010;15:293–9.

100. Castillo JJ, Winer ES, Stachurski D, et al. HIV-negative plasmablastic lymphoma: not in the mouth. Clin Lymphoma Myeloma Leuk 2011;11: 185–9.

101. Castillo JJ, Winer ES, Stachurski D, et al. Clinical and pathological differences between human immunodeficiency virus-positive and human immunodeficiency virus-negative patients with plasmablastic lymphoma. Leuk Lymphoma 2010;51:2047–53.

102. Cattaneo C, Re A, Ungari M, et al. Plasmablastic lymphoma among human immunodeficiency virus-positive patients: results of a single center's experience. Leuk Lymphoma 2015;56:267–9.

103. Liu JJ, Zhang L, Ayala E, et al. Human immunodeficiency virus (HIV)-negative plasmablastic lymphoma: a single institutional experience and literature review. Leuk Res 2011;35:1571–7.

The Expanding Spectrum of Follicular Lymphoma

Yuri Fedoriw, MD[a], Ahmet Dogan, MD, PhD[b],*

KEYWORDS

- Follicular lymphoma • Non-Hodgkin lymphoma • Hematopathology

Key points

- Follicular lymphoma (FL) is a common B-cell lymphoma of germinal center origin, with classically associated clinical, histomorphologic, and genetic features.
- Grading of classic, nodal FL has undergone substantial shifts, and it is important to differentiate grades 1 to 2 disease from grades 3A and 3B.
- FL variants include those associated with age (pediatric FL) and anatomic site (primary intestinal FL and primary cutaneous follicle center cell lymphoma) and are associated with generally good prognosis.

ABSTRACT

Follicular lymphoma is a far more heterogeneous entity than originally appreciated. Clinical and biological variants are increasingly more granularly defined, expanding the spectrum of disease. Some variants associate with age, whereas others with anatomic site. Identification of these biologically distinct diseases has real prognostic and predictive value for patients today and likely will be more relevant in the future. Understanding of follicular lymphoma precursors has also made their identification both scientifically and clinically relevant. This review summarizes the features and understanding of follicular lymphoma, variants, and precursor lesions.

OVERVIEW

Classic nodal FL is commonly encountered in diagnostic practice and most often associated with typical morphologic and cytogenetic features (**Table 1**). Histologically, the nodular pattern is readily identified from low power by light microscopy, in part recapitulating expected follicular architecture (**Fig. 1A, B**). In most cases, the tumor cells express markers of germinal center B cells (CD10 and the master regulator of the germinal center reaction, BCL6) and harbor the t(14;18)(q32;q21) rearrangement. The translocation is associated with overexpression of BCL2, in distinct contrast to the germinal centers of reactive follicular hyperplasia (see **Fig. 1C, D**). Also in contrast to their reactive counterparts, low-grade FL typically shows low Ki-67 expression, a helpful diagnostic immunohistochemical feature (see **Fig. 1E, F**). Bone marrow involvement at presentation is identified in approximately 40% of patients.[1] The infiltrate is often composed of nodules adjacent to the trabecular bone, but paratrabecular localization is not specific for FL and similar patterns are seen in other morphologically low-grade non-Hodgkin lymphomas, including lymphoplasmacytic and mantle cell lymphoma.

Histologic grade can be assigned to FL based on the average number of large cells (centroblasts) per malignant follicle based on the 3-grade scheme originally adopted by the World Health Organization.[2,3] Grading has undergone revision because no clear meaningful prognostic significance was appreciated between grades 1 and 2 FL. Thus, distinguishing between grades 1 and 2 is not necessary in practice.[4–7] The division of grade 3 disease into grades 3A and 3B based on

[a] University of North Carolina School of Medicine, Department of Pathology and Laboratory Medicine, NC Cancer Hospital C3162-D, 101 Manning Drive, Chapel Hill, NC 27599, USA; [b] Hematopathology Service, Department of Pathology, Memorial Sloan Kettering Cancer Center, 1275 York Avenue, New York, NY 10065, USA
* Corresponding author.
E-mail address: dogana@mskcc.org

Surgical Pathology 9 (2016) 29–40
http://dx.doi.org/10.1016/j.path.2015.11.001
1875-9181/16/$ – see front matter © 2016 Elsevier Inc. All rights reserved.

Table 1
Classic diagnostic features of nodal follicular lymphoma

Morphology	Back-to-back follicles lacking polarization
Grading	Grade 1–2: ≤15 centroblasts/high-power field Grade 3A: >15 centroblasts/high-power field; centrocytes present in the background Grade 3B: >15 centroblasts/high-power field; sheets of centroblasts without centrocytes present
Genetics	t(14;18)(q32;q21); *BCL2;* IGH rearrangement in majority of grades 1–2, decreasing in frequency in grade 3A and negative in grade 3B
Immunophenotype	Positive: CD19, CD20, CD10, BCL6, BCL2 Follicular dendritic cell meshworks: CD21, CD23, CD35

the presence or absence of centrocytes, respectively, seems clinically and biologically relevant (**Fig. 2**).[8] Grade 3B FL infrequently harbors the t(14;18) and typically lacks expression of CD10 or BCL2. Expression of other germinal center makers, however, including LMO2 and HGAL GCET2, seem preserved in grade 3FL and may be useful for disease classification.[9,10] In contrast, expression of the postgerminal center transcription factor, IRF4/MUM1, is common in grade 3B FL.[8] In many respects, the biology of grade 3B FL more closely aligns with that of diffuse large B-cell lymphoma (DLBCL) rather than lower grades of FL. A large retrospective study showed that grades 1, 2, and 3A followed a similar and indolent clinical course, whereas patients with grade 3B FL had a lower overall survival.[11] Anthracycline-containing therapies seem to improve overall survival of patients with grade 3B FL to that associated with grades 1 and 2 FL.[11]

A majority of low-grade FL are indolent, but approximately 20% to 30% follow an aggressive clinical course with transformation to DLBCL and refractoriness to therapy.[12] (See Montgomery, Mathews: Transformation in low-grade B-cell neoplasms, in this issue). To date, there is no robust and well-established biomarker to identify this subset. Prognostic parameters, however, including age, lactate dehydrogenase, β_2-microglobulin, and extent of disease are commonly used and incorporated into clinical scoring systems.[13] Apart from grade, histopathologic markers have been investigated, but they have not been uniformly adopted. Ki-67 expression by immunohistochemistry seems to correlate with histologic grade. Nonetheless, there are conflicting published data as to the independent prognostic implications of Ki-67 expression.[11,14] Markers characterizing the tumor microenviroment, including expression of PD1 and CD14, are also being studied and show promise in better predicting disease course.[15,16] (See Mina Xu: Lymphoma microenvironment and

immunotherapy, in this issue). Genetic and molecular factors that relate to FL development have also been the focus of recent study. Mutations in *MLL2*, *EZH2*, and *IRF4* and deletions of EPHA7, for example, are frequent in the genetic landscape of FL, but further study is necessary to assess prognostic and predictive significance.[17–19]

In patients with FL, diffuse areas composed of large cells are diagnostic of transformation/progression to DLBCL and should be reported as such. Diffuse areas of small, mature-appearing lymphocytes, however, are not infrequently identified in low-grade cases of FL and do not represent transformation of disease. The degree of "follicularity" can be assessed by immunostains highlighting the follicular dendritic cell meshworks (CD21 or CD23) and the pattern reported as follicular (<25% diffuse), follicular and diffuse (25%–75% diffuse), or diffuse (<25% follicular). The diffuse pattern alone (ie, in the absence of large cell morphology) does not inherently have an impact on prognosis. As discussed later, however, unique biological subtypes may be associated more frequently with variant histologic appearances, including decreased follicularity.

FOLLICULAR LYMPHOMA VARIANTS

Although a majority of nodal FLs follow the clinical and biological paradigm (discussed previously), variations in clinical presentation, morphology, immunophenotype, and molecular underpinnings have been documented (**Table 2**). Appropriate identification and classification of these FL variants is clinically important, because they often have significant prognostic implications. Some variants associate with age, whereas others, somewhat uniquely, with anatomic location. In contrast to the expected clinical behavior imparted by histologic grade in classic FL, many of the FL variants are indolent, despite appearing histologically aggressive.

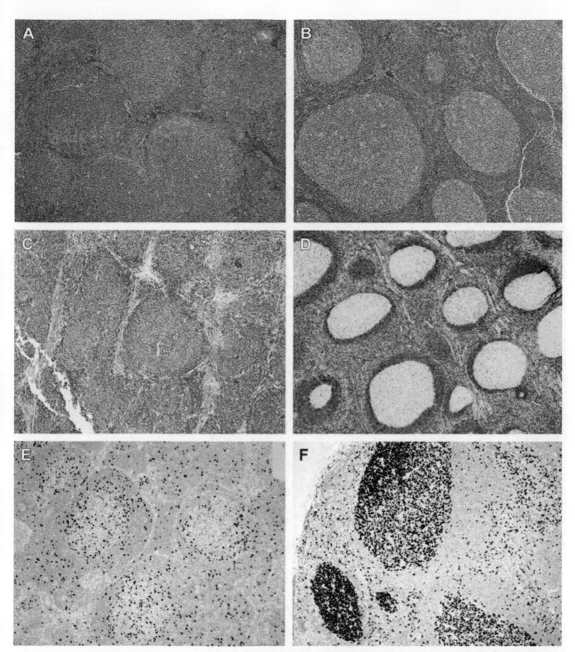

Fig. 1. Classic nodal FL in comparison with reactive follicular hyperplasia. (*A*) Low-power appearance of classic, low-grade FL composed of back-to-back follicles with attenuated/absent mantle zones (H&E). (*B*) In contrast, reactive follicular hyperplasia showing numerous expanded germinal centers with scattered tingible-body macrophages and preserved mantle zones. (*C*) BCL2 expression in FL compared with (*D*) reactive follicular hyperplasia. (*E*) Ki-67 staining, highlighting follicles of low-grade FL in comparison with (*F*) intense, polarized expression in reactive follicular hyperplasia (original objective magnification, ×10).

PEDIATRIC FOLLICULAR LYMPHOMA

Pediatric FL was originally described more than 3 decades ago, but classification of these rare tumors continues to evolve.[20,21] Distinct classes of pediatric FL have seemed to associate with specific anatomic localization. Although immunohistochemical and genetic features are variable, pediatric FL presents as high-grade but low-stage disease with an exceptionally favorable prognosis.[21]

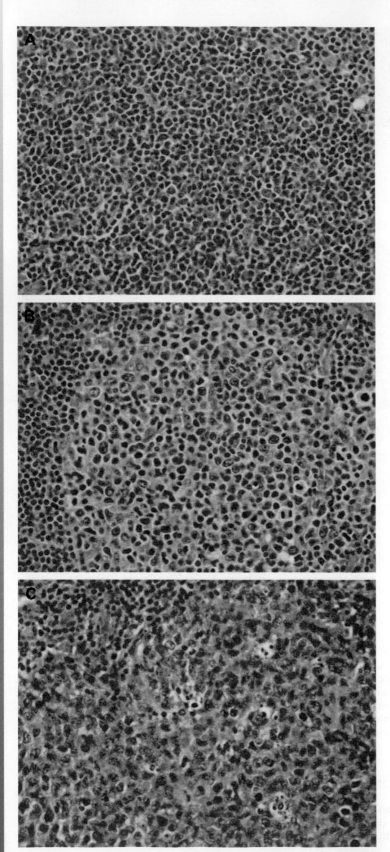

Fig. 2. Grading of FL. High-power images of malignant follicles in grades (*A*) 1 to 2, (*B*) 3A, and (*C*) 3B FL (H&E, original objective magnifications, ×40). Increasing numbers of centroblasts can be appreciated, with virtually no centrocytes seen in the grade 3B follicle.

Table 2
Summary of follicular lymphoma and variants

	Classical Follicular Lymphoma, Grades 1-3A	Follicular Lymphoma, Grade 3B	Pediatric Follicular Lymphoma—Nodal	Waldeyer Ring Follicular Lymphoma	Testicular Follicular Lymphoma	del1p36, Inguinal Follicular Lymphoma	Primary Intestinal Follicular Lymphoma	Primary Cutaneous Follicle Center Cell
t(14;18)—BCL2 rearranged	Frequent (early event)	Negative	Negative	Negative	Negative	Negative	Positive	Mostly Negative
Immunohistochemistry								
CD20	Positive	Positive	Positive	Positive	Positive	Positive	Positive	Positive
CD10	Positive	Negative	Positive	Positive	Positive	Positive	Positive	Positive if follicular, Negative if diffuse
BCL2	Positive	Negative	Negative	Positive	Negative	Positive—consistently in diffuse areas	Positive	Dim/negative more common than positive
MUM1	Negative	Often Positive	Negative	Positive	Negative	?	Negative	Negative
Grade	1-3	3	High	High	High	Low	Variable	Variable
Stage	bone marrow involvement common	Variable	Low	Low	Low	Low	Low	Low
Site	Peripheral lymph node	Anywhere	Head and neck	Waldeyer ring	Testis	inguinal region or axilla	Duodenum	Head or trunk
Prognosis	Variable but indolent	Aggressive	Indolent	Indolent	Indolent	Indolent	Indolent	Indolent
Other genetics	del1(p36) is common and a poor prognostic indicator, BCL6 rearranged	BCL6 abnormalities common	TNFRSF14 deletions or mutations	IRF4 rearranged	Nothing recurrent	del 1(p36)	—	

Pediatric FL occurs primarily in the cervical lymph nodes and shows a marked male predominance. Although the histologic appearance is that of classic, typically grade 3, FL in adults, these lymphomas in the pediatric population lack the t(14;18) and accompanying BCL2 overexpression (Fig. 3).[22] Cases of FL in children and young adults, however, particularly in Waldeyer ring, are enriched for cytogenetically cryptic translocations between the *IRF4* oncogene (on the short arm of chromosome 6) and the immunoglobulin heavy chain (IGH), with overexpression of MUM1.[18,23] Although MUM1 expression is typical of grade 3B adult FL (discussed previously) and predicts poor outcome even in low-grade adult FL, this is not the case in the pediatric population, where an indolent course remains the rule.[24] In pediatric FL lacking the *IRF4* rearrangement, mutations or deletions of *TNFRSF14* have been identified as recurrent aberrations.[25] Pediatric cases with conventionally adult features, including BCL2 expression and t(14;18), are thought to represent classic nodal FL occurring in children rather than pediatric FL and associated with an inferior outcome.[22] Identifying clonal, CD10-positive B cell populations by flow cytometry in the context of reactive follicular hyperplasia does not warrant a diagnosis of pediatric FL. Complicating matters is that these clonal populations are identified in a similar demographic group to that of pediatric FL, namely young men.[26]

Testicular FL occurring in the pediatric population is also accompanied by discordance between histologic grade and clinical behavior. These cases present as a unilateral testicular mass, isolated to the testis. The histologic appearance is that of grade 3 FL and with expression of CD10 and BCL6. *BCL2* rearrangement is not identified, however, and expression of the bcl2 protein is infrequent, similar to other pediatric FLs. High-grade morphology, including areas of DLBCL, are not associated with a worse outcome.[27,28] Conservative therapeutic approaches, including surgery alone, seem curative in most cases.[27,29]

ANATOMIC VARIANTS OF FOLLICULAR LYMPHOMA IN ADULTS

The anatomic site of lymphoma involvement may affect morphologic appearance. Low-grade FL involving the retroperitoneum, for example, can show a diffuse growth pattern with extensive sclerosis (Fig. 4). Particularly in small biopsies, these cases mimic other low-grade lymphoproliferative disorders or nonhematopoietic processes, including retroperitoneal fibrosis and inflammatory pseudotumors. In more typical nodal sites, a diffuse, morphologically low-grade FL may be suggestive of unique biology with impact on prognosis.

Besides the growth pattern, most cases of nodal, diffuse, low-grade FL share immunophentoypic and genetic features of conventional nodal FL. A series of diffuse FL has been reported, however, with a unique constellation of immunophenotypic, genetic, and clinical features.[30] This diffuse variant typically presents as bulky, low-stage disease in the inguinal region. Although expression of CD10, BCL6, and BCL2 is

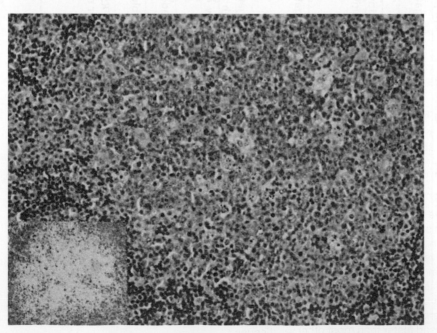

Fig. 3. Pediatric FL. Morphologically high-grade FL in a cervical lymph node biopsy from an adolescent boy (H&E, original objective magnification, ×20). Inset shows lack of BCL2 expression in the malignant follicle.

Fig. 4. FL with abundant sclerosis. Retroperitoneal lymph node biopsy with a diffuse infiltrate of small, mature-appearing lymphocytes. A majority of cells had the classic immunophenotypic features of FL but without appreciable follicular architecture. Sclerotic bands are present throughout (H&E, original objective magnification, ×10).

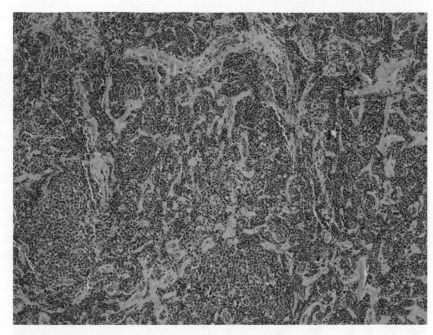

maintained, the neoplastic cells coexpress CD23 in some cases (**Fig. 5**). Unlike other nodal, low grade FL, this variant is negative for the t(14;18) translocation but uniformly harbors deletions of chromosome 1p36.[30] Overall, these patients have an excellent prognosis, with most achieving remission with limited therapy. Loss of 1p36 is not specific for the "inguinal diffuse" FL and is a frequent secondary event in classic FL, where it is associated with an inferior outcome.[31]

Primary intestinal FL represents a truly localized and indolent lymphoproliferation, sharing many of the histologic, immunophenotypic, and cytogenetic features of classic, low-grade, nodal FL (**Fig. 6**).[32,33] The lymphoma appears as expanded, nonpolarized follicles, composed of predominantly small, mature-appearing lymphocytes with a low Ki-67 staining fraction. Although the typical endoscopic appearance is that of multiple, small nodules, typically in the second part of

Fig. 5. Diffuse low-grade FL with 1p36 deletion. Biopsy from an inguinal lymph node of an elderly man showing a diffuse proliferation of small, mature-appearing lymphocytes. The immunophenotype was characteristic of FL with additional CD23 expression identified by flow cytometric analysis. Routine karyotype identified a deletion of 1p36 without the *BCL2* rearrangement (H&E, original objective magnification, ×10).

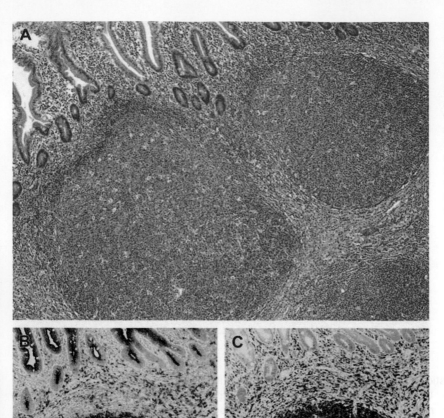

Fig. 6. Primary intestinal FL. (A) Large follicles composed primarily of small, mature-appearing lymphocytes with irregular nuclear contours are evident directly below the small intestinal mucosa (H&E). The neoplastic follicles show expression of (B) CD10, BCL6, and (C) BCL2 diagnostic of follicular lymphoma (original objective magnification, ×10).

the duodenum, the disease is uniformly low stage. It is important to distinguish widespread nodal FL secondarily involving the intestine, which may be difficult in the absence of complete clinical data. There is evidence to suggest that although the typical immunohistochemical pattern of intestinal FL mirrors that of nodal FL with expression of CD10, BCL6, and BCL2, primary intestinal FL is a molecularly distinct neoplasm. Expression of the germinal center program markers, AID and BACH2, and immunoglobulin heavy chains show promise as potential discriminators between nodal and intestinal FL, but definitive validation studies are not yet available nor are the antibodies widely used in clinical practice.[33–35]

More uniquely, primary cutaneous follicle center lymphomas (PCFCLs) exhibit histopathologic and molecular features disparate from those of nodal FLs (Fig. 7). PCFCLs represent the majority of primary B-cell lymphomas of the skin.[36] Virtually any pattern from diffuse to follicular can be appreciated,

and expression of BCL6 is uniform and consistent.[3,37] The cytologic features are variable, with some cases composed of small, mature-appearing lymphocytes and others of numerous large centroblasts. The prognosis is excellent, however, even in cases with numerous large cells, and some cases can be treated with local radiation therapy.[38–40] BCL2 and CD10 expression is an inconsistent finding, but the bcl2 translocation is identified in a few PCFCL cases.[3,37,41] Cases of CD10 and BCL2 coexpression are more likely to harbor the t(14;18) and represent cutaneous involvement by nodal FL rather than PCFCL.

EARLY AND PRECURSOR LESIONS

Perhaps the addressed topic receiving most recent attention is that of early and precursor lesions of FL. Although discussed in the 2008 World Health Organization Classification, challenges in reporting and diagnostic pitfalls have since been appreciated.[3]

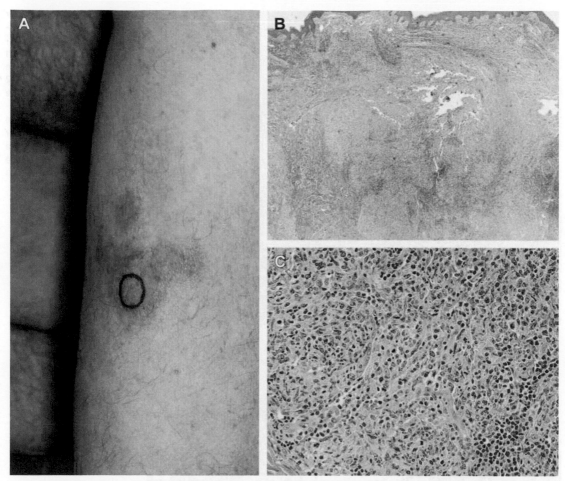

Fig. 7. Primary cutaneous follicle center lymphoma. (*A*) Clinical image of PCFCL. (*B*) The excisional biopsy shows a nodule proliferation of neoplastic lymphocytes in the dermis (H&E, original objective magnification, ×2). (*C*) The neoplastic cells are characterized by large nuclei with irregular contours and abundant cytoplasm (H&E, original objective magnification, ×40).

The diagnosis of intrafollicular neoplasia/in situ FL (ISFL) was warranted when a subset or all of the cells within a morphologically reactive-appearing germinal center expressed CD10 and distinctly bright BCL2 (Fig. 8). These cases, incidentally identified, also harbored the canonical t(14;18).[42] Few cases seem to progress to overt FL and markers predicting such progression have not been identified.[43,44] Because the risk of developing FL is low, discussions over nomenclature, specifically with respect to the use of the word, *lymphoma*, in these cases, is ongoing.[45] Although cells harboring the t(14;18) can be identified in the peripheral blood of more than 50% of the adult population, an even smaller percentage develop FL than those with identifiable ISFL. Thus, although ISFL is an incidental finding, the cells likely represent the next genetic step toward true FL.[46]

Distinguishing ISFL from partial involvement of FL (PFL), however, becomes a more important distinction, because PFL more readily progresses to systemic disease.[43,44] In contrast to ISFL, the malignant follicles of PFL are larger than those typically identified in reactive lymph nodes, and there is a tendency for them to cluster toward to one area of the lymph node. The CD10/BCL2 coexpressing neoplastic population can be identified outside the germinal center, unlike those of ISFL.[47] Both ISFL and PFL are associated with genetic aberrations beyond the t(14;18), including familiar deletions of 1p36, and gains of EZH2 and MLL2.[48] Finally, PFL should be differentiated from systemic, overt FL partially colonizing the lymph node. Clinical evaluation, including imaging studies, may be helpful to assess for systemic involvement.

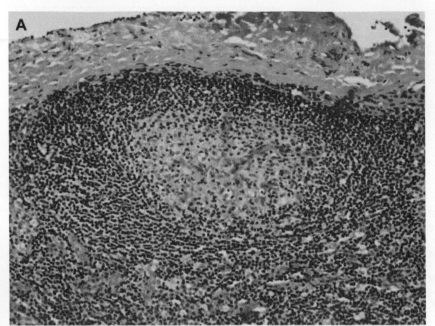

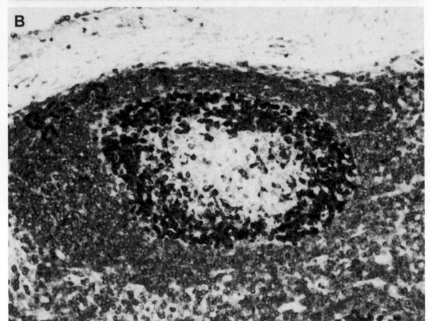

Fig. 8. In situ follicular lymphoma. (*A*) Benign-appearing reactive germinal center with preserved mantle zone (H&E). (*B*) Intense BCL2 expression within the germinal center periphery, in contrast to the appreciably fainter staining in the mantle zone (original objective magnification, ×20).

REFERENCES

1. A clinical evaluation of the International Lymphoma Study Group classification of non-Hodgkin's lymphoma. The Non-Hodgkin's Lymphoma Classification Project. Blood 1997;89(11):3909–18.

2. Mann RB, Berard CW. Criteria for the cytologic sub-classification of follicular lymphomas: a proposed alternative method. Hematol Oncol 1983;1(2):187–92.

3. Swerdlow SH, International Agency for Research on Cancer, World Health Organization. WHO classification of tumours of haematopoietic and lymphoid tissues. 4th edition. Lyon (France): International Agency for Research on Cancer; 2008.

4. Bosga-Bouwer AG, van Imhoff GW, Boonstra R, et al. Follicular lymphoma grade 3B includes 3 cytogenetically defined subgroups with primary t(14;18), 3q27, or other translocations: t(14;18) and 3q27 are mutually exclusive. Blood 2003; 101(3):1149–54.

5. Guo Y, Karube K, Kawano R, et al. Low-grade follicular lymphoma with t(14;18) presents a

homogeneous disease entity otherwise the rest comprises minor groups of heterogeneous disease entities with Bcl2 amplification, Bcl6 translocation or other gene aberrances. Leukemia 2005;19(6): 1058–63.

6. Ott G, Katzenberger T, Lohr A, et al. Cytomorphologic, immunohistochemical, and cytogenetic profiles of follicular lymphoma: 2 types of follicular lymphoma grade 3. Blood 2002;99(10):3806–12.

7. Piccaluga PP, Califano A, Klein U, et al. Gene expression analysis provides a potential rationale for revising the histological grading of follicular lymphomas. Haematologica 2008;93(7):1033–8.

8. Horn H, Schmelter C, Leich E, et al. Follicular lymphoma grade 3B is a distinct neoplasm according to cytogenetic and immunohistochemical profiles. Haematologica 2011;96(9):1327–34.

9. Gratzinger D, Zhao S, West R, et al. The transcription factor LMO2 is a robust marker of vascular endothelium and vascular neoplasms and selected other entities. Am J Clin Pathol 2009;131(2):264–78.

10. Younes SF, Beck AH, Lossos IS, et al. Immunoarchitectural patterns in follicular lymphoma: efficacy of HGAL and LMO2 in the detection of the interfollicular and diffuse components. Am J Surg Pathol 2010; 34(9):1266–76.

11. Wahlin BE, Yri OE, Kimby E, et al. Clinical significance of the WHO grades of follicular lymphoma in a population-based cohort of 505 patients with long follow-up times. Br J Haematol 2012;156(2): 225–33.

12. Link BK, Maurer MJ, Nowakowski GS, et al. Rates and outcomes of follicular lymphoma transformation in the immunochemotherapy era: a report from the University of Iowa/MayoClinic Specialized Program of Research Excellence Molecular Epidemiology Resource. J Clin Oncol 2013;31(26):3272–8.

13. Federico M, Bellei M, Marcheselli L, et al. Follicular lymphoma international prognostic index 2: a new prognostic index for follicular lymphoma developed by the international follicular lymphoma prognostic factor project. J Clin Oncol 2009;27(27): 4555–62.

14. Koster A, Tromp HA, Raemaekers JM, et al. The prognostic significance of the intra-follicular tumor cell proliferative rate in follicular lymphoma. Haematologica 2007;92(2):184–90.

15. Smeltzer JP, Jones JM, Ziesmer SC, et al. Pattern of CD14+ follicular dendritic cells and PD1+ T cells independently predicts time to transformation in follicular lymphoma. Clin Cancer Res 2014;20(11): 2862–72.

16. Westin JR, Chu F, Zhang M, et al. Safety and activity of PD1 blockade by pidilizumab in combination with rituximab in patients with relapsed follicular lymphoma: a single group, open-label, phase 2 trial. Lancet Oncol 2014;15(1):69–77.

17. Morin RD, Mendez-Lago M, Mungall AJ, et al. Frequent mutation of histone-modifying genes in non-Hodgkin lymphoma. Nature 2011;476(7360): 298–303.

18. Salaverria I, Philipp C, Oschlies I, et al. Translocations activating IRF4 identify a subtype of germinal center-derived B-cell lymphoma affecting predominantly children and young adults. Blood 2011; 118(1):139–47.

19. Oricchio E, Nanjangud G, Wolfe AL, et al. The Eph-receptor A7 is a soluble tumor suppressor for follicular lymphoma. Cell 2011;147(3):554–64.

20. Frizzera G, Murphy SB. Follicular (nodular) lymphoma in childhood: a rare clinical-pathological entity. Report of eight cases from four cancer centers. Cancer 1979;44(6):2218–35.

21. Liu Q, Salaverria I, Pittaluga S, et al. Follicular lymphomas in children and young adults: a comparison of the pediatric variant with usual follicular lymphoma. Am J Surg Pathol 2013; 37(3):333–43.

22. Lorsbach RB, Shay-Seymore D, Moore J, et al. Clinicopathologic analysis of follicular lymphoma occurring in children. Blood 2002;99(6):1959–64.

23. Tamura A, Miura I, Iida S, et al. Interphase detection of immunoglobulin heavy chain gene translocations with specific oncogene loci in 173 patients with B-cell lymphoma. Cancer Genet Cytogenet 2001; 129(1):1–9.

24. Xerri L, Bachy E, Fabiani B, et al. Identification of MUM1 as a prognostic immunohistochemical marker in follicular lymphoma using computerized image analysis. Hum Pathol 2014;45(10):2085–93.

25. Martin-Guerrero I, Salaverria I, Burkhardt B, et al. Recurrent loss of heterozygosity in 1p36 associated with TNFRSF14 mutations in IRF4 translocation negative pediatric follicular lymphomas. Haematologica 2013;98(8):1237–41.

26. Kussick SJ, Kalnoski M, Braziel RM, et al. Prominent clonal B-cell populations identified by flow cytometry in histologically reactive lymphoid proliferations. Am J Clin Pathol 2004;121(4):464–72.

27. Lones MA, Raphael M, McCarthy K, et al. Primary follicular lymphoma of the testis in children and adolescents. J Pediatr Hematol Oncol 2012;34(1): 68–71.

28. Darby S, Hancock BW. Localised non-Hodgkin lymphoma of the testis: the Sheffield Lymphoma Group experience. Int J Oncol 2005;26(4):1093–9.

29. Heller KN, Teruya-Feldstein J, La Quaglia MP, et al. Primary follicular lymphoma of the testis: excellent outcome following surgical resection without adjuvant chemotherapy. J Pediatr Hematol Oncol 2004; 26(2):104–7.

30. Katzenberger T, Kalla J, Leich E, et al. A distinctive subtype of t(14;18)-negative nodal follicular non-Hodgkin lymphoma characterized by a predominantly diffuse

growth pattern and deletions in the chromosomal region 1p36. Blood 2009;113(5):1053–61.

31. Cheung KJ, Johnson NA, Affleck JG, et al. Acquired TNFRSF14 mutations in follicular lymphoma are associated with worse prognosis. Cancer Res 2010;70(22):9166–74.

32. Foukas PG, de Leval L. Recent advances in intestinal lymphomas. Histopathology 2015;66(1):112–36.

33. Takata K, Okada H, Ohmiya N, et al. Primary gastrointestinal follicular lymphoma involving the duodenal second portion is a distinct entity: a multicenter, retrospective analysis in Japan. Cancer Sci 2011; 102(8):1532–6.

34. Takata K, Sato Y, Nakamura N, et al. Duodenal follicular lymphoma lacks AID but expresses BACH2 and has memory B-cell characteristics. Mod Pathol 2013;26(1):22–31.

35. Takata K, Sato Y, Nakamura N, et al. Duodenal and nodal follicular lymphomas are distinct: the former lacks activation-induced cytidine deaminase and follicular dendritic cells despite ongoing somatic hypermutations. Mod Pathol 2009;22(7):940–9.

36. Suarez AL, Pulitzer M, Horwitz S, et al. Primary cutaneous B-cell lymphomas: part I. Clinical features, diagnosis, and classification. J Am Acad Dermatol 2013;69(3):329.e1–13 [quiz: 341–2].

37. Pham-Ledard A, Cowppli-Bony A, Doussau A, et al. Diagnostic and prognostic value of BCL2 rearrangement in 53 patients with follicular lymphoma presenting as primary skin lesions. Am J Clin Pathol 2015; 143(3):362–73.

38. Goodlad JR, Krajewski AS, Batstone PJ, et al. Primary cutaneous follicular lymphoma: a clinicopathologic and molecular study of 16 cases in support of a distinct entity. Am J Surg Pathol 2002;26(6):733–41.

39. Wilcox RA. Cutaneous B-cell lymphomas: 2015 update on diagnosis, risk-stratification, and management. Am J Hematol 2015;90(1):73–6.

40. Grange F, Bekkenk MW, Wechsler J, et al. Prognostic factors in primary cutaneous large B-cell lymphomas: a European multicenter study. J Clin Oncol 2001;19(16):3602–10.

41. Swerdlow SH, Quintanilla-Martinez L, Willemze R, et al. Cutaneous B-cell lymphoproliferative disorders: report of the 2011 Society for Hematopathology/European Association for Haematopathology workshop. Am J Clin Pathol 2013;139(4): 515–35.

42. Cong P, Raffeld M, Teruya-Feldstein J, et al. In situ localization of follicular lymphoma: description and analysis by laser capture microdissection. Blood 2002;99(9):3376–82.

43. Jegalian AG, Eberle FC, Pack SD, et al. Follicular lymphoma in situ: clinical implications and comparisons with partial involvement by follicular lymphoma. Blood 2011;118(11):2976–84.

44. Pillai RK, Surti U, Swerdlow SH. Follicular lymphoma-like B cells of uncertain significance (in situ follicular lymphoma) may infrequently progress, but precedes follicular lymphoma, is associated with other overt lymphomas and mimics follicular lymphoma in flow cytometric studies. Haematologica 2013;98(10):1571–80.

45. Fend F, Cabecadas J, Gaulard P, et al. Early lesions in lymphoid neoplasia: Conclusions based on the Workshop of the XV. Meeting of the European Association of Hematopathology and the Society of Hematopathology, in Uppsala, Sweden. J Hematop 2012;5(3).

46. Mamessier E, Broussais-Guillaumot F, Chetaille B, et al. Nature and importance of follicular lymphoma precursors. Haematologica 2014;99(5):802–10.

47. Adam P, Katzenberger T, Eifert M, et al. Presence of preserved reactive germinal centers in follicular lymphoma is a strong histopathologic indicator of limited disease stage. Am J Surg Pathol 2005; 29(12):1661–4.

48. Mamessier E, Song JY, Eberle FC, et al. Early lesions of follicular lymphoma: a genetic perspective. Haematologica 2014;99(3):481–8.

Comprehensive Assessment and Classification of High-Grade B-cell Lymphomas

 CrossMark

Amir Behdad, MD[a],*, Nathanael G. Bailey, MD[b]

KEYWORDS

- Diffuse large B-cell lymphoma • Burkitt lymphoma • Cell of origin • MYC

ABSTRACT

High-grade B-cell lymphomas (HGBCLs) are a heterogeneous group of neoplasms that include subsets of diffuse large B-cell lymphoma, Burkitt lymphoma, and lymphomas with features intermediate between diffuse large B-cell lymphoma and Burkitt lymphoma. Morphologically indistinguishable HGBCLs may demonstrate variable clinical courses and responses to therapy. The morphologic evaluation and classification of these neoplasms must be followed by further genetic and immunophenotypic work-up. These additional diagnostic modalities lead to a comprehensive stratification of HGBCL that determines the prognosis and optimal therapy. This article reviews the well-established and emerging biomarkers that are most relevant to the clinical management of HGBCL.

Key Features

- Determination of cell of origin (COO), GCB vs ABC, is essential in all cases of diffuse large B-cell lymphoma (DLBCL) because it predicts prognosis and may guide treatment.

- Double-hit lymphomas (DHLs) demonstrate aggressive clinical behavior, and evaluation for *MYC*, *BCL2*, and *BCL6* rearrangements by fluorescence in situ hybridization (FISH) should be considered for all cases of high-grade B-cell lymphoma (HGBCL).

- Using proliferative index or MYC expression by immunohistochemistry (IHC) as a surrogate for FISH testing misses a subset of cases with rearrangement.

- MYC and BCL2 expression by IHC has shown prognostic value in DLBCL but currently is not clinically actionable.

- Evaluation for *IGH-IRF4* rearrangement should be considered in cases of DLBCL or high-grade follicular lymphoma (FL) in young patients.

- Evaluation for aberrations of chromosome 11q and *ID3* mutation should be considered for Burkitt lymphomas (BLs) that lack *IGH-MYC*.

OVERVIEW

HGBCL encompasses a broad group of B-cell neoplasms that are histologically characterized by proliferation of intermediate to large B-cells. The morphology-based diagnostic entities in this group include DLBCL, BL, and the more recently described B-cell lymphoma, unclassifiable, with features intermediate between DLBCL and BL

Authors have no conflict of interest. No funding was received for this project.
[a] Division of Hematopathology, Department of Pathology, Northwestern Memorial Hospital, Northwestern University, Feinberg School of Medicine, 251 East Huron, Feinberg 7-210, Chicago, IL 60611, USA; [b] Division of Hematopathology, Department of Pathology, University of Michigan, 5242 Med Sci I, 1301 Catherine Street, Ann Arbor, MI 48109, USA
* Corresponding author.
E-mail address: amir.behdad@northwestern.edu

Surgical Pathology 9 (2016) 41–54
http://dx.doi.org/10.1016/j.path.2015.09.008

surgpath.theclinics.com

(BCLU). BCLU is a provisional category in the World Health Organization (WHO) 2008 lymphoma classification, and as the name implies, it was created to identify tumors that have overlapping morphologic and immunophenotypic features between DLBCL and BL (Fig. 1A, B).[1] Insight into the molecular pathogenesis of HGBCLs in recent years has provided biomarkers that can be integrated in the diagnostic work-up to predict the clinical course and response to various therapies. This article focuses on highlighting the ancillary diagnostic studies that are currently the standard of care for evaluation of HGBCL. Morphologic and site-specific subclasses of DLBCL (including T-cell/histiocyte-rich large B-cell lymphoma, primary effusion lymphoma,

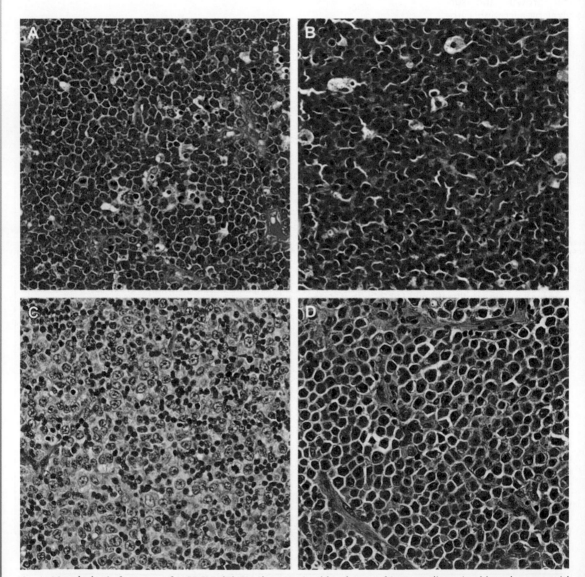

Fig. 1. Morphologic features of HGBCLs. (*A*) BL, characterized by sheets of intermediate-sized lymphocytes with round, fairly monotonous nuclei and multiple indistinct nucleoli. A starry-sky background is present, with numerous apoptotic bodies and mitotic figures. (*B*) BCLU. This tumor exhibits a starry-sky background, with somewhat more nuclear pleomorphism than is present in prototypical BL. This example had rearrangements of both *MYC* and *IGH-BCL2*. (*C*) DLBCL, with centroblastic morphology. The large B cells have ovoid nuclei and multiple small nucleoli, reminiscent of cells in the dark zone of the germinal center. (*D*) DLBCL, with immunoblastic morphology. Greater than 90% of the lymphoma cells exhibit prominent central nucleoli or features suggestive of plasmacytic differentiation, such as eccentric nuclei and amphophilic cytoplasm. All images ×400, hematoxylin-eosin stain.

lymphomatoid granulomatosis, and so forth) and mantle cell lymphoma and its aggressive variants (blastoid and pleomorphic) are beyond the scope of this review. This article focuses on reviewing the current ancillary diagnostic studies that are currently the standard of care for evaluation of HGBCLs, a summary of which is highlighted in Table 1.

MORPHOLOGIC RISK STRATIFICATION

DLBCL is the most common non-Hodgkin lymphoma (NHL) worldwide, constituting 30% to 35% of all NHLs.[2] Although a biologically aggressive lymphoma, DLBCL can be cured in more than 50% of patients,[3] typically using a combination of rituximab with anthracycline-based regimens (rituximab, cyclophosphamide, doxorubicin, vincristine, and prednisone [R-CHOP]).[4–6] Despite improved overall survival, up to a third of patients do not respond to this treatment and require salvage therapy.

The heterogeneity of DLBCL has been recognized for decades. Cases that now are grouped together as DLBCL, not otherwise specified, in the WHO classification schema may previously have been diagnosed as different entities under prior lymphoma classifications due to their morphologic features. In particular, many historic lymphoma classifications considered large cell lymphomas with centroblastic morphology separately from large cell lymphomas with more immunoblastic or plasmacytic differentiation (see Fig. 1C, D).[7–10] This morphologic distinction was de-emphasized at the time of the Revised European-American Lymphoma Classification

due to concerns regarding interobserver reproducibility and therapeutic significance.[11] Recent studies have led to a renaissance in the appreciation of the potential prognostic significance of immunoblastic/plasmacytic differentiation in DLBCL, because this feature is a negative independent prognostic factor, correlating with non-GCB IHC profile and enriched for IGH-MYC–rearranged cases.[12–15]

CELL-OF-ORIGIN DETERMINATION

In 2000, Alizadeh and colleagues[16] demonstrated that distinct subgroups of DLBCL could be recognized through gene expression profiling (GEP) using cDNA microarrays. This seminal work identified that many DLBCL specimens exhibited a profile similar to that of germinal center B-cell like (GCB DLBCL), exhibiting high expression of BCL6, MME (CD10), LMO2, SERPINA9, MYBL1, and others. Other cases expressed genes associated with in vitro activation of peripheral blood B cells (ABC DLBCL) and plasmacytic differentiation, such as IRF4, FOXP1, CCND2, CD44, BLNK, and so forth. These 2 COO groups had markedly disparate outcomes with CHOP-like regimens with significantly better overall survival in patients with GCB DLBCL, a finding confirmed both in other DLBCL cohorts and using other microarray platforms.[17,18] The addition of rituximab to CHOP chemotherapy improved outcomes in both GCB and ABC DLBCL; however, the COO classifier continued to divide DLBCL into prognostic groups even in patients treated with R-CHOP.[19] In addition to the GCB and ABC subtypes, a third, smaller group of DLBCL was

Table 1
Ancillary work-up for high-grade B-cell lymphomas

Test/Biomarker	Type of Lymphoma	Clinical Testing
COO by IHC	DLBCL	Recommended
MYC, BCL2, BCL6 rearrangements by FISH	DLBCL, BCLU	Recommended
MYC and BCL2 expression by IHC	DLBCL, BCLU	Should be considered
IGH-IRF4 rearrangements by FISH	DLBCL, FL	Recommended[a]
Aberrations of chromosome 11q	BL	Recommended[b]
ID3 mutation	BL, BCLU	Investigational
EZH2 mutation	GCB DLBCL	Investigational
MYD88 mutation	ABC DLBCL	Investigational
CD79B mutation	ABC DLBCL	Investigational
CARD11 mutation	ABC DLBCL	Investigational

[a] Recommended only in DLBCL and FL in young patients.
[b] Recommended in BLs that are negative for IGH-MYC rearrangement—not widely clinically available.

recognized by GEP that did not express either GCB-associated or ABC-associated genes at a high level and that had survival intermediate between the other groups.[17,18]

Because GEP technologies of the early 2000s were not readily applicable to routine patient samples, immunohistochemical (IHC) algorithms using protein expression as a surrogate for gene expression were developed to allow for COO classification in diagnostic material. The most widely used algorithm was reported by Hans and colleagues[20] in 2004. In this algorithm, 3 IHC stains are used: CD10, BCL6, and IRF4/MUM1, interpreted sequentially. The investigators designated cases either with CD10 expression or with BCL6 expression without expression of MUM1 as GCB DLBCL. Other staining results led to classification of a DLBCL case as non-GCB (Fig. 2). The IHC results showed reasonably good correlation with the classification established by GEP in their cohort of cases. Non-GCB terminology was used for the IHC classifier as opposed to ABC DLBCL because the binary IHC classification did not allow for an unclassified category as is present when GEP was used to characterize cases. The investigators

of the Hans algorithm, along with other groups, subsequently published multiple other IHC algorithms in an attempt to improve the correlation between IHC and GEP COO results.[21–23] Although several studies, including those that established the algorithms, have shown their prognostic significance, others have not, and the reproducibility and concordance of these algorithms have been called into question.[12,13,24–27]

Although the original microarray platforms used for GEP are not suitable for use with routine formalin-fixed, paraffin-embedded (FFPE) tissue, other gene expression platforms have been developed and are likely to become widely clinically available in the near future. Assessing expression of a subset of genes through reverse transcription–polymerase chain reaction (PCR)[28,29] or digital gene expression methods (NanoString, Seattle, WA)[30,31] has been shown to perform well in FFPE material and correlate with traditional GEP results. It is hoped that GEP platforms will overcome laboratory-to-laboratory variation and interobserver variability that is inherent in IHC assays because clinical practice is becoming ever more reliant on COO status in the treatment of

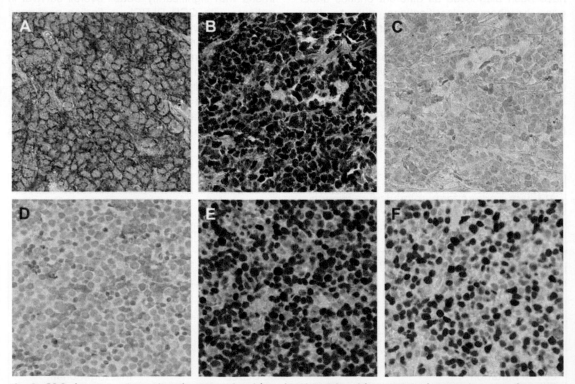

Fig. 2. COO determination using the Hans algorithm. (*A–C*) DLBCL with a germinal center immunophenotype, exhibiting expression of (*A*) CD10 and (*B*) BCL6, without expression of (*C*) IRF4/MUM1. (*D–F*) DLBCL with a non-germinal center immunophenotype, lacking expression of (*D*) CD10, with expression of both (*E*) BCL6 and (*F*) IRF4/MUM1. All images ×400.

patients with DLBCL. This is particularly important because the COO will be a requirement in the diagnosis of DLBCL in the new iteration of the WHO classification.

Many ongoing studies are examining alternatives to R-CHOP that are tailored to the COO subtype of a given lymphoma. Several studies have suggested that regimens that include etoposide (DA-EPOCH-R and R-CHOEP) exhibit greater benefit in GCB DLBCL than in the ABC subtype.[32–34] A randomized phase III study comparing the efficacy of DA-EPOCH-R versus standard R-CHOP is ongoing (NCT00118209). Because ABC DLBCL is characterized by chronic B-cell receptor signaling and nuclear factor (NF)-κB activation,[35,36] agents targeting these pathways are being assessed in ABC DLBCL in the frontline and relapsed/refractory setting. Bortezomib is a proteasome inhibitor that has effects on NF-κB signaling. Its addition to conventional chemotherapy seems to lead to survival benefits in patients with ABC DLBCL.[37,38] A phase III clinical trial is exploring the effect of bortezomib plus R-CHOP (RB-CHOP) versus R-CHOP in molecularly classified DLBCL (NCT01324596). Similarly, the BTK inhibitor ibrutinib would be postulated to be most effective in ABC DLBCL given its greater dependence on BCR signaling than GCB DLBCL. This seems to be the case, because patients with relapsed/refractory ABC DLBCL exhibit better responses to single-agent ibrutinib than do those with GCB DLBCL.[39] Ibrutinib plus R-CHOP is now being compared with R-CHOP alone in patients with ABC DLBCL in a phase III clinical trial (NCT01855750). Lenalidomide (Revlimid), an immunomodulatory agent, reduces NF-κB activation and decreases IRF4/MUM1 expression.[40] Several studies have suggested that lenalidomide is effective in ABC DLBCL,[41–44] and a phase III trial is ongoing to compare lenalidomide plus R-CHOP (R2-CHOP) to R-CHOP alone in DLBCL (NCT02285062). This trial is using the Lymph2Cx COO classifier[31] to categorize DLBCL patients, and the platform is being considered for submission as a companion in vitro diagnostic, which may have regulatory implications for routine COO classification of DLBCL in the near future.

MYC/BCL2/BCL6 REARRANGEMENTS AND DOUBLE-HIT LYMPHOMAS

The *MYC* gene located on chromosome 8q24 encodes the proto-oncogene MYC, which regulates 10% to 15% of all human genes.[45] In B cells, MYC is only transiently expressed in the germinal center B cells, where it plays a role in follicle formation and is later suppressed by expression of BCL6 and PRDM1/BLIMP1.[46]

MYC translocation is the hallmark genetic abnormality in BL, and its identification is a critical component of diagnosis. *MYC* translocations also occur in a subset of morphologic DLBCL and BCLU.[47,48] *MYC* is most frequently translocated to *IGH* or less commonly the immunoglobulin light chain genes (*IGK* and *IGL*) in BL, whereas in DLBCL and BCLU, the partner translocations are often nonimmunoglobulin genes.[49]

In contrast to BL, where *MYC* translocation is present within a simple karyotype,[50,51] *MYC* rearrangements in DLBCL and BCLU sometimes co-occur with *BCL6* and/or *BCL2* translocations that are believed to have synergistic actions in causing the aggressive behavior of HGBCLs. Dysregulation of BCL2, an antiapoptotic protein, through translocation of *IGH-BCL2*, is a major pathogenetic mechanism in FL. As expected, *IGH-BCL2* is frequently seen in DLBCL that has transformed from an underlying FL, but it is also present in 15% to 20% of de novo DLBCL and has been associated with adverse outcomes in some studies.[52,53] Translocation of *BCL6*, a master regulator of the germinal center reaction, is the most common gene rearrangement in DLBCL, encountered in approximately 30% of the cases with an uncertain isolated prognostic significance.[54–58]

Most studies have suggested that the adverse clinical outcomes observed in association with *MYC*-rearranged DLBCL are limited to the cases that concurrently harbor *BCL2* (or uncommonly, *BCL6*) rearrangements: so-called DHL.[47,48,59,60] DHL can show a spectrum of morphologic features that includes BCLU, DLBCL, and, less frequently, FL.[61] It remains unclear whether the morphologic features (that is, BCLU vs DLBCL) are significant in the setting of DHL.[59,62] The frequency of DHL in DLBCL is approximately 5% to 15%, whereas a high percentage of BCLUs harbor double-hit rearrangements.[62–65] Because *IGH-BCL2* occurs almost exclusively in GCB DLBCL, from a phenotypic standpoint, a majority of DHL demonstrate a GC phenotype. The rare DHLs with *BCL6* rearrangements more commonly are nongerminal center type.[53,59,66] The prognostic significance of isolated *MYC* rearrangement is somewhat unclear because many older studies did not assess for the possibility of DHL; however, a few recent publications have identified a poor prognosis of *MYC*-rearranged DLBCL independent of *BCL2* or *BCL6* rearrangements.[67,68]

Identification of DHL is critical, because these patients are clearly insufficiently treated when given R-CHOP.[59,69–71] A standard of care has not been identified, and treatment of DHL patients is an area of active investigation. In general, more-intensive regimens are used,[72] and results with regimens effective in GCB DLBCL, such as DA-EPOCH-R, seem promising.[73]

IDENTIFICATION OF DOUBLE-HIT LYMPHOMAS

Conventional cytogenetic analysis could be considered the gold standard for the identification of MYC rearrangements, because it can identify the translocation partners. Cytogenetic analysis, however, is cumbersome, time consuming, and not routinely performed in the work-up of lymphomas at many centers. The utility of PCR-based assays in detection of these sorts of rearrangements is limited, and FISH is the standard technique for detection of MYC/BCL6/BCL2 rearrangements given its high sensitivity and specificity as well as usability on FFPE tissue.

Given the cost associated with FISH studies, testing strategies to evaluate for the presence of DHL may vary by institution. It would be tempting to use features, such as MYC IHC expression or high Ki-67 proliferative index, as screens for DHL. This strategy, however, misses a significant fraction of DHLs with a low proliferative index or decreased MYC expression (Fig. 3).[65,74] The authors' institution's practices vary: at Northwestern,

MYC FISH is performed on all cases of newly diagnosed DLBCL or BCLU in which there is therapeutic implication, whereas at Michigan, MYC FISH is performed on all GCB DLBCLs or BCLU or ABC cases with concerning clinical or pathologic features. If MYC rearrangement is detected in either algorithm, FISH for BCL6 and BCL2 is performed. From a technical standpoint, to test for the MYC rearrangements in DLBCL or BCLU, break-apart probes and not MYC-IGH dual-fusion probes are typically used to account for the non-IGH translocation partners of MYC. Although break-apart probes are more sensitive in isolation than IGH-MYC fusion probes, IGH-MYC fusion probes detect rare rearrangements that break-apart probes miss.[75] In the event of a MYC break, some laboratories proceed to determine whether it is fused to an IG locus, because a few studies have suggested that non-IG MYC fusions are not prognostically significant in DHL,[59,76] although other investigators have not corroborated this result.[68] For BCL6 translocations, break-apart probes are used, whereas for BCL2, either break-apart or IGH-BCL2 dual-fusion testing strategy can be used.

Another important issue with regard to the interpretation of the FISH results is evaluation for increased copy number or amplification. Several studies have demonstrated similar prognostic impacts for MYC and/or BCL2 copy number increases as are present in rearrangements.[67,77–79] The most appropriate threshold for determining positive

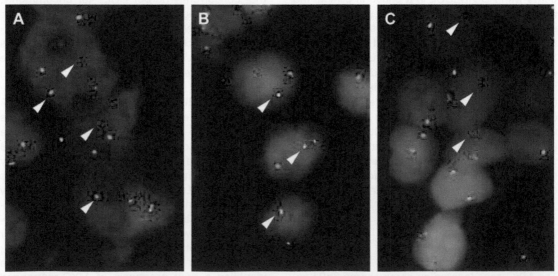

Fig. 3. FISH for (A) MYC rearrangement, (B) IGH-BCL2 fusion, and (C) BCL6 rearrangement. This lymphoma exhibited rearrangements of all 3 genes. The MYC and BCL6 assays are a break-apart probe design, where single red or green or split signals indicate translocation (abnormal signals indicated by *arrowheads*). The IGH-BCL2 assay is a dual-color, dual-fusion design, where the fused red/green (*yellow*) signals indicate rearrangement (*arrowheads*). All images ×1000.

cases, however, has yet has to be fully determined, and the utility of reporting copy number changes by clinical laboratories remains controversial.

IMMUNOHISTOCHEMISTRY FOR EXPRESSION OF MYC AND BCL2

Assessing the expression of MYC and BCL2 by IHC is attractive, because this should identify patients whose lymphomas are driven by increased MYC and/or BCL2 activity secondary to a variety of mechanisms, not solely translocations. Evaluation of MYC expression by IHC has recently become possible, because a novel monoclonal anti-MYC antibody suitable on FFPE tissue has become available.[69,80] The clinical significance of BCL2 expression in DLBCL remains controversial in the postrituximab era.[81–83] Although *IGH-BCL2* is seen nearly exclusively in GCB DLBCL, BCL2 expression is more commonly encountered in ABC DLBCL, consistent with alternative mechanisms of *BCL2* upregulation.[84]

Several recent studies have demonstrated that, as with translocations, MYC expression by IHC in DLBCL is not predictive of an inferior prognosis alone and requires the synergistic effect of BCL2 expression.[69,71,85] MYC/BCL2 coexpression is more common in ABC DLBCL and it may account for much of the inferior prognosis of ABC DLBCL compared with GCB DLBCL.[69–71]

There is a demand to incorporate IHC for these 2 proteins into the routine diagnostic work-up of DLBCL to identify these poor-prognosis, double-expressor lymphomas (DELs). To utilize IHC in the clinical setting, there is a need for uniform interpretation of results. Most DEL studies have used thresholds of greater than 30% to 40% and 50% to 70% positive tumor cells for MYC and BCL2, respectively.[69,70,74,80,85] In addition to the difficulty in scoring cases near these thresholds, a significant interpretive challenge is to define a cutoff for the intensity. MYC staining may be heterogeneous, rendering accurate quantification challenging (Fig. 4), and hematopathologists scored 39% of cases discordantly using a greater than or equal to 40% threshold in 1 study.[86] These concerns make routine application of MYC IHC challenging in the clinical setting. Although DEL cases are not adequately treated by R-CHOP, preliminary data suggest their response to regimens, such as DA-EPOCH-R, may not be as significant as is seen in genetically defined DHL.[73] This may not be surprising given that many DELs have an ABC phenotype, and ultimately further studies are needed to determine the most appropriate therapy for this group of patients.

OTHER CLINICALLY RELEVANT BIOMARKERS IN DIFFUSE LARGE B-CELL LYMPHOMA

CD5 is a pan–T-cell marker that is aberrantly expressed in mantle cell lymphoma and chronic lymphocytic leukemia/small lymphocytic lymphoma (CLL/SLL). Approximately 10% of de novo DLBCLs (not a result of transformation from CLL/SLL) express CD5.[87,88] De novo CD5+ DLBCL, has been shown to have unique clinicopathologic features, including older age, female predominance, frequent involvement of extranodal sites, and an aggressive clinical course.[88–90] Large-scale studies of de novo CD5+ DLBCL are mostly conducted in Japan; a recent study in a Western population showed lower (approximately 5%) frequency but similar adverse clinical outcomes.[91] Patients with CD5+ DLBCL seem to be at high risk of central nervous system relapse, suggesting that central nervous system prophylaxis may be indicated in this group.[92]

CD30, a member of the tumor necrosis factor receptor superfamily, is characteristically expressed on Reed-Sternberg cells in classic Hodgkin lymphoma as well as in other lymphomas but is also expressed in reactive B immunoblasts and T immunoblasts. The prognostic significance of CD30 expression in DLBCL has been controversial, but a recent large-scale study of patients with uniform treatment regimen (R-CHOP) showed superior survival in Epstein-Barr virus–negative, CD30+ DLBCL patients.[93] Additionally, brentuximab vedotin, an anti-CD30 monoclonal antibody-drug conjugate, has shown promising results in refractory Hodgkin lymphoma and anaplastic large cell lymphoma and has been approved by the US Food and Drug Administration for these malignancies.[94,95] This agent may have a role in the treatment of CD30+ DLBCL in the future that would warrant testing by IHC or flow cytometry.

Recently, a novel rearrangement juxtaposing the *IRF4/MUM1* oncogene to the *IGH* locus in GCB DLBCL and FL grade 3 has been identified.[96] The lymphomas harboring this translocation are more common in younger patients, often located in Waldeyer ring, and are associated with favorable outcomes.[96] Additionally, they have unique pathologic features, including *BCL6* aberrations, expression of IRF4 (MUM1) and BCL6 while lacking PRDM1 (BLIMP1) expression and *BCL2* rearrangement. This translocation is cytogenetically cryptic and may be missed by conventional cytogenetic studies and is best detected by FISH. Testing for *IG-IRF4* rearrangements is perhaps only warranted for pediatric and young adult patients with diagnosis of DLBCL and FL and not

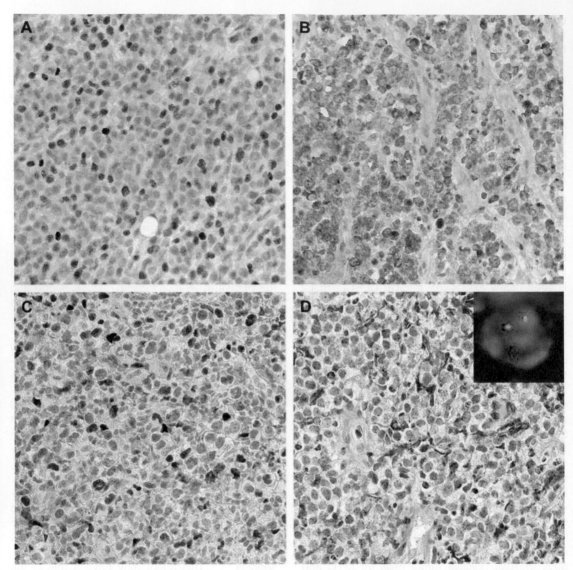

Fig. 4. IHC for MYC and BCL2. (*A–B*) A double-expressor DLBCL exhibiting nuclear expression of (*A*) MYC in greater than 40% of cells, along with strong expression of (*B*) BCL2. (*C*) DLBCL stained for MYC. This case exhibits marked variation in the intensity of MYC staining, and interpretation using a 40% threshold for positivity could depend on whether the very weak cells are counted. (*D*) A rare case of BL exhibiting no staining with anti-MYC antibody. Rare background cells exhibit reactivity, but no staining was present in the tumor on repeat testing. The inset demonstrates the presence of *MYC* rearrangement, detected by FISH. All IHC images ×400; inset ×1000.

necessary for older patients given its age-limited distribution.

OTHER CLINICALLY RELEVANT BIOMARKERS IN BURKITT LYMPHOMA

IGH-MYC translocation is the genetic hallmark of BLs; however, rare cases of morphologic and immunophenotypic characteristics of BL may lack this rearrangement.[51,97] Recently, aberrations of

chromosome 11q, including interstitial gains and telomeric losses, have been described in a subset of lymphomas with BL-like morphology.[97,98] This BL variant has been proposed to be included in the forthcoming WHO classification as "Burkitt-like lymphoma with 11q aberrations." A recent study showed that 11q aberrations are particularly frequent in BL of immune-deficient hosts, such as patients after organ transplantation.[99]

Recurrent mutations of *ID3*, a negative regulator of transcription factor *TCF3 (E2A)* are seen in approximately 30% of BL and implicate this gene as tumor suppressor with a major pathogenic role in this neoplasm.[100–102] Although the original publications suggested that the *ID3* mutations are specific to the BL, a recent study showed that these mutations are comparably high in both BL and BCLU and may be seen in *MYC*-rearranged DLBCL.[103] Evaluation of ID3 by IHC can be performed and its lack of expression can be demonstrated in *ID3*-mutated cases BL as a surrogate marker; however, its clinical utility remains to be determined.[104]

NEW HORIZONS/FUTURE DIRECTIONS

With the advent of massive parallel sequencing technologies, several new mutations have been described in DLBCLs. Compared with the other B-cell lymphomas and acute leukemias, DLBCL has a more complex genome with higher frequency of somatic mutations.[105]

Somatic mutations within exon 15 of the *EZH2* gene that encodes histone-lysine N-methyltransferase (EZH2), are detected in approximately 20% of GCB DLBCL and approximately 7% of FL.[106] These activating point mutations result in the replacement of a single tyrosine (Y641) in the SET domain of the protein, which increases the histone methyltransferase activity of the protein and show an increase in trimethylation of H3K27.[106,107] Inhibition of EZH2 in lymphoma cell lines results in apoptotic cell killing of these cells[108] and has shown promising results in an animal model.[109] Consequently, an oral EZH2 histone methyltransferase inhibitor, E7438, has been developed and is in clinical testing for relapsed DLBCL.[110]

Mutational activation of the NF-κB pathway through alterations of *CARD11*, *MALT1*, *MYD88*, *CD79B*, and *TNFAIP3* plays a role in the pathogenesis of ABC DLBCL[36,111–114] As discussed previously, BCR signaling and the downstream NF-κB pathway is a viable therapeutic target in ABC DLBCL. The mutational status of an individual tumor may predict response to NF-κB inhibition. For instance, ABC DLBCLs with *TNFAIP3* inactivation or *MYD88* mutation without concurrent mutation of *CD79 A/CD79 B* lacked response to ibrutinib, whereas other genotype combinations showed benefit with this therapy.[39] It is unclear whether genetic markers predict response to other ABC-directed therapies currently being evaluated.

If identifying these somatic aberrations gains clinical relevance, comprehensive genetic testing in HGBCL using massive parallel sequencing technologies (next-generation sequencing) may be clinically available in the near horizon. Such platforms will allow simultaneous analysis for various mutations, which also enables the study of tumor heterogeneity and quantitative trending of variant allele frequency, and perhaps allow for more tailored care.

REFERENCES

1. Swerdlow SHN, Jaffe E, Pileri S, et al, editors. WHO classification of tumours of the haematopoietic and lymphoid tissues. 4th edition. Lyon (France): IARC; 2008.
2. Siegel R, Naishadham D, Jemal A. Cancer statistics, 2013. CA Cancer J Clin 2013;63(1):11–30.
3. Armitage JO. My treatment approach to patients with diffuse large B-cell lymphoma. Mayo Clin Proc 2012;87(2):161–71.
4. Fisher RI, Gaynor ER, Dahlberg S, et al. Comparison of a standard regimen (CHOP) with three intensive chemotherapy regimens for advanced non-Hodgkin's lymphoma. N Engl J Med 1993; 328(14):1002–6.
5. Coiffier B, Lepage E, Brière J, et al. CHOP chemotherapy plus rituximab compared with CHOP alone in elderly patients with diffuse large-B-cell lymphoma. N Engl J Med 2002;346(4):235–42.
6. Vose JM, Link BK, Grossbard ML, et al. Phase II Study of rituximab in combination with CHOP chemotherapy in patients with previously untreated, aggressive non-Hodgkin's lymphoma. J Clin Oncol 2001;19(2):389–97.
7. Bennett M, Farrer-Brown G, Henry K, et al. Classification of non-Hodgkin's lymphomas. Lancet 1974; 304(7877):405–8.
8. Lukes RJ, Collins RD. Immunologic characterization of human malignant lymphomas. Cancer 1974;34(S8):1488–503.
9. Stansfeld AG, Diebold J, Kapanci Y, et al. Updated kiel classification for lymphomas. Lancet 1988; 331(8580):292–3.
10. National Cancer Institute sponsored study of classifications of non-Hodgkin's lymphomas. Summary and description of a working formulation for clinical usage. Cancer 1982;49(10):2112–35.
11. Harris N, Jaffe E, Stein H, et al. A revised European-American classification of lymphoid neoplasms: a proposal from the International Lymphoma Study Group [see comments]. Blood 1994;84(5):1361–92.
12. De Paepe P, Achten R, Verhoef G, et al. Large cleaved and immunoblastic lymphoma may represent two distinct clinicopathologic entities within the group of diffuse large B-cell lymphomas. J Clin Oncol 2005;23(28):7060–8.
13. Ott G, Ziepert M, Klapper W, et al. Immunoblastic morphology but not the immunohistochemical GCB/nonGCB classifier predicts outcome in diffuse

large B-cell lymphoma in the RICOVER-60 trial of the DSHNHL. Blood 2010;116(23):4916–25.

14. Horn H, Staiger AM, Vöhringer M, et al. Diffuse large B-cell lymphomas of immunoblastic type are a major reservoir for MYC-IGH translocations. Am J Surg Pathol 2015;39(1):61–6.

15. Horn H, Ziepert M, Wartenberg M, et al. Different biological risk factors in young poor-prognosis and elderly patients with diffuse large B-cell lymphoma. Leukemia 2015;29(7):1564–70.

16. Alizadeh AA, Eisen MB, Davis RE, et al. Distinct types of diffuse large B-cell lymphoma identified by gene expression profiling. Nature 2000; 403(6769):503–11.

17. Rosenwald A, Wright G, Chan WC, et al. The use of molecular profiling to predict survival after chemotherapy for diffuse large-B-cell lymphoma. N Engl J Med 2002;346(25):1937–47.

18. Wright G, Tan B, Rosenwald A, et al. A gene expression-based method to diagnose clinically distinct subgroups of diffuse large B cell lymphoma. Proc Natl Acad Sci U S A 2003; 100(17):9991–6.

19. Lenz G, Wright G, Dave SS, et al. Stromal gene signatures in large-B-cell lymphomas. N Engl J Med 2008;359(22):2313–23.

20. Hans CP, Weisenburger DD, Greiner TC, et al. Confirmation of the molecular classification of diffuse large B-cell lymphoma by immunohistochemistry using a tissue microarray. Blood 2004; 103(1):275–82.

21. Choi WWL, Weisenburger DD, Greiner TC, et al. A new immunostain algorithm classifies diffuse large B-cell lymphoma into molecular subtypes with high accuracy. Clin Cancer Res 2009;15(17): 5494–502.

22. Meyer PN, Fu K, Greiner TC, et al. Immunohistochemical methods for predicting cell of origin and survival in patients with diffuse large B-cell lymphoma treated with rituximab. J Clin Oncol 2011; 29(2):200–7.

23. Visco C, Li Y, Xu-Monette ZY, et al. Comprehensive gene expression profiling and immunohistochemical studies support application of immunophenotypic algorithm for molecular subtype classification in diffuse large B-cell lymphoma: a report from the International DLBCL Rituximab-CHOP Consortium Program Study. Leukemia 2012;26(9):2103–13.

24. Colomo Ls, López-Guillermo A, Perales Ma, et al. Clinical impact of the differentiation profile assessed by immunophenotyping in patients with diffuse large B-cell lymphoma. Blood 2003;101(1): 78–84.

25. Fu K, Weisenburger DD, Choi WWL, et al. Addition of rituximab to standard chemotherapy improves the survival of both the germinal center B-cell–like and non–germinal center B-cell–like subtypes of diffuse large B-cell lymphoma. J Clin Oncol 2008; 26(28):4587–94.

26. Coutinho R, Clear AJ, Owen A, et al. Poor concordance among nine immunohistochemistry classifiers of cell-of-origin for diffuse large B-cell lymphoma: implications for therapeutic strategies. Clin Cancer Res 2013;19(24):6686–95.

27. Gutiérrez-García G, Cardesa-Salzmann T, Climent F, et al. Gene-expression profiling and not immunophenotypic algorithms predicts prognosis in patients with diffuse large B-cell lymphoma treated with immunochemotherapy. Blood 2011; 117(18):4836–43.

28. Collie AMB, Nölling J, Divakar KM, et al. Molecular subtype classification of formalin-fixed, paraffin-embedded diffuse large B-cell lymphoma samples on the ICEPlex® system. Br J Haematol 2014; 167(2):281–5.

29. Xue X, Zeng N, Gao Z, et al. Diffuse large B-cell lymphoma: sub-classification by massive parallel quantitative RT-PCR. Lab Invest 2015;95(1): 113–20.

30. Veldman-Jones MH, Lai Z, Wappett M, et al. Reproducible, quantitative, and flexible molecular subtyping of clinical DLBCL samples using the nanostring nCounter system. Clin Cancer Res 2015;21(10):2367–78.

31. Scott DW, Wright GW, Williams PM, et al. Determining cell-of-origin subtypes of diffuse large B-cell lymphoma using gene expression in formalin-fixed paraffin-embedded tissue. Blood 2014;123(8):1214–7.

32. Gang AO, Pedersen MØ, Knudsen H, et al. Cell of origin predicts outcome to treatment with etoposide-containing chemotherapy in young patients with high-risk diffuse large B-cell lymphoma. Leuk Lymphoma 2015;56(7):2039–46.

33. Wilson WH, Jung S-H, Porcu P, et al. A cancer and leukemia group B multi-center study of DA-EPOCH-rituximab in untreated diffuse large B-cell lymphoma with analysis of outcome by molecular subtype. Haematologica 2012;97(5): 758–65.

34. Wilson WH, Dunleavy K, Pittaluga S, et al. Phase II study of dose-adjusted EPOCH and rituximab in untreated diffuse large B-cell lymphoma with analysis of germinal center and post-germinal center biomarkers. J Clin Oncol 2008;26(16): 2717–24.

35. Davis RE, Brown KD, Siebenlist U, et al. Constitutive nuclear factor kappaB activity is required for survival of activated B cell-like diffuse large B cell lymphoma cells. J Exp Med 2001;194(12): 1861–74.

36. Davis RE, Ngo VN, Lenz G, et al. Chronic active B-cell-receptor signalling in diffuse large B-cell lymphoma. Nature 2010;463(7277):88–92.

37. Dunleavy K, Pittaluga S, Czuczman MS, et al. Differential efficacy of bortezomib plus chemotherapy within molecular subtypes of diffuse large B-cell lymphoma. Blood 2009;113(24): 6069–76.

38. Ruan J, Martin P, Furman RR, et al. Bortezomib plus CHOP-rituximab for previously untreated diffuse large B-cell lymphoma and mantle cell lymphoma. J Clin Oncol 2011;29(6):690–7.

39. Wilson WH, Young RM, Schmitz R, et al. Targeting B cell receptor signaling with ibrutinib in diffuse large B cell lymphoma. Nat Med 2015;21(8): 922–6 advance online publication.

40. Zhang L-H, Kosek J, Wang M, et al. Lenalidomide efficacy in activated B-cell-like subtype diffuse large B-cell lymphoma is dependent upon IRF4 and cereblon expression. Br J Haematol 2013; 160(4):487–502.

41. Nowakowski GS, LaPlant B, Macon WR, et al. Lenalidomide combined with R-CHOP overcomes negative prognostic impact of non–germinal center B-cell phenotype in newly diagnosed diffuse large B-cell lymphoma: a phase II study. J Clin Oncol 2015;33(3):251–7.

42. Vitolo U, Chiappella A, Franceschetti S, et al. Lenalidomide plus R-CHOP21 in elderly patients with untreated diffuse large B-cell lymphoma: results of the REAL07 open-label, multicentre, phase 2 trial. Lancet Oncol 2014;15(7):730–7.

43. Witzig TE, Vose JM, Zinzani PL, et al. An international phase II trial of single-agent lenalidomide for relapsed or refractory aggressive B-cell non-Hodgkin's lymphoma. Ann Oncol 2011;22(7): 1622–7.

44. Chiappella A, Tucci A, Castellino A, et al. Lenalidomide plus cyclophosphamide, doxorubicin, vincristine, prednisone and rituximab is safe and effective in untreated, elderly patients with diffuse large B-cell lymphoma: a phase I study by the Fondazione Italiana Linfomi. Haematologica 2013; 98(11):1732–8.

45. Ott G, Rosenwald A, Campo E. Understanding MYC-driven aggressive B-cell lymphomas: pathogenesis and classification. Hematology Am Soc Hematol Educ Program 2013;2013: 575–83.

46. Calado DP, Sasaki Y, Godinho SA, et al. The cell-cycle regulator c-Myc is essential for the formation and maintenance of germinal centers. Nat Immunol 2012;13(11):1092–100.

47. Savage KJ, Johnson NA, Ben-Neriah S, et al. MYC gene rearrangements are associated with a poor prognosis in diffuse large B-cell lymphoma patients treated with R-CHOP chemotherapy. Blood 2009; 114(17):3533–7.

48. Barrans S, Crouch S, Smith A, et al. Rearrangement of MYC is associated with poor prognosis in patients with diffuse large B-cell lymphoma treated in the era of rituximab. J Clin Oncol 2010;28(20): 3360–5.

49. Salaverria I, Siebert R. The gray zone between Burkitt's lymphoma and diffuse large B-cell lymphoma from a genetics perspective. J Clin Oncol 2011; 29(14):1835–43.

50. Dave SS, Fu K, Wright GW, et al. Molecular diagnosis of Burkitt's lymphoma. N Engl J Med 2006; 354(23):2431–42.

51. Hummel M, Bentink S, Berger H, et al. A biologic definition of Burkitt's lymphoma from transcriptional and genomic profiling. N Engl J Med 2006;354(23): 2419–30.

52. Barrans SL, Evans PA, O'Connor SJ, et al. The t(14;18) is associated with germinal center-derived diffuse large B-cell lymphoma and is a strong predictor of outcome. Clin Cancer Res 2003;9(6):2133–9.

53. Copie-Bergman C, Gaulard P, Leroy K, et al. Immuno-fluorescence in situ hybridization index predicts survival in patients with diffuse large B-cell lymphoma treated with R-CHOP: a GELA study. J Clin Oncol 2009;27(33):5573–9.

54. Offit K, Lo Coco F, Louie DC, et al. Rearrangement of the bcl-6 gene as a prognostic marker in diffuse large-cell lymphoma. N Engl J Med 1994;331(2): 74–80.

55. Lo Coco F, Ye BH, Lista F, et al. Rearrangements of the BCL6 gene in diffuse large cell non-Hodgkin's lymphoma. Blood 1994;83(7):1757–9.

56. Ohno H, Fukuhara S. Significance of rearrangement of the BCL6 gene in B-cell lymphoid neoplasms. Leuk Lymphoma 1997;27(1–2):53–63.

57. Barrans SL, O'Connor SJM, Evans PAS, et al. Rearrangement of the BCL6 locus at 3q27 is an independent poor prognostic factor in nodal diffuse large B-cell lymphoma. Br J Haematol 2002; 117(2):322–32.

58. Akasaka T, Ueda C, Kurata M, et al. Nonimmunoglobulin (non-Ig)/BCL6gene fusion in diffuse large B-cell lymphoma results in worse prognosis than Ig/BCL6. Blood 2000;96(8):2907–9.

59. Johnson NA, Savage KJ, Ludkovski O, et al. Lymphomas with concurrent BCL2 and MYC translocations: the critical factors associated with survival. Blood 2009;114(11):2273–9.

60. Horn H, Ziepert M, Becher C, et al. MYC status in concert with BCL2 and BCL6 expression predicts outcome in diffuse large B-cell lymphoma. Blood 2013;121(12):2253–63.

61. Li S, Lin P, Young KH, et al. MYC/BCL2 double-hit high-grade B-cell lymphoma. Adv Anat Pathol 2013;20(5):315–26.

62. Cook JR, Goldman B, Tubbs RR, et al. Clinical significance of MYC expression and/or "high-grade" morphology in non-Burkitt, diffuse aggressive

B-cell lymphomas: a SWOG S9704 correlative study. Am J Surg Pathol 2014;38(4):494–501.

63. Swerdlow SH. Diagnosis of 'double hit' diffuse large B-cell lymphoma and B-cell lymphoma, unclassifiable, with features intermediate between DLBCL and Burkitt lymphoma: when and how, FISH versus IHC. Hematology Am Soc Hematol Educ Program 2014;2014(1):90–9.

64. Perry AM, Crockett D, Dave BJ, et al. B-cell lymphoma, unclassifiable, with features intermediate between diffuse large B-cell lymphoma and burkitt lymphoma: study of 39 cases. Br J Haematol 2013; 162(1):40–9.

65. Foot NJ, Dunn RG, Geoghegan H, et al. Fluorescence in situ hybridisation analysis of formalin-fixed paraffin-embedded tissue sections in the diagnostic work-up of non-Burkitt high grade B-cell non-Hodgkin's lymphoma: a single centre's experience. J Clin Pathol 2011;64(9):802–8.

66. Pillai RK, Sathanoori M, Van Oss SB, et al. Double-hit B-cell lymphomas with BCL6 and MYC translocations are aggressive, frequently extranodal lymphomas distinct from BCL2 double-hit B-cell lymphomas. Am J Surg Pathol 2013;37(3): 323–32.

67. Valera A, Lopez-Guillermo A, Cardesa-Salzmann T, et al. MYC protein expression and genetic alterations have prognostic impact in patients with diffuse large B-cell lymphoma treated with immunochemotherapy. Haematologica 2013;98(10): 1554–62.

68. Aukema SM, Kreuz M, Kohler CW, et al. Biological characterization of adult MYC-translocation-positive mature B-cell lymphomas other than molecular Burkitt lymphoma. Haematologica 2014; 99(4):726–35.

69. Green TM, Young KH, Visco C, et al. Immunohistochemical double-hit score is a strong predictor of outcome in patients with diffuse large B-cell lymphoma treated with rituximab plus cyclophosphamide, doxorubicin, vincristine, and prednisone. J Clin Oncol 2012;30(28):3460–7.

70. Hu S, Xu-Monette ZY, Tzankov A, et al. MYC/BCL2 protein coexpression contributes to the inferior survival of activated B-cell subtype of diffuse large B-cell lymphoma and demonstrates high-risk gene expression signatures: a report from the International DLBCL Rituximab-CHOP Consortium Program. Blood 2013;121(20): 4021–31 [quiz: 250].

71. Johnson NA, Slack GW, Savage KJ, et al. Concurrent expression of MYC and BCL2 in diffuse large B-cell lymphoma treated with rituximab plus cyclophosphamide, doxorubicin, vincristine, and prednisone. J Clin Oncol 2012;30(28):3452–9.

72. Petrich AM, Gandhi M, Jovanovic B, et al. Impact of induction regimen and stem cell transplantation on outcomes in double-hit lymphoma: a multicenter retrospective analysis. Blood 2014;124(15): 2354–61.

73. Dunleavy K, Fanale M, LaCasce A, et al. Preliminary report of a multicenter prospective phase II study of DA-EPOCH-R in MYC-rearranged aggressive B-cell lymphoma. Blood 2014;124(21):395.

74. Wang XJ, Medeiros LJ, Lin P, et al. MYC cytogenetic status correlates with expression and has prognostic significance in patients with MYC/BCL2 protein double-positive diffuse large B-cell lymphoma. Am J Surg Pathol 2015;39(9): 1250–8.

75. Tzankov A, Xu-Monette ZY, Gerhard M, et al. Rearrangements of MYC gene facilitate risk stratification in diffuse large B-cell lymphoma patients treated with rituximab-CHOP. Mod Pathol 2014;27(7): 958–71.

76. Pedersen MØ, Gang AO, Poulsen TS, et al. MYC translocation partner gene determines survival of patients with large B-cell lymphoma with MYC- or double-hit MYC/BCL2 translocations. Eur J Haematol 2014;92(1):42–8.

77. Li S, Seegmiller AC, Lin P, et al. B-cell lymphomas with concurrent MYC and BCL2 abnormalities other than translocations behave similarly to MYC/BCL2 double-hit lymphomas. Mod Pathol 2015;28(2): 208–17.

78. Yoon SO, Jeon YK, Paik JH, et al. MYC translocation and an increased copy number predict poor prognosis in adult diffuse large B-cell lymphoma (DLBCL), especially in germinal centre-like B cell (GCB) type. Histopathology 2008;53(2):205–17.

79. Stasik CJ, Nitta H, Zhang W, et al. Increased MYC gene copy number correlates with increased mRNA levels in diffuse large B-cell lymphoma. Haematologica 2010;95(4):597–603.

80. Kluk MJ, Chapuy B, Sinha P, et al. Immunohistochemical detection of MYC-driven diffuse large B-cell lymphomas. PLoS One 2012;7(4):e33813.

81. Tang SC, Visser L, Hepperle B, et al. Clinical significance of bcl-2-MBR gene rearrangement and protein expression in diffuse large-cell non-Hodgkin's lymphoma: an analysis of 83 cases. J Clin Oncol 1994;12(1):149–54.

82. Mounier N, Briere J, Gisselbrecht C, et al. Rituximab plus CHOP (R-CHOP) overcomes bcl-2–associated resistance to chemotherapy in elderly patients with diffuse large B-cell lymphoma (DLBCL). Blood 2003;101(11):4279–84.

83. Iqbal J, Meyer PN, Smith LM, et al. BCL2 predicts survival in germinal center B-cell-like diffuse large B-cell lymphoma treated with CHOP-like therapy and rituximab. Clin Cancer Res 2011;17(24): 7785–95.

84. Iqbal J, Sanger WG, Horsman DE, et al. BCL2 translocation defines a unique tumor subset within

the germinal center B-cell-like diffuse large B-cell lymphoma. Am J Pathol 2004;165(1):159–66.

85. Perry AM, Alvarado-Bernal Y, Laurini JA, et al. MYC and BCL2 protein expression predicts survival in patients with diffuse large B-cell lymphoma treated with rituximab. Br J Haematol 2014;165(3):382–91.

86. Mahmoud AZ, George TI, Czuchlewski DR, et al. Scoring of MYC protein expression in diffuse large B-cell lymphomas: concordance rate among hematopathologists. Mod Pathol 2015;28(4):545–51.

87. Harada S, Suzuki R, Uehira K, et al. Molecular and immunological dissection of diffuse large B cell lymphoma: CD5+, and CD5- with CD10+ groups may constitute clinically relevant subtypes. Leukemia 1999;13(9):1441–7.

88. Kroft SH, Howard MS, Picker LJ, et al. De novo CD5+ diffuse large B-cell lymphomas. A heterogeneous group containing an unusual form of splenic lymphoma. Am J Clin Pathol 2000;114(4):523–33.

89. Yamaguchi M, Ohno T, Oka K, et al. De novo CD5-positive diffuse large B-cell lymphoma: clinical characteristics and therapeutic outcome. Br J Haematol 1999;105(4):1133–9.

90. Yamaguchi M, Seto M, Okamoto M, et al. De novo CD5+ diffuse large B-cell lymphoma: a clinicopathologic study of 109 patients. Blood 2002; 99(3):815–21.

91. Xu-Monette ZY, Tu M, Jabbar KJ, et al. Clinical and biological significance of de novo CD5+ diffuse large B-cell lymphoma in Western countries. Oncotarget 2015;6(8):5615–33.

92. Miyazaki K, Yamaguchi M, Suzuki R, et al. CD5-positive diffuse large B-cell lymphoma: a retrospective study in 337 patients treated by chemotherapy with or without rituximab. Ann Oncol 2011;22(7):1601–7.

93. Hu S, Xu-Monette ZY, Balasubramanyam A, et al. CD30 expression defines a novel subgroup of diffuse large B-cell lymphoma with favorable prognosis and distinct gene expression signature: a report from the International DLBCL Rituximab-CHOP Consortium Program Study. Blood 2013; 121(14):2715–24.

94. Pro B, Advani R, Brice P, et al. Brentuximab vedotin (SGN-35) in patients with relapsed or refractory systemic anaplastic large-cell lymphoma: results of a phase II study. J Clin Oncol 2012;30(18):2190–6.

95. Younes A, Bartlett NL, Leonard JP, et al. Brentuximab vedotin (SGN-35) for relapsed CD30-positive lymphomas. N Engl J Med 2010;363(19):1812–21.

96. Salaverria I, Philipp C, Oschlies I, et al. Translocations activating IRF4 identify a subtype of germinal center-derived B-cell lymphoma affecting predominantly children and young adults. Blood 2011; 118(1):139–47.

97. Salaverria I, Martin-Guerrero I, Wagener R, et al. A recurrent 11q aberration pattern characterizes

a subset of MYC-negative high-grade B-cell lymphomas resembling Burkitt lymphoma. Blood 2014;123(8):1187–98.

98. Pienkowska-Grela B, Rymkiewicz G, Grygalewicz B, et al. Partial trisomy 11, dup(11)(q23q13), as a defect characterizing lymphomas with Burkitt pathomorphology without MYC gene rearrangement. Med Oncol 2011;28(4):1589–95.

99. Ferreiro JF, Morscio J, Dierickx D, et al. Post-transplant molecularly defined Burkitt lymphomas are frequently MYC-negative and characterized by the 11q-gain/loss pattern. Haematologica 2015; 100(7):e275–9.

100. Schmitz R, Young RM, Ceribelli M, et al. Burkitt lymphoma pathogenesis and therapeutic targets from structural and functional genomics. Nature 2012; 490(7418):116–20.

101. Richter J, Schlesner M, Hoffmann S, et al. Recurrent mutation of the ID3 gene in Burkitt lymphoma identified by integrated genome, exome and transcriptome sequencing. Nat Genet 2012;44(12): 1316–20.

102. Love C, Sun Z, Jima D, et al. The genetic landscape of mutations in Burkitt lymphoma. Nat Genet 2012;44(12):1321–5.

103. Momose S, Weissbach S, Pischimarov J, et al. The diagnostic gray zone between Burkitt lymphoma and diffuse large B-cell lymphoma is also a gray zone of the mutational spectrum. Leukemia 2015; 29(8):1789–91.

104. Schmitz R, Ceribelli M, Pittaluga S, et al. Oncogenic mechanisms in Burkitt lymphoma. Cold Spring Harb Perspect Med 2014;4(2).

105. Lawrence MS, Stojanov P, Polak P, et al. Mutational heterogeneity in cancer and the search for new cancer-associated genes. Nature 2013;499(7457): 214–8.

106. Morin RD, Johnson NA, Severson TM, et al. Somatic mutations altering EZH2 (Tyr641) in follicular and diffuse large B-cell lymphomas of germinal-center origin. Nat Genet 2010;42(2):181–5.

107. Yap DB, Chu J, Berg T, et al. Somatic mutations at EZH2 Y641 act dominantly through a mechanism of selectively altered PRC2 catalytic activity, to increase H3K27 trimethylation. Blood 2011;117(8): 2451–9.

108. Knutson SK, Wigle TJ, Warholic NM, et al. A selective inhibitor of EZH2 blocks H3K27 methylation and kills mutant lymphoma cells. Nat Chem Biol 2012;8(11):890–6.

109. McCabe MT, Ott HM, Ganji G, et al. EZH2 inhibition as a therapeutic strategy for lymphoma with EZH2-activating mutations. Nature 2012;492(7427): 108–12.

110. Study of EPZ-6438 formerly known as E7438 (EZH2 histone methyl transferase [HMT] inhibitor) as a single agent in subjects with advanced solid tumors

or with B-cell lymphomas. ClinicalTrials.gov: US National Library of Medicine; 2013.

111. Compagno M, Lim WK, Grunn A, et al. Mutations of multiple genes cause deregulation of NF-kappaB in diffuse large B-cell lymphoma. Nature 2009; 459(7247):717–21.

112. Honma K, Tsuzuki S, Nakagawa M, et al. TNFAIP3/ A20 functions as a novel tumor suppressor gene in several subtypes of non-Hodgkin lymphomas. Blood 2009;114(12):2467–75.

113. Lenz G, Davis RE, Ngo VN, et al. Oncogenic CARD11 mutations in human diffuse large B cell lymphoma. Science 2008;319(5870):1676–9.

114. Ngo VN, Young RM, Schmitz R, et al. Oncogenically active MYD88 mutations in human lymphoma. Nature 2011;470(7332):115–9.

B-cell Lymphoproliferative Disorders Associated with Primary and Acquired Immunodeficiency

Lawrence K. Low, MD, PhD, Joo Y. Song, MD*

KEYWORDS

- Primary immunodeficiency • Acquired immunodeficiency • B-Cell lymphoma
- Post-transplant lymphoproliferative disorder

ABSTRACT

The diagnosis of lymphoproliferative disorders associated with immunodeficiency can be challenging because many of these conditions have overlapping clinical and pathologic features and share similarities with their counterparts in the immunocompetent setting. There are subtle but important differences between these conditions that are important to recognize for prognostic and therapeutic purposes. This article provides a clinicopathologic update on how understanding of these B-cell lymphoproliferations in immunodeficiency has evolved over the past decade.

Key Features

- Knowledge of the clinical history is an important step in the evaluation of lymphoproliferative disorders associated with immunodeficiency.

- There is some overlap in morphologic and phenotypic features between lymphoproliferative disorders in immunedeficient versus immunocompetent settings. Viral infection by Epstein-Barr virus (EBV) and/or human herpes virus 8 (HHV8), however, seems more commonly associated with immunodeficiency.

- EBV-positive mucocutaneous ulcer (EBV MCU) is an important entity to recognize due to its indolent nature compared with other EBV-positive lymphoproliferations.

- Newer genomic approaches have revealed that the expression of key viral genes can alter the normal function of cell survival and proliferation pathways. Additional knowledge of how these pathways are altered may play an integral role in the future diagnosis and treatment of immunodeficiency-associated lymphomas.

OVERVIEW

B-cell lymphoproliferative disorders represent a heterogeneous group of diseases. Epidemiologic and experimental studies in the past 40 years have revealed a correlation between the development of a subset of B-cell lymphoproliferative disorders and a defect in immune surveillance. These defects in immune surveillance often occur as a result of an inherited or acquired immunodeficiency. Primary causes of inherited immunodeficiency include common variable immunodeficiency, severe combined immunodeficiency, and Wiskott-Aldrich syndrome; their associations with various types of lymphoproliferative processes are listed (**Table 1**). Acquired immunodeficiencies, on the other hand, can arise in the settings of HIV infection (**Table 2**), post-transplant, or iatrogenic-associated immune

Disclosure Statement: The authors have nothing to disclose.
Department of Pathology, City of Hope National Medical Center, 1500 East Duarte Road, Duarte, CA 91010, USA
* Corresponding author.
E-mail address: josong@coh.org

Table 1
Primary immunodeficiency and associated lymphoproliferative disorders

Disease	Genetic/Protein Defect	Immune Deficiency	Lymphoproliferative Disorders/Lymphomas
Combined B-cell and T-cell immunodeficiencies			
Severe combined immunodeficiency syndrome[118,119]	Many subtypes	Decreased T-cells, B-cells, and Ig depends on subtype	EBV-associated lesions (DLBCL and HL), mostly B-cell NHL, fatal infectious mononucleosis
Hyper-IgM syndrome[120]	CD40 ligand or CD40	Neutropenia	EBV-associated lesions (DLBCL and HL) and LGL leukemia
Wiskott-Aldrich syndrome[121]	WAS	Progressive decrease of T-cells, B-cells, low IgM, increased IgE	EBV-associated lesions (DLBCL and HL) and mostly B-cell NHLs; may involve CNS
Antibody deficiency			
Common variable immune deficiency[122]	Unknown	Decreased IgG, IgA, and/or IgM; decreased B-cells	EBV-associated lesions (DLBCL and HL), MALT lymphoma, SLL, LPL, and PTCL (rare)
DNA repair defects			
Ataxia-telangiectasia[123]	ATM	Progressive decrease of T-cells and B-cells; increased IgM and decreased IgA, IgE, IgG	HL, DLBCL, BL, nonleukemic clonal T-cell proliferations, T-PLL (children), T-ALL (young adults)
Nimegen breakage syndrome[124]	NBN	Progressive decrease of T-cells, normal/reduced B-cells; decreased IgA, IgE, and IgG	B-cell and T-cell NHL, T-LBL/ALL, and HL
Immune dysregulation			
X-linked lymphoproliferative syndrome[125]	SH2D1A	Normal/reduced B-cells, normal/reduced immunoglobulin	EBV-associated lesions (DLBCL and BL)
Autoimmune lymphoproliferative syndrome[126]	FAS (type 1a), FASL (type 1b), CASP10 (type 2a) or CASP8 (type 2b)	Increased CD4−/CD8− T-cells	HL, DLBCL, BL, and PTCL (rare)
Chédiak-Higashi syndrome[127]	LYST	No immune deficiency	EBV-associated lesions

Abbreviations: Ig, immunoglobulin; LGL, large granulocyte lymphocyte; LPL, lymphoplasmacytic lymphoma; MALT, mucosa-associated lymphoid tissue; PTCL, peripheral T-cell lymphoma; SLL, small lymphocytic lymphoma; T-ALL, T-cell acute lymphoblastic leukemia; T-LBL, T-cell lymphoblastic lymphoma; T-PLL, T-cell prolymphocytic leukemia.

Table 2
Differential diagnosis of lymphoproliferative disorders specifically associated with HIV

Disease	Infection	Location	Morphology	Phenotype
PEL				
Classic PEL	HIV, HSHV, EBV	Body cavity	Blastic, anaplastic	CD45+, CD30+, IRF4/MUM1+, CD138+, B-cell antigens±, clonal
Solid PEL (extracavitary KSHV positive solid lymphoma)	HIV, KSHV, EBV	Extracavitary solid mass	Plasmablastic, immunoblastic	CD45+, CD30+, IRF4/MUM1+, CD138+, B-cell antigens±, clonal
Early PEL	HIV, KSHV, EBV	Lymph node follicle	Plasmablastic, immunoblastic	CD45+, CD30+, IRF4/MUM1+, CD138+, B-cell antigens±, clonal
MCD				
MCD, plasmablastic variant	HIV±, KSHV, EBV−/+	Lymph node, spleen	Scattered plasmablasts in follicle mantle zones	IgM lambda+, polyclonal, B-cell antigens−/+
MCD-associated plasmablastic microlymphoma	HIV±, KSHV	Lymph node, spleen	Clusters of plasmablasts in follicles	CD20±, CD79a−, CD138−, CD38−/+, IRF4/MUM1+, cIgM, clonal (lambda light chain restriction)
LBL arising in MCD	HIV±, KSHV	Lymph node, spleen	Confluent expansion of plasmablasts	CD20±, CD79a−, CD138−, CD38−/+, IRF4/MUM1+, cIgM, clonal (lambda light chain restriction)
PBL of the oral cavity	HIV±, EBV	Oral cavity or extranodal mucosal sites	Plasmablastic, immunoblastic	CD45−, CD20−, PAX5−, CD79a−/+, CD38+, CD138+, IRF4/MUM1+

Abbreviations: −/+, usually negative; ±, usually positive; KSHV, Kaposi sarcoma herpesvirus.

suppression (**Table 3**). There are some important distinctions between the source of immune suppression, the onset of disease, and the spectrum of lymphoproliferative processes that develop (see **Tables 1–3**). Another characteristic feature that seems to be shared among primary and acquired immunodeficiencies is that reduced immune surveillance can result in the proliferation of viruses, such as EBV HHV8.[1] EBV and HHV8 have been linked or are known to cause certain lymphoproliferative disorders. This article describes some of the more common B-cell lymphoproliferative disorders associated with primary and acquired immunodeficiencies. Important clinicopathologic features of each entity are highlighted because several of these lymphomas can pose different diagnostic challenges for the clinician.

DIFFUSE LARGE B-CELL LYMPHOMA

OVERVIEW

Diffuse large B-cell lymphoma (DLBCL) represents one of the more common lymphoproliferative disorders that occur in the immunocompromised setting.[2–5] DLBCL in immunocompromised states closely resembles DLBCL in the immunocompetent setting, except EBV infection is more commonly observed in the immunocompromised setting. In immunosuppressed states, such as HIV infection, post-transplant, or after iatrogenic treatment of autoimmune conditions, DLBCL can be systemic or involve the central nervous system (CNS).[2,5–10] In addition, these cases can be further subdivided based on morphologic subtypes

Table 3
Iatrogenic causes of immunodeficiencies and associated lymphoproliferative disorders

Drug	Underlying Disorder	Duration of Therapy	Type of Lymphoproliferative Disorder
Methotrexate[10]	Autoimmune diseases, psoriasis	3 y (0.5–5 y)	DLBCL, HL, polymorphic LPD, and PTCL
TNF-α antagonists[128–131]			
Infliximab (MAb)	Autoimmune diseases	6 wk (2–44 y)	DLBCL and other B-cell NHLs
	Crohn disease (young patients)	1–58 mo	HSTL and other T-cell NHLs
Adalimumab (Mab)	Autoimmune diseases	NA	Any type
Etanercept (fusion protein with p75)	Autoimmune diseases	8 wk (2–52 wk)	Any type
Thiopurine analogs[132,133]			
Azathioprine	Inflammatory bowel disease	6–24 mo	Any type
6-mercaptopurine	Inflammatory bowel disease	6–24 mo	Any type

Abbreviations: HSTL, hepatosplenic T-cell lymphoma; LPD, lymphoproliferative disorder; PTCL, peripheral T-cell lymphoma.

(immunoblastic vs centroblastic) and cell-of-origin gene expression signatures[11–13]; however, the significance of these additional subclassifications is unclear in immunosuppressed states.

CLINICAL FEATURES

DLBCL in immunocompromised patients is similar in clinical presentation to DLBCL in immunocompetent persons.[2] Patients can present with nodal or extranodal disease (gastrointestinal tract, bone, testis, spleen, liver, and so forth). Symptoms vary and are usually due to secondary mass effect from a rapidly growing tumor.

DIAGNOSIS

The neoplastic cells can have a germinal center or non–germinal center phenotype. Morphologically, the neoplastic lymphoid cells with the non-germinal center phenotype tend to have an immunoblastic or plasmablastic appearance (**Fig. 1**). In these subsets of cases, B-cell markers, such as CD20, may be weak or negative, whereas the expression of plasma cell markers, such as CD138, are expressed. Transcription factors that are associated with germinal center B cells (ie, BCL6) are down-regulated, and terminal differentiation toward a plasma cell is characterized by expression of IRF4/MUM1, XBP1, and BLIMP1.[14–16] Approximately one-third of these cases are driven by EBV infection, and colocalization of EBV-encoded small RNA (EBER) or latent

membrane protein 1 (LMP1) can be observed in the tumor cells.[2–4] EBV-induced dysregulation of transcription may contribute toward the plasmablastic differentiation of cells. Recent genomic studies have also suggested that activation of the nuclear factor (NF)-κB pathway via loss of A20 (tumor necrosis factor, alpha-induced protein 3 [TNFAIP3]) and LMP1 expression may play an important role in the pathogenesis of this disease.[17]

PROGNOSIS

Although clinical outcomes vary depending on the underlying cause of immune suppression, a majority of cases require cytotoxic therapy to achieve remission.

IMMUNODEFICIENCY-ASSOCIATED BURKITT LYMPHOMA

OVERVIEW

HIV-associated Burkitt lymphoma (HIV BL) is a highly aggressive lymphoma. Compared with other HIV-related non-Hodgkin lymphomas (NHLs), its clinical presentation is unpredictable and clinical changes are rapid if left untreated. Burkitt lymphoma (BL) seems more common in HIV than in other forms of immunosuppression.[2–4,18,19] The lymphoma occurs earlier in HIV infection when CD4 counts are higher, suggesting other mechanisms besides immune suppression

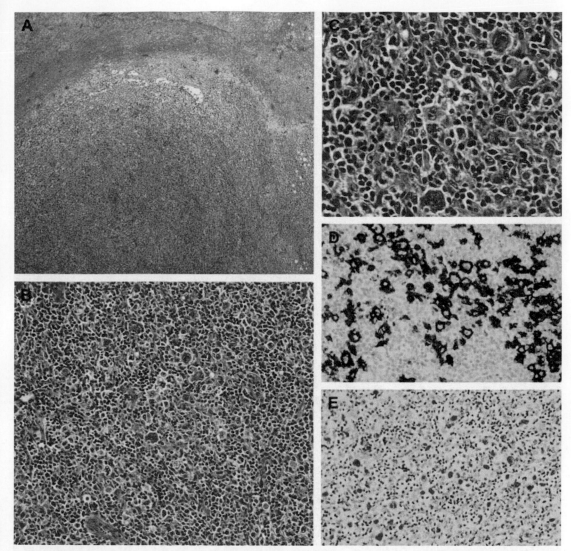

Fig. 1. DLBCL after iatrogenic treatment of rheumatoid arthritis. The lymph node architecture is replaced by a diffuse infiltrate composed of medium-to-large pleomorphic cells hematoxylin-eosin ([A] H&E, ×50; [B] H&E, ×200). Extensive necrosis is observed. (C) Several larger cells resemble RS cells (H&E, ×400). The atypical medium and large cells express (D) CD20 (×200) and (E) EBER ISH (×200).

are critical for lymphomagenesis.[2] HIV BL is nowadays treated with intensive chemotherapy regimens that are effective in achieving remission and long-term survival.[20,21]

CLINICAL FEATURES

HIV BL presents either as nodal or extranodal disease in the abdomen and has a higher frequency for bone marrow involvement.[4,19] Signs and symptoms may include abdominal pain, bowel obstruction, jaundice, or gastrointestinal bleeding. A rapid decline in clinical status is not uncommon. The tumors are often large at presentation and may have

disseminated to secondary sites due to reduced immune surveillance.

DIAGNOSIS

HIV BL is indistinguishable from the HIV-negative counterparts (**Fig. 2**).[2,4,22,23] HIV BL cases may also develop plasmacytoid features with larger pleomorphic cells, eccentric nuclei, and prominent nucleoli. EBV-infected cells are more common in cases of plasmacytoid differentiation (up to 50%–70%).[24] The phenotype of HIV BL is similar to non–HIV BL because the neoplastic cells express pan B-cell antigens, CD10, and BCL6. BCL2 and TDT are negative. EBV infection

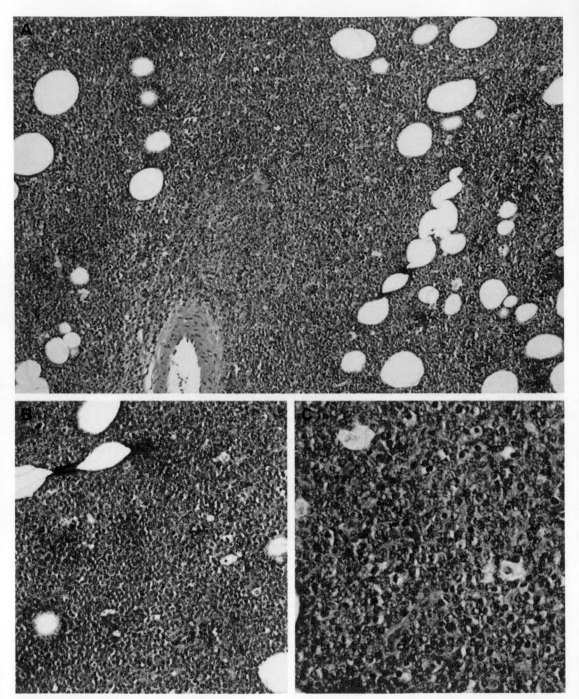

Fig. 2. HIV BL extensively involving the small bowel. The submucosa is replaced by a diffuse and monomorphic population of medium-sized lymphoid cells with evenly distributed chromatin and occasional small nucleoli ([*A*] hematoxylin-eosin [H&E], ×100; [*B*] H&E, ×200; and [*C*], H&E, ×400).

exhibits a latency type I phenotype, and the infected cells can be detected by in situ hybridization (ISH) for EBER whereas EBV LMP1 and Epstein-Barr nuclear antigen 2 (EBNA-2) are usually absent. The proliferation index is nearly 100% with Ki67. The background is nearly devoid of T cells. At the genetic level, there are similarities as well. *MYC* translocations are common but can be absent in cases where dysregulation of microRNA pathways may be more important.[25] In addition to *MYC* gene rearrangements, recent studies have shown that other genetic alterations are common, such as loss of *TP53* as well as mutations in *TCF3 (E2A)* or its negative regulator *ID3* and *CCND3*.[26]

PROGNOSIS

Before combined antiretroviral therapy (cART) was introduced, HIV BL outcomes were dismal.[27–30] Clinical awareness of the disease's variable presentation and rapid clinical course has had a dramatic impact on improving patient survival. In addition, newer and more aggressive chemotherapy regimens have resulted in better outcomes.

HUMAN IMMUNODEFICIENCY VIRUS-ASSOCIATED CLASSIC HODGKIN LYMPHOMA

OVERVIEW

Hodgkin lymphoma (HL) is one of the most common types of lymphoma in HIV-infected patients.[2,31–33] Despite cART therapy, the incidence of HIV-associated classic HL (HIV HL) seems to be increasing. HIV HL differs from non-HIV HL because patients have a poorer prognosis that is associated with tumor subtype, EBV infection, and B symptoms (see below). Clinical outcomes have improved with multiple therapeutic regimens that combine chemotherapy with timed intervention with retroviral agents. More intense chemotherapy and the option of hematopoietic stem cell transplantation (HSCT) have improved survival.

CLINICAL FEATURES

Most patients with HIV HL present with B symptoms (ie, fever, night sweats, and weight loss). There is a higher percentage of patients who present with stage IV disease (Ann Arbor classification) and involvement with extranodal sites (bone marrow, liver, and spleen) compared with non-HIV HL.[34,35] Bone marrow involvement is not uncommon and has been reported in up to 50% of cases in 1 series.[36]

DIAGNOSIS

Although HIV-infected patients can acquire any subtype of HL, they are more likely to present with subtypes, such as the mixed cellularity (>50% of cases) and lymphocyte-depleted variants, which are associated with a poorer prognosis (**Fig. 3**).[2,37] Reed-Sternberg (RS) cells are more prevalent in these cases. In addition, coinfection with EBV is present in a majority of cases (>80%).[6,37] These cells are positive for PAX5 (weak), CD15 (variable), CD30, IRF4/MUM1, and CD138 and are usually negative for CD20, CD45, and BCL6.[38] When CD20 is present, there is usually a variable level of expression in the RS cells. The B-cell activation markers Oct-2 and Bob.1 are decreased or absent. EBV-infected RS cells can be detected by ISH for EBER as well as LMP1.

PROGNOSIS

Although HIV HL is considered more aggressive compared with non-HIV HL, the prognosis of HIV HL has greatly improved once cART therapy was combined with current chemotherapy regimens.[39,40]

LYMPHOMATOID GRANULOMATOSIS

OVERVIEW

Lymphomatoid granulomatosis (LYG) is a B-cell lymphoproliferative disorder with a predilection for vessels and vascular invasion that was first reported by Liebow and colleagues[41] in 1972.[2,42] LYG is a rare condition that usually affects extranodal locations, in particular the lungs, CNS, and skin. In addition, there is a strong association with EBV infection.[43,44] An increased risk for LYG is seen in immunocompromised patients and predisposed conditions include allogeneic organ transplantation, Wiskott-Aldrich syndrome, HIV infection, and X-linked lymphoproliferative syndrome. Now proved to be a B-cell proliferation driven by EBV, several of the early reported cases of LYG were misclassified as a T-cell or natural killer (NK)-cell lymphoma. Recent studies suggest that defective immune surveillance by CD8-positive T cells may contribute to the pathogenesis of the disease.[42,45]

CLINICAL FEATURES

LYG is usually seen in adults but it can affect children with an underlying immunodeficiency. It affects men more often than women (male:female ratio ≥2:1) and appears more frequently in western countries.[2] The most common sites involved include the lung (>90%), skin (25%–50%), kidney (32%), liver (29%), and CNS (26%).[2,42] Most patients are symptomatic and present with one or more of the following: cough (60%), fever (60%), rash/nodules (40%), weight loss (35%), dyspnea (30%), neurologic abnormalities (30%), and chest pain (15%).[2,42] Imaging studies typically show bilateral lung nodules of varying size. Necrosis may be observed in the larger nodules. Skin lesions can vary in appearance. Subcutaneous nodules

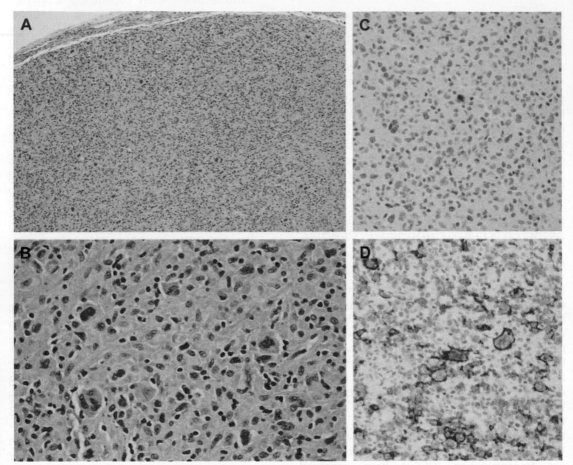

Fig. 3. HIV HL, lymphocyte depleted. The architecture of the lymph node is effaced by a diffuse infiltrate composed of several RS cells and scattered histiocytes ([A] hematoxylin-eosin [H&E], ×100; [B] H&E, ×400). The RS cells express PAX5 (weak, not shown) and (D) CD30 (×200), and are negative for (C) CD15 (×200).

and dermal necrosis/ulceration seem more common than superficial rashes and plaques.

DIAGNOSIS

LYG is associated with an angiocentric and angiodestructive polymorphous infiltrate.[42,43,46] The lesions often have a patchy distribution and are well circumscribed. The degree of vessel involvement can vary immensely. Vascular lesions can be prominent and vascular integrity may sometimes become compromised, resulting in large areas of coagulative necrosis (Fig. 4). The polymorphous infiltrate is composed of numerous small T cells, histiocytes, and occasional plasma cells. Neutrophils, eosinophils, or granulomas are not usually seen. Large atypical B cells are seen that are EBV positive and may resemble immunoblasts or have Hodgkin-like morphology; however, the presence of RS cells should raise suspicion of HL. Skin lesions are also rich in small

T cells with variable numbers of large EBV-positive B cells and may contain granulomatous inflammation.

The EBV-positive B cells are positive for CD20 and variably express CD30 (see Fig. 4). CD15 is usually negative. LMP1 may be positive in the larger cells. CD4-positive T cells predominate in the background and within the vessel walls. Molecular studies show evidence of immunoglobulin gene rearrangement in the higher-grade cases (43%).[42] Rare T-cell receptor gene rearrangements have been reported (6%); therefore, a T-cell lymphoma should be excluded.[42]

Grading of LYG is important for treatment and is based on the density of EBV-positive cells within the polymorphous infiltrate.[2] LYG grade 1 typically has fewer than 5 EBV-positive B cells per high-power field (HPF) whereas higher-grade lesions (LYG grades 2 and 3) are associated with increased numbers of large EBV-positive B cells per HPF (5–50/HPF for grade 2 and >50/HPF for

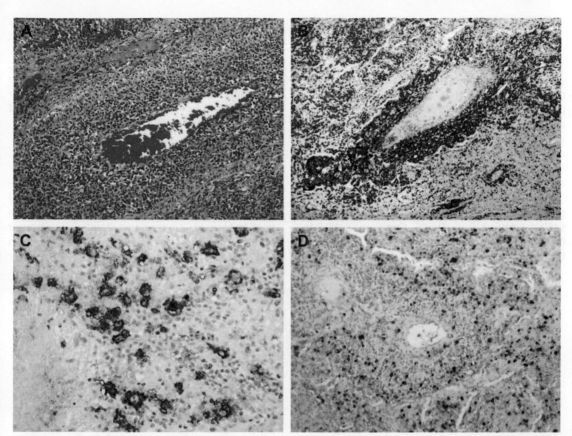

Fig. 4. LYG, grade 2. The lung contains an (*A*) angiocentric infiltrate (hematoxylin-eosin [H&E], ×100) composed of numerous medium-to-large cells that express (*B*) CD20 (×100), (C) (×200), and (*D*) EBER ISH (<50/HPF) (×200).

grade 3) and larger areas of necrosis. Confluent sheets of large atypical B-cells are not seen and suggest the possibility of an EBV-positive DLBCL.

PROGNOSIS

Most cases are characterized by aggressive disease with a median survival of 2 years after initial diagnosis. Immunochemotherapy (ie, dose-adjusted EPOCH-R (Etoposide, Prednisolone, Oncovin-Vincristine, Cyclophosphamide, Hydroxydaunorubicin-Doxorubicin, Rituximab)) has proved useful as some recent series have reported a response for grade 3 lesions.[47] Grades 1 to 2 lesions usually respond to interferon alpha-2b treatment.[45]

EPSTEIN-BARR VIRUS–POSITIVE MUCOCUTANEOUS ULCER

OVERVIEW

EBV MCU is a rare B-cell lymphoproliferative disorder recently described.[48,49] It is associated with immunosuppression after iatrogenic drug therapy, post-transplant, and in elderly individuals where immunesenescence can arise.[48–50] The lymphoproliferative lesions present as isolation mucosal and/or skin lesions. EBV MCU is an important clinicopathologic entity to recognize and differentiate from other EBV-positive lymphoproliferative disorders because the clinical course is usually benign and self-limited.

CLINICAL FEATURES

The clinical background of most patients is variable but the affected persons (median age of 77 years) have some form of immune suppression, either from iatrogenic immunosuppression (methotrexate, azathioprine, or cyclosporin A) for autoimmune conditions or solid organ transplantation (ie, kidney, heart, or lung). Immunosenescence as a result of advanced age (median age of 80 years) may contribute to the occurrence in a subset of patients who are not immunosuppressed.[48] Patients present with isolated slow-growing indurated ulcers that most commonly involve the oropharyngeal mucosa. Other sites of involvement include the tongue, tonsils, palate, gastrointestinal tract, and skin. Although localized lymphadenopathy may be observed, generalized lymphadenopathy is not present.

DIAGNOSIS

Shallow, well-circumscribed ulcers are detected and patchy necrosis can be seen (**Fig. 5**).[48,49] An underlying polymorphous infiltrate is composed of small lymphocytes, histiocytes, eosinophils, plasma cells, and a variable numbers of large atypical lymphocytes, which can be prominent in some cases. The large atypical lymphoid cells can resemble RS cells. In rare cases, the large lymphoid cells are angioinvasive with surrounding areas of necrosis.

The large atypical lymphoid cells have a B-cell phenotype (see **Fig. 5**).[48] The cells coexpress CD20, PAX5, CD30, CD45, Oct-2, and MUM1. CD15, Bob.1, BCL2, and BCL6 are variable. CD3, CD10, and CD138 are negative. The small lymphocytes and large atypical B-cells are nearly always positive for EBV, which can be detected by ISH for EBER or LMP1 immunohistochemistry. The background is comprised of a predominance of CD4-positive T cells. Molecular studies can be clonal for immunoglobulin or T-cell receptor gene rearrangements in approximately a third of cases.

PROGNOSIS

Most patients require minimal therapeutic intervention. In the post-transplant setting, EBV MCU may be difficult to discern from a more aggressive post-transplant lymphoproliferative disorder (PTLD).[49] It may be challenging to distinguish EBV MCU from polymorphic PTLDs or HL;

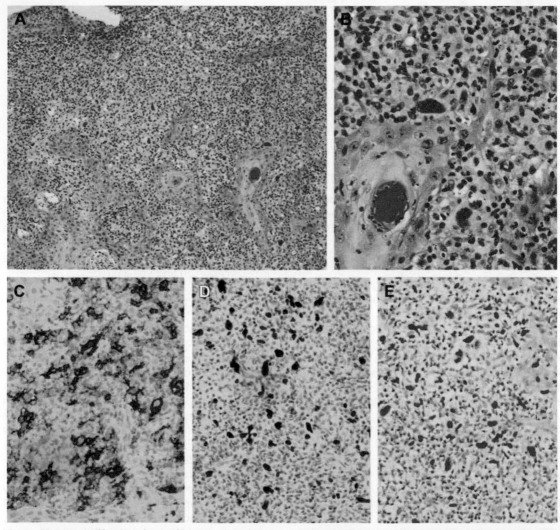

Fig. 5. EBV MCU affecting the oral cavity. (*A*) Low-power (hematoxylin-eosin [H&E], ×100) and (*B*) high-power (H&E, ×400) images showing ulcerated mucosa with an underlying diffuse polymorphous infiltrate. Some of the larger cells resemble RS cells. The large cells express (*C*) CD20 (×200), (*D*) Oct-2 (×200), and (*E*) EBER ISH (×200).

therefore, morphologic, immunophenotypic, and clinical findings must be correlated. This distinction is important because the clinical course of EBV MCU is indolent in both immunosuppressed and nonimmunosuppressed patients.[48,51]

PLASMABLASTIC LYMPHOMA

OVERVIEW

Plasmablastic lymphoma (PBL) was first described in 1997 and is considered a subtype of DLBCL in the setting of immunosuppression.[2,52,53] PBL is commonly associated with HIV infection. It has also been observed in patients with other immunodeficiencies and rarely in immunocompetent individuals.[54] PBL is seen more often in male adults (median age, 50 years) but it can also rarely be seen in children.[2] Iatrogenic causes of immune suppression for autoimmune disease and treatment of post-transplant allograft rejection have also been implicated.[54] HIV-negative cases of PBL have a tendency to affect elderly individuals and arise as a result of transformation from previous lymphoproliferative disorders.[55,56]

CLINICAL FEATURES

PBL usually involves the oral cavity but it may occur in other extranodal locations, such as bone, gastrointestinal tract, nasal cavity, orbit, and soft tissues.[53] Lymph node involvement is uncommon in the setting of HIV.[53] Most patients have advanced disease and a high international prognostic index (IPI) score at presentation.

DIAGNOSIS

PBL can be a difficult diagnosis because of its rare incidence and overlapping morphologic and immunophenotypic features with other entities, especially plasma cell myeloma with plasmablastic morphology or lymphomas with plasmablastic differentiation (see Table 2).[2,53,55] The tumor cells are organized in a diffuse pattern, often with effacement of extranodal and nodal sites (Fig. 6). Tingible body macrophages may be scattered in the field of tumor cells and produce a starry sky appearance. The tumor cells resemble large immunoblasts and are composed of central round-to-oval nuclei with a prominent nucleolus and abundant cytoplasm. In the oral mucosa and nasal cavity, in the setting of underlying HIV infection, prominent immunoblasts are the norm. In cases of non-HIV PBL, however, the neoplastic cells may present with plasmacytic differentiation

(eccentric large nucleus, perinuclear hof, basophilic cytoplasm, and so forth) in other extranodal and nodal sites.[53]

Neoplastic cells have a phenotype similar to neoplastic plasma cells, and it can be a challenge to distinguish the 2 entities (see Fig. 6).[53,57] PBL cells express CD38, CD79a, CD138, IRF4/MUM1, and BLIMP1. Most cases have a high proliferative index seen with Ki67 (>90%). Only weak or negative CD45, CD20, and PAX5 expression is seen. CD56 is uncommon but it may be seen in cases with plasmacytic differentiation. Cytoplasmic immunoglobulins are expressed in up to 50% to 70% of cases. ISH for EBER can be detected in up to 70% of cases and is more often seen in HIV-associated cases; however, EBV LMP1 is usually negative but the latency type I pattern is most common.[53] The latency pattern type III can be seen in HIV and post-transplant patients with PBL. HHV8 is negative. The presence of CD56 and lack of EBER staining should raise concern for possible myeloma rather than PBL.

MYC expression is observed in up to 50% of cases and may be helpful in distinguishing PBL from plasmablastic myeloma (see Fig. 6).[53] In addition, two-thirds of PBL cases harbor MYC gene rearrangements whereas a minor subset have MYC amplification.[58,59] Additional comparative genomic hybridization studies have also demonstrated that PBL is more closely related to DLBCL compared with myeloma.[60]

PROGNOSIS

For the most part, PBL is associated with poor clinical outcomes and most patients die within the first year of diagnosis.[2] The most predictive factors associated with poor outcomes are high IPI scores and the presence of MYC gene rearrangement.[53,55]

PRIMARY EFFUSION LYMPHOMA

OVERVIEW

Primary effusion lymphoma (PEL) is a rare lymphoma that was recognized as a distinct clinical entity in the WHO in 2001.[2,61–64] It is always associated with HHV8 and coinfection with EBV is usually present.[65] In addition, PEL usually occurs in the setting of immunodeficiency. PEL usually occurs in young to middle-aged male adults with HIV infection or underlying non–HIV-associated severe immunodeficiency. PEL can occur in solid organ transplant patients as well as in elderly patients in the absence of immunodeficiency.[66] In

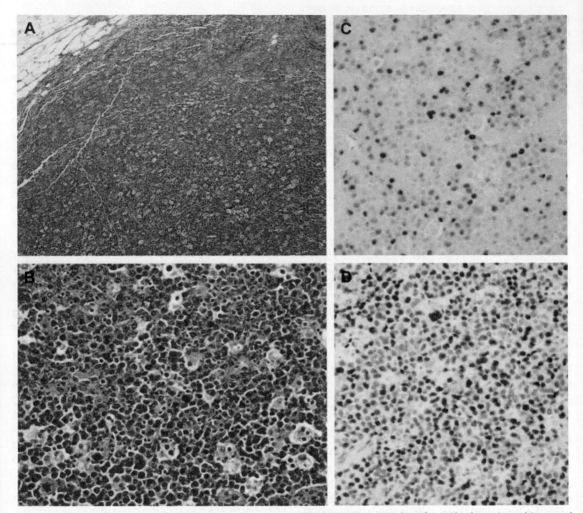

Fig. 6. Lymph node involved by PBL. (*A*) At low power (hematoxylin-eosin [H&E], ×50), there is architectural effacement by a diffuse lymphoid infiltrate with a starry sky pattern. (*B*) At higher power (H&E, ×200), many cells resemble large immunoblasts. The neoplastic cells express (*C*) EBER ISH (×200) and (*D*) MYC (×200).

elderly patients, there is no male or female predilection, and the prevalence of HHV8 infection is high.[66,67] Occasionally, HHV8-positive lymphomas with similar features to PEL may present as solid tumor masses and have been labeled as extracavitary PEL.[68]

ETIOLOGY

The neoplastic cells of PEL are positive for HHV8. HHV8 encodes several genes that are involved in regulating cell proliferation and apoptosis.[69,70] Loss of HHV8 in PEL neoplastic cells in cell culture studies results in apoptosis, implying the significance of HHV8 genes in promoting cell survival.[71] Some of the molecular pathways that may be disrupted due to interactions with HHV8 genes, including NF-κB, p53, retinoblastoma protein,

and transforming growth factor β pathway signaling.[72–75]

CLINICAL FEATURES

PELs originate in the pleura, pericardium, peritoneum, joint spaces, and, rarely, the meninges.[2,64,68] In most cases, affected patients present with serous effusion in the absence of a mass lesion. Serous effusion usually occurs in one location. Symptoms develop as a result of the mass effect imparted by accumulation of fluid. Extracavitary solid masses that are morphologically and phenotypically indistinguishable from PEL have been reported in the gastrointestinal tract (most common), skin, lung, lymph nodes, and CNS.[64] Comorbidities include Kaposi sarcoma in approximately half of patients with PEL. In addition, some cases have been associated with multicentric Castleman disease (MCD).[70]

DIAGNOSIS

The morphology of the neoplastic cells is variable, ranging from immunoblastic, to plasmablastic to anaplastic in appearance (Fig. 7; see Table 2).[2,62,76] Cytologic specimens typically reveal large cells with round to irregular nuclei and prominent nucleoli. The cytoplasm is often abundant and can be deeply basophilic with occasional vacuolization. Neoplastic cells may have plasmacytoid features or resemble RS cells. In histologic sections, the morphology is more uniform compared with cytologic preparations.

The neoplastic cells exhibit a null lymphocyte phenotype (see Fig. 7).[62,77] CD45 is positive but the pan B-cell markers (CD19, CD20, and CD79a) and T-cell markers (CD3, CD4, and CD8) are negative. Surface and cytoplasmic immunoglobulins are absent as well. Rather, lymphocyte activation, plasma cell–specific, and nonlineage-specific markers are often expressed

(ie, CD30, CD38, CD138, HLA-DR, and EMA). Cells are usually negative for BCL6. Definitive diagnosis rests on the ability to demonstrate the presence of HHV8 in the neoplastic cells. Evidence of HHV8 infection can be elicited via immunohistochemical staining for the presence of latency-associated nuclear antigen 1 (LANA-1), which is characterized by nuclear dotlike staining.[62] ISH for EBER can be used to detect EBV; however, EBV LMP1, and EBNA-2 are usually absent, consistent with a latency type I phenotype.[78] Neoplastic cells of the extracavitary variant of PEL may express B-cell associated antigens and immunoglobulins more often than the classic types of PEL.

Immunoglobulin gene rearrangements and somatic hypermutation are common and are supportive of a postgerminal center B-cell cell origin.[79,80] In rare cases, T-cell gene rearrangements have been observed.[80] Recurrent chromosomal abnormalities have not been identified. HHV8 viral genomes have been associated with all cases of reported PEL. The key viral gene products seem to be LANA, vCYC, and vFLIP, which

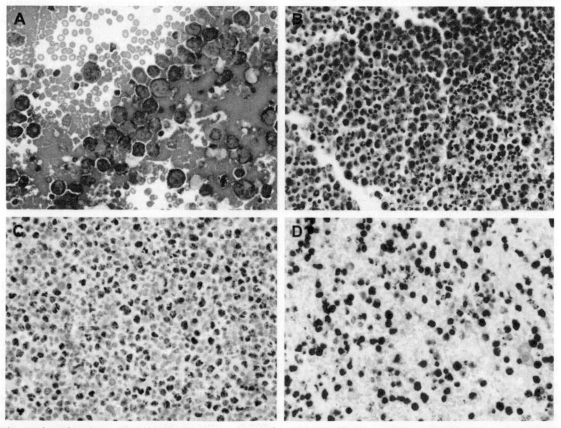

Fig. 7. Pleural cavity involved by PEL. Numerous large pleomorphic cells are observed in the (*A*) pleural fluid smear (Diff-Quik, ×400) and (*B*) clot section (hematoxylin-eosin, ×200). The tumor cells express (*C*) EBER ISH (×200) and (*D*) HHV8 (×200).

are important for regulating host cell survival and proliferation pathways. LANA can interact with Rb1, p53, and MYC proteins.[73,74,81] vCYC can bypass regulatory cell cycle checkpoints by interacting with CDK6 (leading to phosphorylation of RB1) to promote degradation of CDKN1B and prevent cell cycle arrest.[82,83] vFLIP can activate NF-κB through multiple pathways.[84,85]

PROGNOSIS

The prognosis is poor with unfavorable clinical outcomes. In most cases, overall survival is less than 6 months.[86,87]

*LARGE B-CELL LYMPHOMA ARISING IN HUMAN HERPES VIRUS 8–ASSOCIATED MULTICENTRIC CASTLEMAN DISEASE

OVERVIEW

Large B-cell lymphoma (LBL) arising in HHV8-associated MCD (HHV8 MCD) is a rare subtype of LBL. The clonal B cells are always associated with HHV8 and underlying HIV infection.[2,88,89] Interleukin (IL)-6 and IL-10 dysregulation seem to play an important role in development of HHV8 MCD and the associated LBL.[90] The lymphoma is characterized by sheets of plasmablastic cells that have features resembling plasma cells. The frequency of HHV8 infection correlates with increased numbers of MCD and LBLs.[91] Approximately 1% to 10% of infected persons occur in developed countries but the percentage increases to 75% in endemic areas in equatorial Africa.[92,93]

CLINICAL FEATURES

The presentation of MCD is variable but patients who develop HHV8-associated LBL (HHV8 LBL) usually have profound immunodeficiency.[2,94] Generalized lymphadenopathy and splenomegaly are observed as the lymph nodes and spleen are primary sites of involvement. In rare cases, the HHV8 neoplastic cells may manifest as leukemia. Kaposi sarcoma lesions may be seen concurrently.

DIAGNOSIS

The lymphoma arises in the background of MCD (see Table 2). In the spleen and lymph nodes, the features of MCD include follicles with varying degrees of involution and hyalinization of germinal centers. Prominent mantle zones with an onion skin appearance may be seen (Fig. 8).[88] Large scattered plasmablastic cells with eccentric nuclei, prominent nucleoli, and abundant amphophilic cytoplasm may be scattered in the mantle zones and interfollicular areas. In addition, the interfollicular areas contain sheets of plasma cells. As the disease progresses, aggregates of plasmablastic cells may form in the germinal center forming a so-called *microlymphoma.[88,95–97] Lymphoma that develops in the background of HHV8 MCD resembles PBL (Fig. 9) with nodal effacement. *Nomenclature for HHV8 MCD and microlymphoma may be updated in the next edition of the WHO classification of tumours of hematopoietic and lymphoid tissues.

The neoplastic plasmablasts are positive for LANA-1, viral IL-6, cytoplasmic IgM, and lambda light chain restriction. CD20 and CD38 may be positive in some cases. CD79a and CD138 are usually negative. The plasma cells within the interfollicular areas are polytypic for immunoglobulin light chains and are negative for HHV8.

There are some key distinctions between HHV8 LBL and PBL. Molecular studies have shown that the plasmablasts that arise from HHV8 PL are monoclonal for immunoglobulin gene rearrangements but the variable genes in the immunoglobulin genes are unmutated, which corresponds to a naïve IgM-producing plasma cell without immunoglobulin somatic hypermutation.[89,92] In addition, HHV8 PL is negative for EBER ISH and positive for HHV8 LANA-1.

PROGNOSIS

The prognosis of patients with HHV8 PL in the setting of MCD is poor and patient survival is usually less than a year.[92,98]

POST-TRANSPLANT LYMPHOPROLIFERATIVE DISORDER

OVERVIEW

PTLD is a heterogeneous clinicopathologic group and represents a spectrum of benign proliferations to malignant lymphomas that arise after solid organ transplantation (SOT) or HSCT. There are several risk factors for developing PTLD, including EBV infection, recipient age, transplanted organ type, type of immunosuppression, and underlying genetics.[99–101] Transplanting an organ from an EBV-seropositive donor to an EBV-seronegative recipient increases the incidence of PTLD 10-fold to 75-fold.[102] Children who are usually EBV seronegative tend to have a higher incidence of PTLD compared with adults. In EBV-positive PTLD, EBV-positive cells proliferate in the absence of immune surveillance whereas in EBV-negative PTLD, the pathogenesis may be

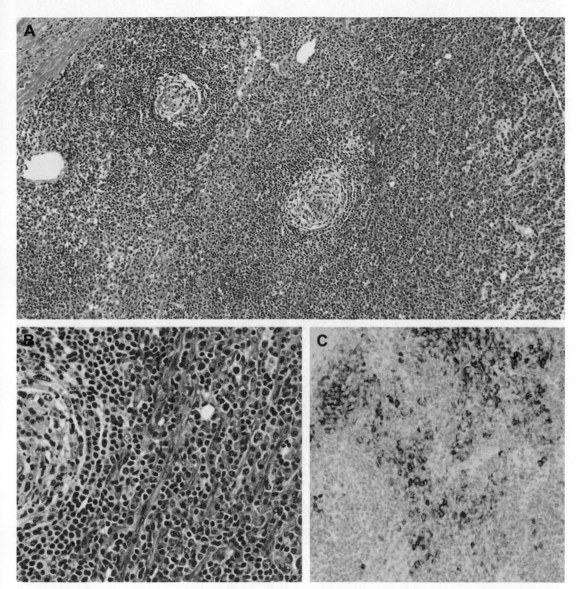

Fig. 8. MCD involving a lymph node. (*A*) Low-power (hematoxylin-eosin [H&E], ×100) and (*B*) high-power (H&E, ×400) views show (*C*) small, hyalinized follicles surrounded by sheets of plasma cells (CD138, ×200).

related to NHLs in the general population. Although it has been hypothesized that the EBV-negative PTLDs may have a nonviral etiology, recent gene expression profiling could not distinguish between EBV-positive and EBV-negative cases.[103] Four subclasses of PTLD have been described by the World Health Organization (WHO)[2]: early lesions, polymorphic PTLD, monomorphic PTLD, and classic HL.

CLINICAL FEATURES

Clinical presentation of PTLD depends on the organ system and degree of organ involvement.

PTLD may present at any time after transplantation. There is a short interval typically in young patients and in patients with bone marrow, lung, or heart transplant. Extranodal involvement is common. Symptoms are often related to dysfunction of the organ involved, but patients can also develop constitutional symptoms. Extranodal sites may include the gastrointestinal tract, lungs, kidneys, skin, CNS, and bone marrow.[104,105] In addition, there are many similarities and differences between the epidemiology of PTLD in SOT and allogenic-HSCT (listed). The most important risk factor for developing PTLD is EBV seronegativity at the time of transplantation.[106]

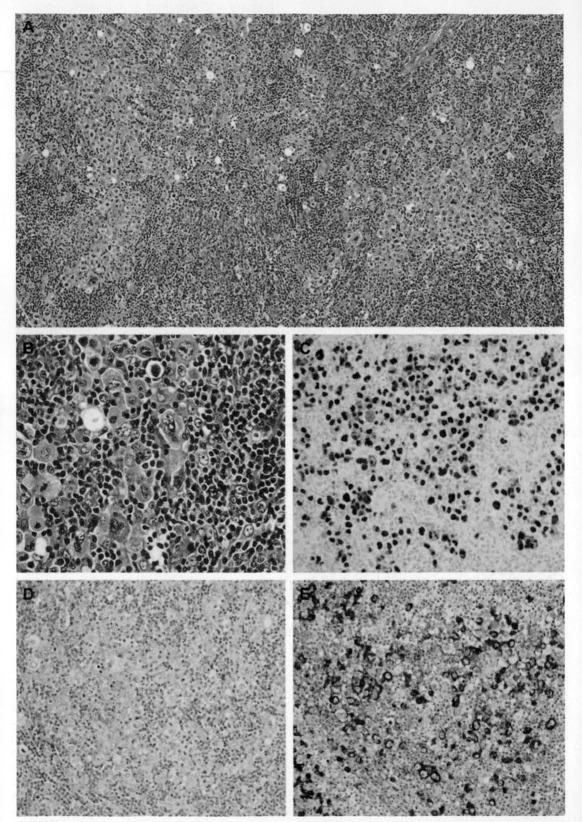

Fig. 9. LBL arising in a background of MCD (see Fig. 8). (*A*) Low-power (hematoxylin-eosin [H&E], ×100) and (*B*) high-power (H&E, ×100) images showing partial effacement of the lymph node by large aggregates of plasmablasts. The plasmablasts express (*C*) HHV8 (×200) and (*E*) lambda light chains (×200) but are negative for (*D*) kappa light chains (×200).

Solid Organ Transplantation

- PTLD affects 10% to 15% of adult SOT recipients (highest incidence after small bowel transplant followed by lung, heart, liver, and renal transplants).[105,107]
- Incidence of PTLD in children is higher than in adults.[108]
- Median time of onset of PTLD after SOT is 30 to 40 months.
- Risk of PTLD is highest in those who develop a primary EBV infection after transplantation.
- Cyclosporine, tacrolimus, antithymocyte globulin, and the T-cell depleting agent (OKT3) are associated with increased risk of PTLD,[109]
- Other risk factors include hepatitis C, cytomegalovirus, HHV8, and age younger than 10 or older than 60 years.[109–112]

Allogeneic Hematopoietic Cell Transplantation

- Incidence of PTLD after allogeneic HSCT is much lower (2.5%) compared with SOT.[106]
- Median time of onset of PTLD after allogeneic HCT is 2 to 6 months.[106]
- T-cell depletion of the donor marrow or peripheral blood stem cell product is the most important risk factor.[113]

- EBV infection, degree of HLA mismatch, and age above 50 at time of transplant are additional risk factors.[113]

DIAGNOSIS

Current diagnosis and classification of PTLD are based on the 2008 WHO classification.[2,114] Four histologic subtypes have been described and are summarized (Table 4).

EARLY LESIONS

Early lesions appear within the first year of transplantation. Lymphoid tissue architecture is preserved but 1 of 2 histologic patterns is present—plasmacytic hyperplasia or infectious mononucleosis-like lesion. Plasmacytic hyperplasia is characterized by sheets of polytypic and mature plasma cells with scattered EBV-positive immunoblasts. The infectious mononucleosis-like lesion is composed of an expanded paracortical region comprised of variable numbers of EBV-infected immunoblasts and small lymphocytes.

POLYMORPHIC POST-TRANSPLANT LYMPHOPROLIFERATIVE DISORDER

Polymorphic PTLD is characterized by effacement of the tissue architecture by lymphoid proliferation

---

Table 4
Pathologic spectrum of post-transplant lymphoproliferative disorders

Post-Transplant Lymphoproliferative Disorder Subtype	Effacement of Architecture	Histology	Phenotype	Genetics
Early lesions	No	Small lymphocytes, plasma cells, follicular hyperplasia (±), immunoblasts (±)	Polyclonal B-cells and T-cells, usually EBV+	Polyclonal, rare small monoclonal B-cells
Polymorphic PTLD	Yes	Polymorphous population of small-to-medium lymphocytes and plasma cells with occasional atypia	Polyclonal or monoclonal B-cells and T-cells, usually EBV+	Monoclonal B-cells; nonclonal T-cells; occasional BCL6 somatic hypermutations
Monomorphic PTLD	Yes	Fulfills WHO criteria for B-cell, T-cell NHL, or plasma cell neoplasm	Varies and depends on type of neoplasm, EBV+ is more variable	Clonal B-cells or T-cells; other genetic abnormalities usually present
HL-like PTLD	Yes	Fulfills WHO criteria for CHL	Similar to other CHL; EBV+	Unknown

Abbreviation: ±, may or may not be present; CHL, classic Hodgkin lymphoma.
Adapted from Swerdlow SH, Campo E, Harris NL, et al. WHO classification of tumours of haematopoietic and lymphoid tissues. 4th edition. Lyon (France): IARC Press; 2008:348; and Nalesnik MA. The diverse pathology of post-transplant lymphoproliferative disorders: the importance of a standardized approach. Transpl Infect Dis 2001;3:88–96.

or the presence of a destructive extranodal mass. The infiltrate is composed of a polymorphous population of cells, including small-to-medium lymphocytes with variable atypia, immunoblasts, and mature plasma cells. Monoclonal detection may or may not be present, which is dependent on the clonal burden. Many cells tend to be positive for EBV. Histologically, the features of polymorphic PTLD do not resemble any of the distinct lymphoproliferative disorders as defined by the WHO 2008 classification.

MONOMORPHIC POST-TRANSPLANT LYMPHOPROLIFERATIVE DISORDER

Monomorphic PTLD is the most common type of PTLD. This subclass represents B-cell and T-cell/NK-cell lymphomas that have also been described in the WHO 2008 classification in nontransplant settings. B-cell PTLDs are most common and include DLBCL (most common), BL, plasma cell myeloma, and plasmacytoma-like PTLD. Although the conventional morphology is seen, on occasion, pleomorphic RS-like cells may be seen in the neoplastic population.

CLASSIC HODGKIN LYMPHOMA

Classic HL is the rarest form of PTLD. It usually presents late after transplantation and is strongly associated with EBV infection. The histology is indistinguishable from the conventional subtypes of classic HL in immunocompetent settings. Like the other subtypes of PTLD can have Hodgkin-like cells, it is important to use ancillary studies to confirm the presence of RS cells, which are typically positive for PAX5 (weak), CD15, and CD30 but negative for CD20 and CD45.

PROGNOSIS

Due to the large variability of disorders encompassed in PTLD, no reliable prognostic scoring system exists.[115,116] Current treatment strategies focus to cure PTLD while maintaining transplanted organ function. Unfortunately, there are no established guidelines for the treatment of PTLD. The first line of treatment in most cases is reduction in immunosuppression, with more recent studies suggesting favorable outcomes with early administration of rituximab. For more aggressive cases of PTLD, addition of chemotherapy may be warranted.

SUMMARY

The 2008 WHO classification provided a much needed foundation for classifying lymphoproliferative disorders associated with immune suppression and recent research has elucidated this topic. A vast majority of the lymphoproliferative disorders are associated with viral infection, especially EBV and HHV8. The relationship between EBV and HHV8 infection and the predominance of disorders associated with B-cell lymphoproliferation is not surprising given that these viruses preferentially target B cells. Newer genomic approaches have provided information about cell survival and proliferation pathways that are regulated by EBV and HHV8 genes in B-cell lymphoma. Whether other viruses play an important role in the pathogenesis of lymphomas in immunodeficiency is unclear, but recent studies have suggested that the tumor-virus landscape is limited, especially in AIDS-related lymphomas, with EBV infection predominating.[117]

Understanding of lymphoproliferative disorders in immunodeficient settings has also shed light on a couple of lesser-known entities. EBV MCUs are now an important entity to recognize and distinguish from morphologically similar-appearing lymphomas because of their indolent behavior. The dysregulation of *MYC* gene expression is increasingly observed in PBLs, which can be used as a helpful diagnostic tool to PBLs from other lymphomas with plasmablastic differentiation.

It is likely that the incorporation of new genomic approaches will allow continued improvement in understanding and classification of immunodeficiency-associated lymphoproliferative disorders in the future. Better treatment outcomes in several HIV-associated lymphomas in the post-cART era are already observed. In the future, the genetic landscape of these entities will be better defined and there will likely be several opportunities to develop more directed therapeutics.

REFERENCES

1. Cesarman E. Gammaherpesviruses and lymphoproliferative disorders. Annu Rev Pathol 2014;9:349–72.
2. Swerdlow SH, Campo E, Harris NL, et al. WHO classification of tumours of haematopoietic and lymphoid tissues. 4th edition. Lyon (France): IARC Press; 2008.
3. Tran H, Nourse J, Hall S, et al. Immunodeficiency-associated lymphomas. Blood Rev 2008;22: 261–81.
4. Gloghini A, Dolcetti R, Carbone A. Lymphomas occurring specifically in HIV-infected patients: from pathogenesis to pathology. Semin Cancer Biol 2013;23:457–67.
5. Ok CY, Li L, Young KH. EBV-driven B-cell lymphoproliferative disorders: from biology, classification and differential diagnosis to clinical management. Exp Mol Med 2015;47:e132.

6. Camilleri-Broet S, Davi F, Feuillard J, et al. AIDS-related primary brain lymphomas: histopathologic and immunohistochemical study of 51 cases. The French Study Group for HIV-Associated Tumors. Hum Pathol 1997;28:367–74.

7. Kamel OW, van de Rijn M, Weiss LM, et al. Brief report: reversible lymphomas associated with Epstein-Barr virus occurring during methotrexate therapy for rheumatoid arthritis and dermatomyositis. N Engl J Med 1993;328:1317–21.

8. Salloum E, Cooper DL, Howe G, et al. Spontaneous regression of lymphoproliferative disorders in patients treated with methotrexate for rheumatoid arthritis and other rheumatic diseases. J Clin Oncol 1996;14:1943–9.

9. Wolfe F, Michaud K. Lymphoma in rheumatoid arthritis: the effect of methotrexate and anti-tumor necrosis factor therapy in 18,572 patients. Arthritis Rheum 2004;50:1740–51.

10. Wolfe F, Michaud K. The effect of methotrexate and anti-tumor necrosis factor therapy on the risk of lymphoma in rheumatoid arthritis in 19,562 patients during 89,710 person-years of observation. Arthritis Rheum 2007;56:1433–9.

11. Scott DW, Wright GW, Williams PM, et al. Determining cell-of-origin subtypes of diffuse large B-cell lymphoma using gene expression in formalin-fixed paraffin-embedded tissue. Blood 2014;123:1214–7.

12. Hans CP, Weisenburger DD, Greiner TC, et al. Confirmation of the molecular classification of diffuse large B-cell lymphoma by immunohistochemistry using a tissue microarray. Blood 2004; 103:275–82.

13. Alizadeh AA, Eisen MB, Davis RE, et al. Distinct types of diffuse large B-cell lymphoma identified by gene expression profiling. Nature 2000;403: 503–11.

14. Montes-Moreno S, Gonzalez-Medina AR, Rodriguez-Pinilla SM, et al. Aggressive large B-cell lymphoma with plasma cell differentiation: immunohistochemical characterization of plasmablastic lymphoma and diffuse large B-cell lymphoma with partial plasmablastic phenotype. Haematologica 2010;95:1342–9.

15. Klein U, Gloghini A, Gaidano G, et al. Gene expression profile analysis of AIDS-related primary effusion lymphoma (PEL) suggests a plasmablastic derivation and identifies PEL-specific transcripts. Blood 2003;101:4115–21.

16. Tarte K, Zhan F, De Vos J, et al. Gene expression profiling of plasma cells and plasmablasts: toward a better understanding of the late stages of B-cell differentiation. Blood 2003;102:592–600.

17. Giulino L, Mathew S, Ballon G, et al. A20 (TNFAIP3) genetic alterations in EBV-associated AIDS-related lymphoma. Blood 2011;117:4852–4.

18. Chadburn A, Abdul-Nabi AM, Teruya BS, et al. Lymphoid proliferations associated with human immunodeficiency virus infection. Arch Pathol Lab Med 2013;137:360–70.

19. Johnson DH, Reske T, Ruiz M. Case report and review of immunodeficiency-associated Burkitt lymphoma. Clin Lymphoma Myeloma Leuk 2015;15: e121–5.

20. Lim ST, Karim R, Tulpule A, et al. Prognostic factors in HIV-related diffuse large-cell lymphoma: before versus after highly active antiretroviral therapy. J Clin Oncol 2005;23:8477–82.

21. Wolf T, Brodt HR, Fichtlscherer S, et al. Changing incidence and prognostic factors of survival in AIDS-related non-Hodgkin's lymphoma in the era of highly active antiretroviral therapy (HAART). Leuk Lymphoma 2005;46:207–15.

22. Ferry JA. Burkitt's lymphoma: clinicopathologic features and differential diagnosis. Oncologist 2006; 11:375–83.

23. Carbone A, Gloghini A, Dotti G. EBV-associated lymphoproliferative disorders: classification and treatment. Oncologist 2008;13:577–85.

24. Davi F, Delecluse HJ, Guiet P, et al. Burkitt-like lymphomas in AIDS patients: characterization within a series of 103 human immunodeficiency virus-associated non-Hodgkin's lymphomas. Burkitt's Lymphoma Study Group. J Clin Oncol 1998;16: 3788–95.

25. Leucci E, Cocco M, Onnis A, et al. MYC translocation-negative classical Burkitt lymphoma cases: an alternative pathogenetic mechanism involving miRNA deregulation. J Pathol 2008;216: 440–50.

26. Schmitz R, Young RM, Ceribelli M, et al. Burkitt lymphoma pathogenesis and therapeutic targets from structural and functional genomics. Nature 2012; 490:116–20.

27. Schommers P, Hentrich M, Hoffmann C, et al. Survival of AIDS-related diffuse large B-cell lymphoma, Burkitt lymphoma, and plasmablastic lymphoma in the German HIV Lymphoma Cohort. Br J Haematol 2015;168:806–10.

28. Rodrigo JA, Hicks LK, Cheung MC, et al. HIV-associated burkitt lymphoma: good efficacy and tolerance of intensive chemotherapy including CODOX-M/IVAC with or without RItuximab in the HAART Era. Adv Hematol 2012;2012:735392.

29. Petrich AM, Sparano JA, Parekh S. Paradigms and controversies in the treatment of HIV-related burkitt lymphoma. Adv Hematol 2012;2012:403648.

30. Blinder VS, Chadburn A, Furman RR, et al. Improving outcomes for patients with Burkitt lymphoma and HIV. AIDS Patient Care STDS 2008; 22:175–87.

31. Shiels MS, Koritzinsky EH, Clarke CA, et al. Prevalence of HIV Infection among U.S. Hodgkin

lymphoma cases. Cancer Epidemiol Biomarkers Prev 2014;23:274–81.

32. Gibson TM, Morton LM, Shiels MS, et al. Risk of non-Hodgkin lymphoma subtypes in HIV-infected people during the HAART era: a population-based study. AIDS 2014;28:2313–8.

33. Gotti D, Danesi M, Calabresi A, et al. Clinical characteristics, incidence, and risk factors of HIV-related Hodgkin lymphoma in the era of combination antiretroviral therapy. AIDS Patient Care STDS 2013; 27:259–65.

34. Vaccher E, Spina M, Tirelli U. Clinical aspects and management of Hodgkin's disease and other tumours in HIV-infected individuals. Eur J Cancer 2001;37:1306–15.

35. Tirelli U, Errante D, Dolcetti R, et al. Hodgkin's disease and human immunodeficiency virus infection: clinicopathologic and virologic features of 114 patients from the Italian Cooperative Group on AIDS and Tumors. J Clin Oncol 1995;13:1758–67.

36. Spina M, Berretta M, Tirelli U. Hodgkin's disease in HIV. Hematol Oncol Clin North Am 2003;17:843–58.

37. Said JW. Immunodeficiency-related Hodgkin lymphoma and its mimics. Adv Anat Pathol 2007; 14:189–94.

38. Carbone A, Gloghini A, Larocca LM, et al. Human immunodeficiency virus-associated Hodgkin's disease derives from post-germinal center B cells. Blood 1999;93:2319–26.

39. Aries J, Montoto S. Managing HIV and Hodgkin lymphoma in the twenty-first century. Curr Hematol Malig Rep 2014;9:227–32.

40. Jacobson CA, Abramson JS. HIV-associated hodgkin's lymphoma: prognosis and therapy in the era of cART. Adv Hematol 2012;2012:507257.

41. Liebow AA, Carrington CR, Friedman PJ. Lymphomatoid granulomatosis. Hum Pathol 1972;3: 457–558.

42. Song JY, Pittaluga S, Dunleavy K, et al. Lymphomatoid granulomatosis–a single institute experience: pathologic findings and clinical correlations. Am J Surg Pathol 2015;39:141–56.

43. Katzenstein AL, Carrington CB, Liebow AA. Lymphomatoid granulomatosis: a clinicopathologic study of 152 cases. Cancer 1979;43:360–73.

44. Guinee D Jr, Jaffe E, Kingma D, et al. Pulmonary lymphomatoid granulomatosis. Evidence for a proliferation of Epstein-Barr virus infected B-lymphocytes with a prominent T-cell component and vasculitis. Am J Surg Pathol 1994;18:753–64.

45. Wilson WH, Kingma DW, Raffeld M, et al. Association of lymphomatoid granulomatosis with Epstein-Barr viral infection of B lymphocytes and response to interferon-alpha 2b. Blood 1996;87:4531–7.

46. Koss MN, Hochholzer L, Langloss JM, et al. Lymphomatoid granulomatosis: a clinicopathologic study of 42 patients. Pathology 1986;18:283–8.

47. Dunleavy K, Little RF, Pittaluga S, et al. The role of tumor histogenesis, FDG-PET, and short-course EPOCH with dose-dense rituximab (SC-EPOCH-RR) in HIV-associated diffuse large B-cell lymphoma. Blood 2010;115:3017–24.

48. Dojcinov SD, Venkataraman G, Raffeld M, et al. EBV positive mucocutaneous ulcer–a study of 26 cases associated with various sources of immunosuppression. Am J Surg Pathol 2010;34:405–17.

49. Hart M, Thakral B, Yohe S, et al. EBV-positive mucocutaneous ulcer in organ transplant recipients: a localized indolent posttransplant lymphoproliferative disorder. Am J Surg Pathol 2014;38: 1522–9.

50. Di Napoli A, Giubettini M, Duranti E, et al. Iatrogenic EBV-positive lymphoproliferative disorder with features of EBV+ mucocutaneous ulcer: evidence for concomitant TCRgamma/IGH rearrangements in the Hodgkin-like neoplastic cells. Virchows Arch 2011;458:631–6.

51. Cohen JI, Kimura H, Nakamura S, et al. Epstein-Barr virus-associated lymphoproliferative disease in non-immunocompromised hosts: a status report and summary of an international meeting, 8-9 September 2008. Ann Oncol 2009;20:1472–82.

52. Delecluse HJ, Anagnostopoulos I, Dallenbach F, et al. Plasmablastic lymphomas of the oral cavity: a new entity associated with the human immunodeficiency virus infection. Blood 1997;89:1413–20.

53. Castillo JJ, Bibas M, Miranda RN. The biology and treatment of plasmablastic lymphoma. Blood 2015; 125:2323–30.

54. Colomo L, Loong F, Rives S, et al. Diffuse large B-cell lymphomas with plasmablastic differentiation represent a heterogeneous group of disease entities. Am J Surg Pathol 2004;28:736–47.

55. Morscio J, Dierickx D, Nijs J, et al. Clinicopathologic comparison of plasmablastic lymphoma in HIV-positive, immunocompetent, and posttransplant patients: single-center series of 25 cases and meta-analysis of 277 reported cases. Am J Surg Pathol 2014;38:875–86.

56. Teruya-Feldstein J, Chiao E, Filippa DA, et al. CD20-negative large-cell lymphoma with plasmablastic features: a clinically heterogenous spectrum in both HIV-positive and -negative patients. Ann Oncol 2004;15:1673–9.

57. Vega F, Chang CC, Medeiros LJ, et al. Plasmablastic lymphomas and plasmablastic plasma cell myelomas have nearly identical immunophenotypic profiles. Mod Pathol 2005;18:806–15.

58. Bogusz AM, Seegmiller AC, Garcia R, et al. Plasmablastic lymphomas with MYC/IgH rearrangement: report of three cases and review of the literature. Am J Clin Pathol 2009;132:597–605.

59. Valera A, Balague O, Colomo L, et al. IG/MYC rearrangements are the main cytogenetic alteration in

plasmablastic lymphomas. Am J Surg Pathol 2010; 34:1686–94.

60. Chang CC, Zhou X, Taylor JJ, et al. Genomic profiling of plasmablastic lymphoma using array comparative genomic hybridization (aCGH): revealing significant overlapping genomic lesions with diffuse large B-cell lymphoma. J Hematol Oncol 2009;2:47.

61. Jaffe ES, Harris NL, Stein H, et al. Pathology and genetics: tumours of haematopoietic and lymphoid tissues. Lyon (France): IARC Press; 2001.

62. Nador RG, Cesarman E, Chadburn A, et al. Primary effusion lymphoma: a distinct clinicopathologic entity associated with the Kaposi's sarcoma-associated herpes virus. Blood 1996; 88:645–56.

63. Said JW, Tasaka T, Takeuchi S, et al. Primary effusion lymphoma in women: report of two cases of Kaposi's sarcoma herpes virus-associated effusion-based lymphoma in human immunodeficiency virus-negative women. Blood 1996;88: 3124–8.

64. Carbone A, Gloghini A. PEL and HHV8-unrelated effusion lymphomas: classification and diagnosis. Cancer 2008;114:225–7.

65. Patel S, Xiao P. Primary effusion lymphoma. Arch Pathol Lab Med 2013;137:1152–4.

66. Luppi M, Barozzi P, Santagostino G, et al. Molecular evidence of organ-related transmission of Kaposi sarcoma-associated herpesvirus or human herpesvirus-8 in transplant patients. Blood 2000; 96:3279–81.

67. Teruya-Feldstein J, Zauber P, Setsuda JE, et al. Expression of human herpesvirus-8 oncogene and cytokine homologues in an HIV-seronegative patient with multicentric Castleman's disease and primary effusion lymphoma. Lab Invest 1998;78: 1637–42.

68. Chadburn A, Hyjek E, Mathew S, et al. KSHV-positive solid lymphomas represent an extra-cavitary variant of primary effusion lymphoma. Am J Surg Pathol 2004;28:1401–16.

69. Jarviluoma A, Koopal S, Rasanen S, et al. KSHV viral cyclin binds to p27KIP1 in primary effusion lymphomas. Blood 2004;104:3349–54.

70. Carbone A, Gloghini A, Vaccher E, et al. Kaposi's sarcoma-associated herpesvirus/human herpesvirus type 8-positive solid lymphomas: a tissue-based variant of primary effusion lymphoma. J Mol Diagn 2005;7:17–27.

71. Wies E, Mori Y, Hahn A, et al. The viral interferon-regulatory factor-3 is required for the survival of KSHV-infected primary effusion lymphoma cells. Blood 2008;111:320–7.

72. Guasparri I, Keller SA, Cesarman E. KSHV vFLIP is essential for the survival of infected lymphoma cells. J Exp Med 2004;199:993–1003.

73. Friborg J Jr, Kong W, Hottiger MO, et al. p53 inhibition by the LANA protein of KSHV protects against cell death. Nature 1999;402:889–94.

74. Radkov SA, Kellam P, Boshoff C. The latent nuclear antigen of Kaposi sarcoma-associated herpesvirus targets the retinoblastoma-E2F pathway and with the oncogene Hras transforms primary rat cells. Nat Med 2000;6:1121–7.

75. Lei X, Zhu Y, Jones T, et al. A Kaposi's sarcoma-associated herpesvirus microRNA and its variants target the transforming growth factor beta pathway to promote cell survival. J Virol 2012;86:11698–711.

76. Brimo F, Michel RP, Khetani K, et al. Primary effusion lymphoma: a series of 4 cases and review of the literature with emphasis on cytomorphologic and immunocytochemical differential diagnosis. Cancer 2007;111:224–33.

77. Knowles DM, Inghirami G, Ubriaco A, et al. Molecular genetic analysis of three AIDS-associated neoplasms of uncertain lineage demonstrates their B-cell derivation and the possible pathogenetic role of the Epstein-Barr virus. Blood 1989;73:792–9.

78. Fassone L, Bhatia K, Gutierrez M, et al. Molecular profile of Epstein-Barr virus infection in HHV-8-positive primary effusion lymphoma. Leukemia 2000;14:271–7.

79. Matolcsy A, Nador RG, Cesarman E, et al. Immunoglobulin VH gene mutational analysis suggests that primary effusion lymphomas derive from different stages of B cell maturation. Am J Pathol 1998; 153:1609–14.

80. Said JW, Shintaku IP, Asou H, et al. Herpesvirus 8 inclusions in primary effusion lymphoma: report of a unique case with T-cell phenotype. Arch Pathol Lab Med 1999;123:257–60.

81. Fujimuro M, Hayward SD. Manipulation of glycogen-synthase kinase-3 activity in KSHV-associated cancers. J Mol Med (Berl) 2004;82: 223–31.

82. Godden-Kent D, Talbot SJ, Boshoff C, et al. The cyclin encoded by Kaposi's sarcoma-associated herpesvirus stimulates cdk6 to phosphorylate the retinoblastoma protein and histone H1. J Virol 1997;71:4193–8.

83. Ellis M, Chew YP, Fallis L, et al. Degradation of p27(Kip) cdk inhibitor triggered by Kaposi's sarcoma virus cyclin-cdk6 complex. EMBO J 1999; 18:644–53.

84. Chaudhary PM, Jasmin A, Eby MT, et al. Modulation of the NF-kappa B pathway by virally encoded death effector domains-containing proteins. Oncogene 1999;18:5738–46.

85. Matta H, Chaudhary PM. Activation of alternative NF-kappa B pathway by human herpes virus 8-encoded Fas-associated death domain-like IL-1 beta-converting enzyme inhibitory protein (vFLIP). Proc Natl Acad Sci U S A 2004;101:9399–404.

86. Waddington TW, Aboulafia DM. Failure to eradicate AIDS-associated primary effusion lymphoma with high-dose chemotherapy and autologous stem cell reinfusion: case report and literature review. AIDS Patient Care STDS 2004;18:67–73.

87. Ripamonti D, Marini B, Rambaldi A, et al. Treatment of primary effusion lymphoma with highly active antiviral therapy in the setting of HIV infection. AIDS 2008;22:1236–7.

88. Dupin N, Diss TL, Kellam P, et al. HHV-8 is associated with a plasmablastic variant of Castleman disease that is linked to HHV-8-positive plasmablastic lymphoma. Blood 2000;95:1406–12.

89. Miranda RN, Khoury JD, Medeiros LJ. Atlas of lymph node pathology. New York: Springer; 2013.

90. Uldrick TS, Polizzotto MN, Yarchoan R. Recent advances in Kaposi sarcoma herpesvirus-associated multicentric Castleman disease. Curr Opin Oncol 2012;24:495–505.

91. Oksenhendler E, Boulanger E, Galicier L, et al. High incidence of Kaposi sarcoma-associated herpesvirus-related non-Hodgkin lymphoma in patients with HIV infection and multicentric Castleman disease. Blood 2002;99:2331–6.

92. Bhutani M, Polizzotto MN, Uldrick TS, et al. Kaposi sarcoma-associated herpesvirus-associated malignancies: epidemiology, pathogenesis, and advances in treatment. Semin Oncol 2015;42:223–46.

93. Boshoff C, Weiss RA. Epidemiology and pathogenesis of Kaposi's sarcoma-associated herpesvirus. Philos Trans R Soc Lond B Biol Sci 2001;356: 517–34.

94. Goedhals J, Beukes CA, Hardie D. HHV8 in plasmablastic lymphoma. Am J Surg Pathol 2008;32: 172 [author reply: 72–4].

95. Seliem RM, Griffith RC, Harris NL, et al. HHV-8+, EBV+ multicentric plasmablastic microlymphoma in an HIV+ Man: the spectrum of HHV-8+ lymphoproliferative disorders expands. Am J Surg Pathol 2007;31:1439–45.

96. Dargent JL, Lespagnard L, Sirtaine N, et al. Plasmablastic microlymphoma occurring in human herpesvirus 8 (HHV-8)-positive multicentric Castleman's disease and featuring a follicular growth pattern. APMIS 2007;115:869–74.

97. Courville EL, Sohani AR, Hasserjian RP, et al. Diverse clinicopathologic features in human herpesvirus 8-associated lymphomas lead to diagnostic problems. Am J Clin Pathol 2014;142: 816–29.

98. Bower M, Dalla Pria A. What Is the best treatment for HIV-associated multicentric Castleman disease? Clin Adv Hematol Oncol 2012;10:207–9.

99. Al-Mansour Z, Nelson BP, Evens AM. Post-transplant lymphoproliferative disease (PTLD): risk factors, diagnosis, and current treatment strategies. Curr Hematol Malig Rep 2013;8:173–83.

100. Doak PB, Montgomerie JZ, North JD, et al. Reticulum cell sarcoma after renal homotransplantation and azathioprine and prednisone therapy. Br Med J 1968;4:746–8.

101. Penn I, Hammond W, Brettschneider L, et al. Malignant lymphomas in transplantation patients. Transplant Proc 1969;1:106–12.

102. Cockfield S. Identifying the patient at risk for post-transplant lymphoproliferative disorder. Transpl Infect Dis 2001;3:70–8.

103. Vakiani E, Basso K, Klein U, et al. Genetic and phenotypic analysis of B-cell post-transplant lymphoproliferative disorders provides insights into disease biology. Hematol Oncol 2008;26:199–211.

104. Taylor AL, Marcus R, Bradley JA. Post-transplant lymphoproliferative disorders (PTLD) after solid organ transplantation. Crit Rev Oncol Hematol 2005; 56:155–67.

105. Parker A, Bowles K, Bradley JA, et al. Diagnosis of post-transplant lymphoproliferative disorder in solid organ transplant recipients - BCSH and BTS Guidelines. Br J Haematol 2010;149:675–92.

106. Sundin M, Le Blanc K, Ringden O, et al. The role of HLA mismatch, splenectomy and recipient Epstein-Barr virus seronegativity as risk factors in post-transplant lymphoproliferative disorder following allogeneic hematopoietic stem cell transplantation. Haematologica 2006;91:1059–67.

107. Kinch A, Baecklund E, Backlin C, et al. A population-based study of 135 lymphomas after solid organ transplantation: the role of Epstein-Barr virus, hepatitis C and diffuse large B-cell lymphoma subtype in clinical presentation and survival. Acta Oncol 2014;53:669–79.

108. Colita A, Moise L, Arion C, et al. Post-transplant lymphoproliferative disorders after solid organ transplantation in children. Chirurgia (Bucur) 2012;107:431–7.

109. Opelz G, Dohler B. Lymphomas after solid organ transplantation: a collaborative transplant study report. Am J Transplant 2004;4:222–30.

110. Buda A, Caforio A, Calabrese F, et al. Lymphoproliferative disorders in heart transplant recipients: role of hepatitis C virus (HCV) and Epstein-Barr virus (EBV) infection. Transpl Int 2000;13(Suppl 1): S402–5.

111. Manez R, Breinig MC, Linden P, et al. Posttransplant lymphoproliferative disease in primary Epstein-Barr virus infection after liver transplantation: the role of cytomegalovirus disease. J Infect Dis 1997;176:1462–7.

112. Ahmadpoor P, Ilkhanizadeh B, Sharifzadeh P, et al. Seroprevalence of human herpes virus-8 in renal transplant recipients: a single center study from Iran. Transplant Proc 2007;39:1000–2.

113. Landgren O, Gilbert ES, Rizzo JD, et al. Risk factors for lymphoproliferative disorders after allogeneic

hematopoietic cell transplantation. Blood 2009;113: 4992–5001.

114. Nalesnik MA. The diverse pathology of post-transplant lymphoproliferative disorders: the importance of a standardized approach. Transpl Infect Dis 2001;3:88–96.

115. Caillard S, Porcher R, Provot F, et al. Post-transplantation lymphoproliferative disorder after kidney transplantation: report of a nationwide French registry and the development of a new prognostic score. J Clin Oncol 2013;31:1302–9.

116. Evens AM, David KA, Helenowski I, et al. Multicenter analysis of 80 solid organ transplantation recipients with post-transplantation lymphoproliferative disease: outcomes and prognostic factors in the modern era. J Clin Oncol 2010;28:1038–46.

117. Arvey A, Ojesina AI, Pedamallu CS, et al. The tumor virus landscape of AIDS-related lymphomas. Blood 2015;125:e14–22.

118. Shapiro RS. Malignancies in the setting of primary immunodeficiency: implications for hematologists/oncologists. Am J Hematol 2011;86:48–55.

119. Al-Herz W, Bousfiha A, Casanova JL, et al. Primary immunodeficiency diseases: an update on the classification from the international union of immunological societies expert committee for primary immunodeficiency. Front Immunol 2014;5:162.

120. Al-Saud BK, Al-Sum Z, Alassiri H, et al. Clinical, immunological, and molecular characterization of hyper-IgM syndrome due to CD40 deficiency in eleven patients. J Clin Immunol 2013;33:1325–35.

121. Bosticardo M, Marangoni F, Aiuti A, et al. Recent advances in understanding the pathophysiology of Wiskott-Aldrich syndrome. Blood 2009;113: 6288–95.

122. Resnick ES, Moshier EL, Godbold JH, et al. Morbidity and mortality in common variable immune deficiency over 4 decades. Blood 2012; 119:1650–7.

123. Micol R, Ben Slama L, Suarez F, et al. Morbidity and mortality from ataxia-telangiectasia are associated with ATM genotype. J Allergy Clin Immunol 2011; 128:382–9.e1.

124. Gladkowska-Dura M, Dzierzanowska-Fangrat K, Dura WT, et al. Unique morphological spectrum of lymphomas in Nijmegen breakage syndrome (NBS) patients with high frequency of consecutive lymphoma formation. J Pathol 2008;216:337–44.

125. Booth C, Gilmour KC, Veys P, et al. X-linked lymphoproliferative disease due to SAP/SH2D1A deficiency: a multicenter study on the manifestations, management and outcome of the disease. Blood 2011;117:53–62.

126. Neven B, Magerus-Chatinet A, Florkin B, et al. A survey of 90 patients with autoimmune lymphoproliferative syndrome related to TNFRSF6 mutation. Blood 2011;118:4798–807.

127. Merino F, Henle W, Ramirez-Duque P. Chronic active Epstein-Barr virus infection in patients with Chediak-Higashi syndrome. J Clin Immunol 1986; 6:299–305.

128. Heslop HE, Hoffbrand AV, Brenner MK. TNF and chronic B lymphoproliferative disorders. Leukemia 1993;7:1476.

129. Parakkal D, Sifuentes H, Semer R, et al. Hepatosplenic T-cell lymphoma in patients receiving TNF-alpha inhibitor therapy: expanding the groups at risk. Eur J Gastroenterol Hepatol 2011;23: 1150–6.

130. Herrinton LJ, Liu L, Weng X, et al. Role of thiopurine and anti-TNF therapy in lymphoma in inflammatory bowel disease. Am J Gastroenterol 2011;106: 2146–53.

131. Mariette X, Tubach F, Bagheri H, et al. Lymphoma in patients treated with anti-TNF: results of the 3-year prospective French RATIO registry. Ann Rheum Dis 2010;69:400–8.

132. Khan N, Abbas AM, Lichtenstein GR, et al. Risk of lymphoma in patients with ulcerative colitis treated with thiopurines: a nationwide retrospective cohort study. Gastroenterology 2013;145:1007–15.e3.

133. Beaugerie L, Brousse N, Bouvier AM, et al. Lymphoproliferative disorders in patients receiving thiopurines for inflammatory bowel disease: a prospective observational cohort study. Lancet 2009;374:1617–25.

Transformation in Low-grade B-cell Neoplasms

Nathan D. Montgomery, MD, PhD, Stephanie P. Mathews, MD*

KEYWORDS

- Transformation • Low-grade lymphoma • CLL/SLL • Follicular lymphoma • Clonality
- Richter syndrome

ABSTRACT

Low-grade B-cell leukemias/lymphomas are a diverse group of indolent lymphoproliferative disorders that are typically characterized by good patient outcomes and long life expectancies. A subset of cases, however, undergo histologic transformation to a higher-grade neoplasm, a transition associated with a more aggressive clinical course and poor survival. Transformation of follicular lymphoma to diffuse large B-cell lymphoma and Richter transformation of chronic lymphocytic leukemia/small lymphocytic lymphoma are best characterized in the literature. This article reviews clinical and pathologic characteristics of these most common forms of transformation, with an emphasis on salient histologic, immunophenotypic, and genetic features.

Key Features

- Transformation of low grade B-cell neoplasms to higher grade malignancies is a clinically important event that portends a worse prognosis, and pathologic recognition is vital.
- The evolutionary pattern of transformation may be "branched", "linear", or in some cases, show no clonal relationship to the low grade lymphoma.
- Transformation to DLBCL is the most common, but more rare transformations to BCL-U, BLL, and Hodgkin lymphoma may occur.
- In many cases, subtle immunophenotypic, cytogenetic, and molecular differences exist between transformed and de novo lymphomas.
- Mimics of transformation, including the diffuse variant of low grade follicular lymphoma and prolymphocytic progression of CLL/SLL, exist and have a significantly better prognosis than transformed lymphomas.

OVERVIEW

Low-grade B-cell lymphomas are a clinically and biologically heterogeneous group of disorders typically characterized by small cell size, bland cytologic features, and an indolent clinical course. Although most cases do not require chemotherapeutic intervention, histologic transformation (HT) to a high-grade malignancy may occur and is associated with more aggressive clinical behavior and poor outcome.[1-3] The transformation of low-grade follicular lymphoma (FL) and Richter transformation of chronic lymphocytic leukemia (CLL)/small lymphocytic lymphoma (SLL) to diffuse large B-cell lymphoma (DLBCL) are most commonly described. Transformation of FL to other histologic types, however, including B-lymphoblastic leukemia/lymphoma (BLL) and B-cell lymphoma, unclassifiable, with features intermediate between DLBCL and Burkitt lymphoma (BCLU) as well as transformation of CLL to Hodgkin lymphoma (HL) are also reported.[1-9] More rare transformations of FL, CLL, and other low-grade B cell lymphomas, including marginal zone and lymphoplasmacytic lymphomas, have been described but are beyond the scope of this review.[10-12] Due to the prognostic and therapeutic implications of transformation, clinical and pathologic recognition is vital.

Disclosure Statement: The authors have no competing financial conflicts of interest to disclose.
Division of Hematopathology, Department of Pathology and Laboratory Medicine, University of North Carolina School of Medicine, CB #7525, Chapel Hill, NC 27599-7525, USA
* Corresponding author.
E-mail address: Stephanie.Mathews@unchealth.unc.edu

surgpath.theclinics.com

BIOLOGICAL CATEGORIES OF CLINICAL TRANSFORMATION

Although biological concepts of transformation imply clonal evolution of a low-grade lesion by progressive accumulation of secondary mutations, current clinical definitions do not always require a genetic relationship between low-grade and transformed lymphoma. Instead, in some settings, clinical transformation is defined by rapid development of any aggressive lymphoid malignancy in a patient with a pre-existing low-grade lymphoma, clonally related or otherwise.[1,2,5,6] As such, clinical transformation encompasses at least 3 distinct biological relationships between low-grade lesions and their transformed counterparts.

Cases of linear evolution fit within classic biological concepts of transformation, in which the higher-grade lesion evolves from an aggressive subclone of the original low-grade lymphoma by stepwise accumulation of new mutations (**Fig. 1A**).[5] Here, the higher-grade lesion is expected to retain those mutations found in the original lymphoma while gaining additional mutations that drive more aggressive behavior. This pattern predominates in Richter transformation of CLL to DLBCL but is less common in other forms of transformation.[13]

In other cases, low-grade and transformed lymphomas are genetically related but via a less direct relationship, reflecting a pattern of branched evolution (see **Fig. 1B**).[2,14] In this scenario, the original low-grade lymphoma is a temporal but not a direct biological precursor of the subsequent high-grade lymphoma. Here, the 2 lesions share a common progenitor cell, which follows multiple independent evolutionary paths, first leading to development of low-grade disease and later following a parallel path to a more aggressive lesion. Although some early mutations are shared, the initial and subsequent neoplasms should show evidence of their independent evolutionary histories, with mutations present in each that are absent in the other. Emerging data suggest that transformation of FL to DLBCL typically proceeds by such a mechanism, in which low-grade and high-grade components arise separately from a progenitor cell harboring the canonical t(14;18) rearrangement.[2,14]

Finally, in some cases, there is no clonal relationship between the low-grade lymphoma and its more aggressive counterpart (see **Fig. 1C**). This pattern is seen in a minority of Richter transformations of CLL to DLBCL and may reflect underlying immunodeficiency inherent to the leukemic state.[5,6]

CLINICAL FEATURES OF TRANSFORMATION

Because it may be associated with a grave prognosis, transformation should be considered at the time of disease progression and with all relapses. It is often accompanied by a sudden or excessive

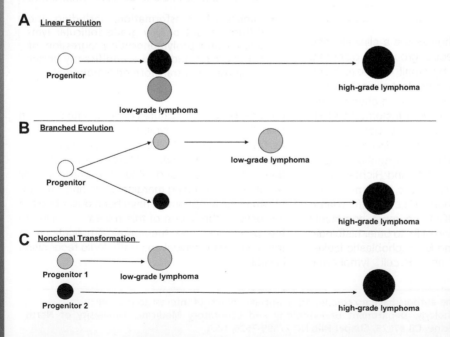

A Linear Evolution
Progenitor
low-grade lymphoma
high-grade lymphoma

B Branched Evolution
Progenitor
low-grade lymphoma
high-grade lymphoma

C Nonclonal Transformation
Progenitor 1   low-grade lymphoma
Progenitor 2   high-grade lymphoma

Fig. 1. Biological categories of clinical transformation. Transformation of low-grade lymphomas may proceed through at least 3 distinct pathways. (*A*) In cases of linear evolution, an aggressive subclone of the low-grade lymphoma becomes more aggressive through the accumulation of additional mutations. In this case, the high-grade lymphoma is a direct descendant of the preceding low-grade lymphoma. (*B*) In cases of branched evolution, the low-grade lymphoma and high-grade lymphoma share a common progenitor, which then follows multiple independent evolutionary paths, first leading to development of low-grade disease and later following a parallel path to a more aggressive lesion. The high-grade lymphoma is a genetic cousin of its low-grade counterpart but not a direct descendant. (*C*) Finally, in some cases, there is no clonal relationship between the low-grade lymphoma and its more aggressive counterpart.

rise in lactate dehydrogenase; rapid or discordant localized lymph node growth; new involvement of an unusual site, such as liver, bone, or central nervous system; development of new B symptoms; or new hypercalcemia.[15] New foci of intense metabolic uptake as visualized by fluorodeoxyglucose (FDG) PET scan can also suggest HT with higher standardized uptake values (SUVs) correlating with more aggressive disease.[16,17] SUVs above 10 in 1 study reliably predicted aggressive or transformed lymphoma with a specificity of 80%.[16] Biopsy, however, remains the gold standard for confirming HT and should be directed at the site of greatest FDG avidity on PET scan when possible. Absence of HT in a given biopsy does not exclude transformation at another site.

FOLLICULAR LYMPHOMA TRANSFORMATION

FL is characterized by mature, clonal B cells arranged in follicles that mimic the morphologic and immunophenotypic features of germinal centers.[18] The neoplastic cells usually coexpress CD20, CD10, and BCL6. Unlike benign germinal centers, however, BCL2 is frequently overexpressed in the malignant follicles, and a corresponding t(14;18) is identified by cytogenetic and/or FISH studies in approximately 85% of cases (FL is reviewed by Fedoriw and Dogan elsewhere in this issue).[19]

FL typically follows an indolent but heterogeneous clinical course. Although some patients may go decades without requiring treatment, others progress rapidly with frequent relapses and short survival. HT to a more aggressive malignancy occurs with a reported frequency of 10% to 60%.[15,20–23] The variability in incidence of higher-grade transformation is likely explained in part by the diagnostic method, rebiopsy protocols, variable duration of follow-up, and definition of transformation used in various studies. Although the International Prognostic Index for FL is a strong predictor of outcome, predicting transformation remains challenging.[24]

Transformation occurs when the follicular architecture of grade 1, 2, or 3a FL becomes diffusely effaced by a population of large cells. Grade 3b FL is often considered a DLBCL equivalent and, as such, progression of grade 3b FL to DLBCL is typically not considered transformation.[18] Similarly, development of high-grade (3a or 3b) FL in a patient previously diagnosed with low-grade (1 or 2) FL is defined as progression, rather than transformation.[22] Although the presence of both FL and DLBCL in the initial diagnostic biopsy implies early transformation and a clonal relationship, the strictest definitions of unequivocal transformation require at least 6 months between the original FL diagnosis and subsequent higher-grade malignancy.[21,25]

Unlike Richter transformation of CLL, a clonal relationship must be established between the original FL and the subsequent higher-grade malignancy.[26,27] This can be accomplished using molecular techniques, or, as is more often the case in clinical practice, a clonal relationship may be inferred by shared cytogenetic or immunophenotypic features. As discussed previously, transformation from FL to DLBCL most often reflects a pattern of branched evolution from a common progenitor cell (see Fig. 1B).

The exact morphologic and immunophenotypic features of transformation may be variable and are dependent on the whether the FL transforms to DLBCL, BCLU, or BLL (Fig. 2). Although the World Health Organization (WHO) criteria should be applied in diagnosing and subclassifying transformed FL, the criteria are largely based on de novo lymphomas, and subtle differences in the transformed counterpart may make classification more challenging.

DLBCL is characterized by sheets of large lymphoid cells with centroblastic or immunoblastic morphology (see Fig. 2B) that typically retain a germinal center immunophenotype (CD10+, BCL6+) when arising in FL.[28,29] Antigenic gains (eg, CD5) and losses (eg, CD10) do occur, but differences in immunophenotype between the original and transformed lymphoma do not preclude a clonal relationship.[28,30] In cases of a subtle nodular appearance that makes identifying a follicular pattern, or lack thereof, difficult, immunohistochemical staining for CD21, CD23, or CD35 may be helpful to highlight follicular dendritic networks and malignant follicles if present (Fig. 3). This technique helps confirm the diffuse nature of transformation or, conversely, identify FL with subtle follicular architecture or composite FL/DLBCL.

BCLU is an aggressive lymphoma with morphologic, immunophenotypic, and/or genetic features of both DLBCL and Burkitt lymphoma.[18] Cases that arise in FL may resemble the starry-sky pattern of Burkitt lymphoma at low power,[18,31] but the cells are often larger with more variation in nuclear size/shape (see Fig. 2C). Like most cases of Burkitt lymphoma and FL, the neoplastic cells have a germinal center immunophenotype, but strong BCL-2, dim CD20 expression, and/or Ki-67 proliferation index of less than 95% typically preclude a straightforward diagnosis of Burkitt lymphoma.[18] Transformed FL should not be classified as Burkitt lymphoma, because the characteristic t(14;18) or complex karyotypic abnormalities usually seen in FL transformation are not found in de novo Burkitt lymphoma.[32,33]

Finally, BLL arising from FL is morphologically identical to its de novo counterpart and

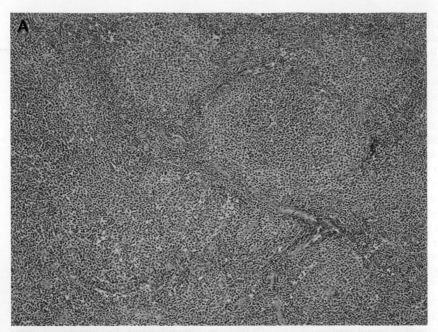

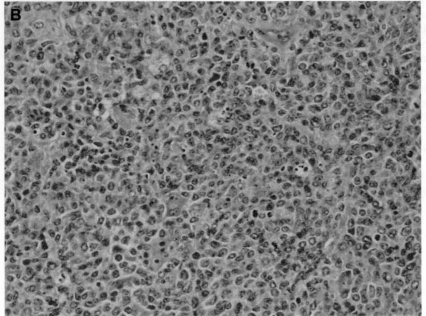

Fig. 2. Transformation of FL. (*A*) Grade 1 to 2 FL, original objective magnification ×10. (*B*) DLBCL, original objective magnification ×40.

characterized by sheets of immature-appearing cells with dispersed chromatin and numerous mitotic figures (see **Fig. 2**D). Tumor cells typically retain expression of CD10 and BCL-2, acquire positivity for TdT and MUM-1, and may lose BCL-6 expression.[34] In contrast to classic cases of de novo BLL, BLL transformed from FL may have bright surface light chain expression and be CD34−.[34] Because these latter features may suggest a more mature phenotype, it is prudent to assess TdT expression by flow cytometry or immunohistochemistry in all large B-cell lymphomas.

MECHANISMS OF TRANSFORMATION IN FOLLICULAR LYMPHOMA

As discussed previously, a majority of FLs harbor a t(14;18).[19] *BCL2* rearrangement is less frequent in higher-grade FLs,[35] however, and its presence is not required for diagnosis. In transformed FL of any histologic subtype, a frequently complex karyotype may also include *MYC* and *BCL6* translocations.[36–38] Cases that show both *MYC* and *BCL2* and/or *BCL6* translocations are considered double-hit lymphomas and are associated with

Fig. 2. (continued). (*C*) BCLU, original objective magnification ×40. (*D*) BLL, original objective magnification ×40.

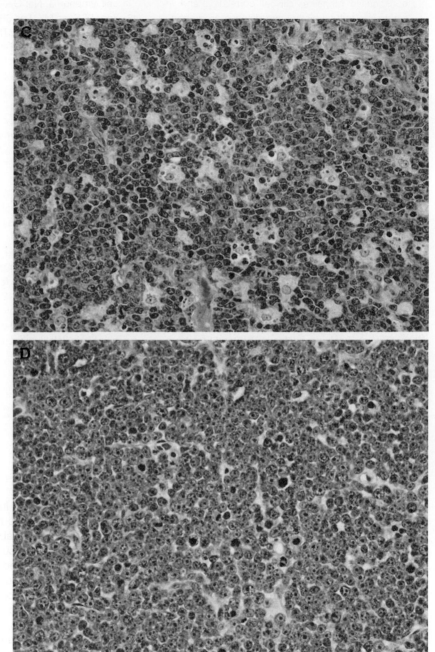

very aggressive clinical behavior.[18] Double-hit cytogenetics may be seen in any transformed FL, but the BCLU category is particularly enriched for this finding.[18]

Paired studies have shown that transformation of FL proceeds through 1 of at least 2 oncogenic mechanisms.[28] The first pathway is characterized by high proliferation. The second is not as well understood but may involve T-cell and follicular dendritic associated genes. Although transformed FL typically maintains a germinal center B-cell expression profile, not surprisingly, the genome is more complex and harbors unique combinations of oncogenic and tumor suppressor genes that may have prognostic and therapeutic implications.[39–42] Some genetic lesions, including those involving genes that encode histone modification enzymes (MLL2) and inhibitors of programmed cell death (BCL2), are shared by FL and transformed FL, suggesting these lesions are acquired early by the common progenitor cell of the branched evolution pattern described previously.[40] Other recurrent aberrations, such as biallelic loss of *CDKN2A/B* and *TP53* mutation or *MYC*

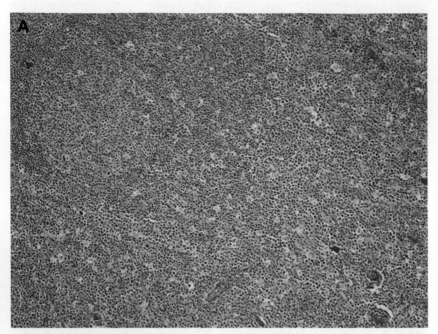

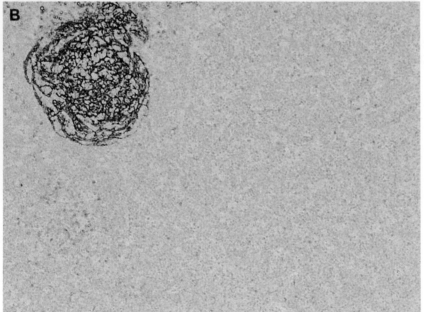

Fig. 3. Loss of follicular dendritic cell networks in DLBCL arising from FL. (*A*) Hematoxylin-eosin–stained section with nodules of FL and sheets of DLBCL. (*B*) CD21 immunohistochemical stain highlights residual follicular dendritic cell networks in areas of FL and loss in DLBCL. All images original objective magnification ×10.

dysregulation, are more specifically associated with transformation and rarely, if ever, seen in non-transformed FL.[28,40] Mutations and deletions of genes involved in the control of immune recognition by cytotoxic T cells and natural killer cells may also be enriched at transformation.[40,43]

Although research efforts have largely focused on genetic alterations in tumor cells, emerging data indicate that several factors in the tumor microenvironment, including loss of follicular dendritic cells, increased microvessel density, and the immunoarchitectural pattern of tumor-associated T cells, also play a crucial role in FL transformation and outcome (see the article by Xu and Fedoriw elsewhere in this issue).

MIMICS OF TRANSFORMED FOLLICULAR LYMPHOMA

Given the poor prognosis of transformed lymphomas, it is important to recognize histologic mimics that should not be confused with transformation. As discussed previously, grade 3b FL is typically considered a DLBCL equivalent, and as such, progression from the former to the latter is not classified as transformation. Similarly, development of higher-grade FL (3a or 3b) in a patient previously diagnosed with low-grade FL (grade 1/2) is considered histologic progression but not transformation.[18] One underappreciated mimic is the diffuse pattern of low-grade FL. This morphologic variant is composed predominantly of small centrocyte-like cells (ie, grade 1–2 cytology) with diffuse pattern growth. Given that diffuse low-grade FL does not seem associated with a worse prognosis, it should not be classified as transformation.[18] By definition, grade 3 lesions with diffuse growth are classified as DLBCL.[18]

RICHTER TRANSFORMATION OF CHRONIC LYMPHOCYTIC LEUKEMIA/SMALL LYMPHOCYTIC LYMPHOMA

CLL is the most common leukemia in the Western world.[44] In straightforward cases, characteristic peripheral blood morphology and immunophenotype are diagnostic.[18] A lymphocytosis is invariably present, consisting predominantly of monomorphic, mature-appearing neoplastic lymphocytes, which typically have scant cytoplasm and so-called soccer ball chromatin (Fig. 4A). Smudge cells may be abundant on smears prepared without albumin. Although not shared by all cases, when present, the classic CD5+, CD23+, CD20 dim, monotypic surface immunoglobulin dim immunophenotype is virtually diagnostic. Cases of fewer than 5000 neoplastic cells per microliter, in the absence of extramedullary tissue or lymph node involvement, should be classified as monoclonal B-cell lymphocytosis.[18]

SLL represents the lymphomatous presentation of CLL.[45] Nodal architecture is effaced by a similarly monotonous population of small lymphocytes with the same immunophenotype seen in the peripheral blood. Cytologic monotony is interrupted only by occasional proliferation centers, which represent pale zones composed predominantly of prolymphocytes and paraimmunoblasts (Fig. 5A).[46–48]

Despite these well-defined diagnostic features, CLL/SLL is a disease with a heterogenous clinical course. Although many patients with CLL/SLL never progress and have near-normal life expectancy, a nearly equal number experience rapid progression and die within a few years of diagnosis.[49,50] It is now understood that prognosis is correlated in large part to the mutational status of the immunoglobulin heavy chain variable region

(IGHV).[49,50] Whereas mutated IGHV (<98% identity to the germline sequence) is associated with favorable outcomes, unmutated cases (>98% identity to the germline sequence) have a poor prognosis, in large part due to an increased risk of transformation to higher-grade disease. In immunophenotyping assays, ZAP70 and CD38 expression are often used as surrogates, albeit imperfect ones, to identify high-risk cases.[50,51]

Transformation of CLL/SLL to an aggressive lymphoma is known as Richter syndrome (RS), in honor of Maurice Richter, an American pathologist who in 1928 first reported rapid development of an aggressive malignant tumor in a patient with "chronic lymphatic leukemia."[52] In most cases of RS, including in Richter's seminal publication, the transformed lymphoma is morphologically similar to DLBCL (DLBCL/RS), with diffuse pattern growth of large, markedly atypical neoplastic cells.[6,52,53] Immunophenotypic differences between DLBCL/RS and the preceding CLL/SLL are common, including bright CD20 expression and a tendency to lack expression of CD5 and CD23.[5,54] A large majority of DLBCL/RS—more than 90% in 1 study—have a nongerminal center immunophenotype using the immunohistochemistry-based Hans classifier.[54,55] Despite earlier speculation, only a small minority of cases are associated with Epstein-Barr virus (EBV) infection.[55–57] Finally, advanced cases may show leukemic involvement, with large neoplastic cells present in the peripheral blood (see Fig. 4C).[53] This latter finding must be distinguished from prolymphocytic progression (see Fig. 4B), which is distinct from transformation (described later).[5,18]

Despite their morphologic similarity and although current classification schema include them under the same DLBCL umbrella, the large cell lymphomas that arise at transformation in patients with CLL/SLL seem biologically and clinically distinct from de novo DLBCL.[13,54,55,58] For instance, whereas the IGH variable region is virtually always mutated in de novo DLBCL, it is mutated in less than 40% of cases of DLBCLs in RS, reflecting a tendency for these lymphomas to arise from high risk cases of CLL/SLL with unmutated IGHV.[54,55] Likewise, although BCL2 and BCL6 translocations are common in de novo DLBCL, they are virtually never seen in DLBCL/RS.[13,55] Finally, common recurrent mutations that have been reported in de novo DLBCL, such as those in CARD11 and NF-κB pathway components, are only rarely identified in DLBCL/RS.[55] In conjunction with dramatic differences in overall mean survival,[18,54–57,59] these observations support the conclusion that DLBCL/RS is a distinct biological and clinical entity. Moreover, given differences in prognosis and potentially therapy, it

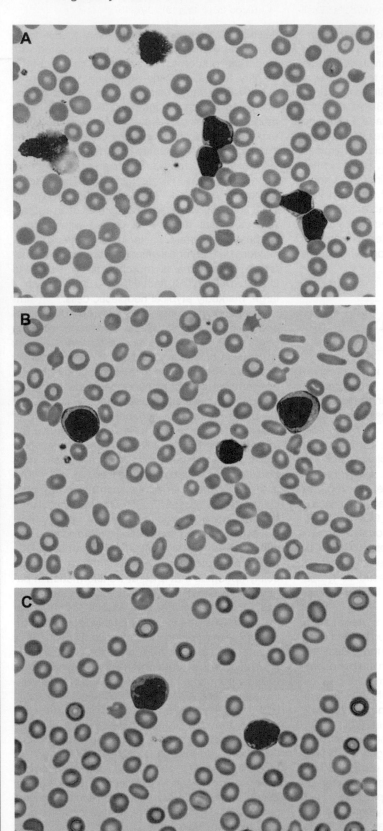

Fig. 4. Peripheral blood findings in CLL, prolymphocytic progression, and large cell transformation. (*A*) CLL. Peripheral blood findings include numerous smudge cells and small intact lymphocytes with condensed, soccer ball–type chromatin (*B*) Prolymphocytic progression of CLL. Circulating prolymphocytes are intermediate-sized lymphoid cells with a moderate amount of cytoplasm and prominent, centrally located nucleoli. (*C*) Large cell transformation of CLL. In advanced cases of RS, there may be leukemic involvement by large neoplastic lymphoid cells, often with marked atypical nuclear features, as shown. All images, original objective magnification ×100.

Fig. 5. Proliferation centers in typical and accelerated phase of SLL. (*A*) Proliferation center in SLL. In most cases of SLL, there are occasional proliferation centers, which appear as pale zones at low power on hematoxylin-eosin–stained sections. Proliferation centers are composed of focal collections of paraimmunoblasts and prolymphocytes. Original magnification ×60. (*B, C*) Accelerated phase of SLL. In the accelerated phase of SLL, proliferation centers are expanded (broader than 1 ×40) field. (*B*) At low power, the expanded proliferation centers may give the lesion a markedly nodular appearance. (*C*) Typical small lymphocytes of CLL/SLL can be seen at higher power (*right*) adjacent to pale cells of the proliferation center (*left*). Original objective magnifications ×4 and ×20, respectively.

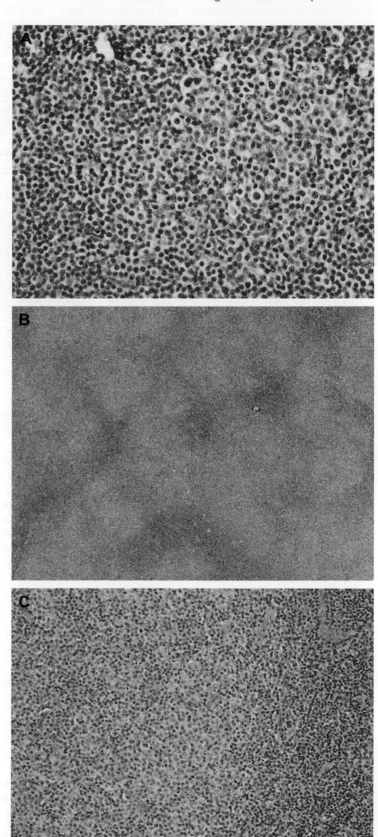

is critical that pathologists distinguish de novo DLBCL and DLBCL/RS, a task that may be more difficult when there is no antecedent history of CLL/SLL (discussed later).

Even among cases of DLBCL/RS, clinical outcomes are heterogenous and historically unpredictable, with some patients dying within weeks of diagnosis and others living more than a decade.[55,56] This variability may reflect, at least in part, diverse mechanisms of transformation. A historical peculiarity of RS is that a clonal relationship is not required between the original CLL/SLL and the subsequent aggressive malignancy. In his original description, Richter wrongly concluded that the secondary tumor was not of lymphoid origin.[52] The modern definition of RS reflects such historical uncertainty and requires only that an aggressive lymphoma develop rapidly in a patient with CLL/SLL.[18]

More recent data, however, have made clear that clonal and nonclonal CLL/SLL transformations are biologically and clinically distinct.[54,55] Whereas clonal cases exhibit stereotyped usage of specific IGH variable chains and frequent TP53 disruption, these features are decidedly less common in nonclonal cases.[55] More importantly, 1 large study has suggested dramatic differences in outcomes between these groups, with a median survival of 14.2 months in clonal RS compared with 62.5 months in nonclonal cases.[55] As a caveat, differences in outcome may be largely explained by differences in the frequency of TP53 disruption between these groups, and it is unclear from multivariate analysis whether clonality remains prognostically informative after correcting for TP53 status. If these observations are replicated in additional studies, it may become appropriate to revisit the definition of RS in the future.[55]

Using the current, less restrictive definition, multiple studies have demonstrated that the secondary malignancy is clonally derived from pre-existing CLL/SLL in approximately 80% of cases,[54,55] with transformation occurring via a linear evolutionary model (see Fig. 1A).[13] In the remaining 20% of cases, the secondary malignancy is unrelated (see Fig. 1C). In the latter cases, patients may be predisposed to development of independent malignancy as a result of underlying immunosuppression caused by CLL/SLL or its treatment.[6]

MECHANISMS OF TRANSFORMATION IN DIFFUSE LARGE B-CELL LYMPHOMA/RICHTER SYNDROME

The single most common anomaly in DLBCL/RS is TP53 inactivation either by point mutation or deletion of 17p, at least 1 of which is seen in

approximately 60% of cases.[13,55] As alluded to previously, TP53 status is an independent predictor of outcome in multivariate analyses. In 1 recent study, median survival in RS/DLBCL patients with wild-type TP53 was 47.1 months, compared with 9.4 months for patients with TP53 mutation or deletion.[55] There is no consensus in the literature as to whether TP53 disruption is more commonly acquired at transformation or already present in antecedent CLL/SLL.[55,58] In either case, TP53 disruption is clearly associated with a loss of genomic integrity, as reflected by an increased propensity for copy number gains and losses relative to cases with intact TP53.[13]

Other common anomalies in DLBCL/RS include NOTCH1 and MYC activating mutations, deletions involving CDKN2A on chromosome 9p21, and trisomy 12.[13,58] Studies attempting to genomically characterize DLBCL/RS have suggested that 2 distinct pathways lead to transformation, 1 involving some combination of TP53 inactivation, CDKN2A loss, MYC activation, and sometimes 13q14 loss, and the other involving NOTCH1 mutation and trisomy 12.[58]

MIMICS OF DIFFUSE LARGE B-CELL LYMPHOMA/RICHTER SYNDROME

As described previously for transformation of FL, it is important to distinguish RS from several mimics, many of which do not carry the same grave prognosis. The most important of these are prolymphocytic progression and the related accelerated phase of CLL/SLL, EBV-positive high-grade lymphomas in patients treated with alemtuzumab (Campath, Genzyme, Boston, MA) for CLL, and de novo CD5+ DLBCL.

Prolymphocytes are intermediate-sized lymphoid cells, with prominent, centrally located nucleoli and a moderate amount of cytoplasm (see Fig. 4B).[18] These cells correspond to one of the cell types present in proliferation centers in lymph nodes involved by CLL/SLL. During the course of disease, the proportion of prolymphocytes in the peripheral blood may increase.[5,60] Prolymphocytic transformation/progression refers to those cases in which prolymphocytes represent greater than 55% of all circulating lymphocytes. An increased proportion of prolymphocytes does not represent RS.[5,18] As such, it is important to distinguish prolymphocytes from true circulating transformed leukemic cells (see Fig. 4C). When morphology is equivocal, immunophenotype may be informative. Unlike DLBCL/RS, prolymphocytes frequently retain CD5/CD23 dual positivity.[5] Finally, it is important to distinguish prolymphocytic progression from B-prolymphocytic leukemia. In the 2008 WHO classification, by definition, the latter disease is not preceded by CLL/SLL.[18]

Accelerated-phase SLL is the tissue equivalent of prolymphocytic progression (Fig. 5B, C). Proliferation centers are expanded (broader than 1 ×20 field, in 1 proposed framework) and show increased mitotic activity. The latter can be ascertained by either mitotic count (>2.4 mitotic figures per proliferation center) or Ki-67 immunohistochemistry (>40% of cells staining).[59] In a small core biopsy, expanded proliferation centers may be mistaken for a diffuse component diagnostic of DLBCL/RS. Accurate distinction is important, given that accelerated phase SLL is associated with much longer median survival compared with DLBCL/RS (34 months vs 4.3 months in 1 study).[59]

In defining RS, some authorities exclude cases of EBV-positive lymphomas that arise in CLL/SLL patients treated with the CD52 monoclonal antibody alemtuzumab, arguing that such cases are biologically more similar to EBV-associated DLBCL of the elderly and other EBV-positive lymphomas arising in immunosuppressed patients.[6]

Fig. 6. Hodgkin-type transformation and its mimics. (A) Rare CD30⁺/EBV-positive cells in low-grade lymphoma. Scattered CD30⁺/EBER-positive cells may be seen in low-grade lymphomas and are not diagnostic of Hodgkin-type transformation when surrounded by typical small neoplastic lymphocytes. (B) Hodgkin-type transformation of low-grade lymphoma. True cases of Hodgkin-type transformation are defined by scattered Hodgkin-type cells in the background milieu seen in de novo cases of CHL, including eosinophils, plasma cells, and histiocytes. Original objective magnification ×100.

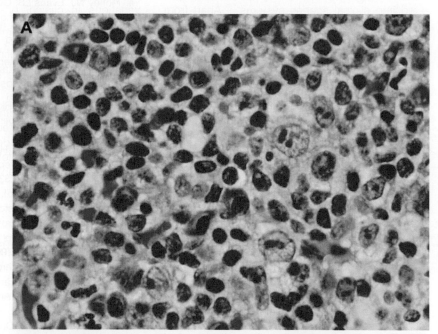

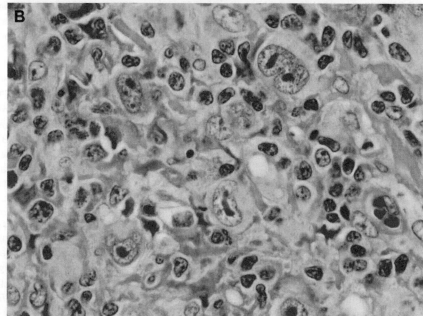

This distinction seems, however, somewhat arbitrary, given that other CLL/SLL therapies, like fludarabine, are similarly T-cell immunosuppressive, and, in general, nonclonal RS may be predisposed to arise due to poor immune function inherent to the leukemic state.

Finally, when there is no prior diagnosis of CLL, it may be difficult to distinguish CD5[+] DLBCL from DLBCL/RS. CD5, however, is often lost in RS,[5,54] and if other immunophenotypic and particularly cytogenetic features do not suggest evolution from CLL/SLL, a modicum of caution is appropriate.

VARIANTS OF RICHTER SYNDROME

Although DLBCL is the most common aggressive lymphoid malignancy that arises in patients with CLL/SLL, secondary classical HL (CHL)/RS, lymphoblastic lymphoma, and even high-grade T-cell lymphoma have been reported.[5–10,61,62] Of these, CHL/RS merits specific mention.

Patients with CLL/SLL have a nearly 8-fold increased risk of CHL.[8] On average, transformation occurs between 2.6 and 6.2 years after CLL/SLL diagnosis, with prior therapy associated with a longer interval until transformation.[8,9] Reported mean survival after CHL/RS diagnosis has varied from 0.8 to 3.9 years in published reports, supporting a more aggressive clinical course than is in seen in de novo CHL.[8,9,56,63]

Consistent with an immunosusceptible state, many cases of CHL/RS are EBV-positive and associated with prior fludarabine exposure.[8,61] Moreover, a clonal relationship to the underlying CLL/SLL seems less common than in DLBCL/RS.[54,64] As in other cases of immunodeficiency-associated CHL, such as that seen in HIV, the mixed cellularity histologic subtype predominates.[8] Irrespective of subtype, attention to the background cellular milieu is critical. Occasional CD30[+] cells may be seen in lymph nodes involved by CLL/SLL, and, in many cases, these cells are even EBV-positive (**Fig. 6A**).[54,65,66] CHL/RS should not, however, be diagnosed unless the background is appropriate for HL (see **Fig. 6B**).

SUMMARY

Almost 90 years after Maurice Richter first reported a case of transformation in a patient with CLL, pathologic evaluation remains the sine qua non for proof of transformation in low-grade B-cell neoplasia. Although historical definitions persist, a modern understanding of transformation involves recognizing not only salient morphologic features but also immunophenotypic and molecular characteristics.

REFERENCES

1. Bernstein SH, Burack WR. The incidence, natural history, biology, and treatment of transformed lymphomas. Hematology Am Soc Hematol Educ Program 2009;532–41.
2. Montoto S, Fitzgibbon J. Transformation of indolent B-cell lymphomas. J Clin Oncol 2011;29(14): 1827–34.
3. Casulo C, Burack WR, Friedberg JW. Transformed follicular non-Hodgkin lymphoma. Blood 2015; 125(1):40–7.
4. Morley NJ, Evans LS, Goepel J, et al. Transformed follicular lymphoma: the 25-year experience of a UK provincial lymphoma treatment centre. Oncol Rep 2008;20(4):953–6.
5. Jain P, O'Brien S. Richter's transformation in chronic lymphocytic leukemia. Oncology (Williston Park) 2012;26(12):1146–52.
6. Rossi D, Gaidano G. Richter syndrome: molecular insights and clinical perspectives. Hematol Oncol 2009;27(1):1–10.
7. Brecher M, Banks PM. Hodgkin's disease variant of Richter's syndrome. Report of eight cases. Am J Clin Pathol 1990;93(3):333–9.
8. Bockorny B, Codreanu I, Dasanu CA. Hodgkin lymphoma as Richter transformation in chronic lymphocytic leukaemia: a retrospective analysis of world literature. Br J Haematol 2012;156(1):50–66.
9. Parikh SA, Habermann TM, Chaffee KG, et al. Hodgkin transformation of chronic lymphocytic leukemia: Incidence, outcomes, and comparison to de novo Hodgkin lymphoma. Am J Hematol 2015;90(4): 334–8.
10. Pistoia V, Roncella S, Di Celle PF, et al. Emergence of a B-cell lymphoblastic lymphoma in a patient with B-cell chronic lymphocytic leukemia: evidence for the single-cell origin of the two tumors. Blood 1991;78(3):797–804.
11. Yoshino T, Omonishi K, Kobayashi K, et al. Clinico-pathological features of gastric mucosa associated lymphoid tissue (MALT) lymphomas: high grade transformation and comparison with diffuse large B cell lymphomas without MALT lymphoma features. J Clin Pathol 2000;53(3):187–90.
12. Lin P, Mansoor A, Bueso-Ramos C, et al. Diffuse large B-cell lymphoma occurring in patients with lymphoplasmacytic lymphoma/Waldenstrom macro-globulinemia. Clinicopathologic features of 12 cases. Am J Clin Pathol 2003;120(2):246–53.
13. Fabbri G, Khiabanian H, Holmes AB, et al. Genetic lesions associated with chronic lymphocytic leukemia transformation to Richter syndrome. J Exp Med 2013;210(11):2273–88.
14. Carlotti E, Wrench D, Matthews J, et al. Transformation of follicular lymphoma to diffuse large B-cell lymphoma may occur by divergent evolution from a

common progenitor cell or by direct evolution from the follicular lymphoma clone. Blood 2009;113(15): 3553–7.

15. Al-Tourah AJ, Gill KK, Chhanabhai M, et al. Population-based analysis of incidence and outcome of transformed non-Hodgkin's lymphoma. J Clin Oncol 2008;26(32):5165–9.

16. Schoder H, Noy A, Gonen M, et al. Intensity of 18fluorodeoxyglucose uptake in positron emission tomography distinguishes between indolent and aggressive non-Hodgkin's lymphoma. J Clin Oncol 2005;23(21):4643–51.

17. Noy A, Schoder H, Gonen M, et al. The majority of transformed lymphomas have high standardized uptake values (SUVs) on positron emission tomography (PET) scanning similar to diffuse large B-cell lymphoma (DLBCL). Ann Oncol 2009;20(3): 508–12.

18. Swerdlow SH, Campo E, Harris NL, et al, editors. WHO classification of tumours of haematopoietic and lymphoid tissues. 4th edition. Lyon (France): IARC; 2008. p. 169–268.

19. Horsman DE, Gascoyne RD, Coupland RW, et al. Comparison of cytogenetic analysis, southern analysis, and polymerase chain reaction for the detection of t(14; 18) in follicular lymphoma. Am J Clin Pathol 1995;103(4):472–8.

20. Risdall R, Hoppe RT, Warnke R. Non-Hodgkin's lymphoma: a study of the evolution of the disease based upon 92 autopsied cases. Cancer 1979; 44(2):529–42.

21. Bastion Y, Sebban C, Berger F, et al. Incidence, predictive factors, and outcome of lymphoma transformation in follicular lymphoma patients. J Clin Oncol 1997;15(4):1587–94.

22. Montoto S, Davies AJ, Matthews J, et al. Risk and clinical implications of transformation of follicular lymphoma to diffuse large B-cell lymphoma. J Clin Oncol 2007;25(17):2426–33.

23. Link BK, Maurer MJ, Nowakowski GS, et al. Rates and outcomes of follicular lymphoma transformation in the immunochemotherapy era: a report from the University of Iowa/MayoClinic specialized program of research excellence molecular epidemiology resource. J Clin Oncol 2013;31(26):3272–8.

24. Solal-Celigny P, Roy P, Colombat P, et al. Follicular lymphoma international prognostic index. Blood 2004;104(5):1258–65.

25. Hubbard SM, Chabner BA, DeVita VT Jr, et al. Histologic progression in non-Hodgkin's lymphoma. Blood 1982;59(2):258–64.

26. Lossos IS, Alizadeh AA, Diehn M, et al. Transformation of follicular lymphoma to diffuse large-cell lymphoma: alternative patterns with increased or decreased expression of c-myc and its regulated genes. Proc Natl Acad Sci U S A 2002;99(13): 8886–91.

27. Lossos IS, Levy R. Higher grade transformation of follicular lymphoma: phenotypic tumor progression associated with diverse genetic lesions. Semin Cancer Biol 2003;13(3):191–202.

28. Davies AJ, Rosenwald A, Wright G, et al. Transformation of follicular lymphoma to diffuse large B-cell lymphoma proceeds by distinct oncogenic mechanisms. Br J Haematol 2007;136(2):286–93.

29. Lossos IS, Gascoyne RD. Transformation of follicular lymphoma. Best Pract Res Clin Haematol 2011; 24(2):147–63.

30. Maeshima AM, Omatsu M, Nomoto J, et al. Diffuse large B-cell lymphoma after transformation from low-grade follicular lymphoma: morphological, immunohistochemical, and FISH analyses. Cancer Sci 2008;99(9):1760–8.

31. Carbone A, Gloghini A, Aiello A, et al. B-cell lymphomas with features intermediate between distinct pathologic entities. From pathogenesis to pathology. Hum Pathol 2010;41(5):621–31.

32. Hummel M, Bentink S, Berger H, et al. A biologic definition of Burkitt's lymphoma from transcriptional and genomic profiling. N Engl J Med 2006; 354(23):2419–30.

33. Boerma EG, Siebert R, Kluin PM, et al. Translocations involving 8q24 in Burkitt lymphoma and other malignant lymphomas: a historical review of cytogenetics in the light of todays knowledge. Leukemia 2009;23(2):225–34.

34. Geyer JT, Subramaniyam S, Jiang Y, et al. Lymphoblastic transformation of follicular lymphoma: a clinicopathologic and molecular analysis of 7 patients. Hum Pathol 2015;46(2):260–71.

35. Ott G, Katzenberger T, Lohr A, et al. Cytomorphologic, immunohistochemical, and cytogenetic profiles of follicular lymphoma: 2 types of follicular lymphoma grade 3. Blood 2002;99(10):3806–12.

36. Macpherson N, Lesack D, Klasa R, et al. Small noncleaved, non-Burkitt's (Burkit-Like) lymphoma: cytogenetics predict outcome and reflect clinical presentation. J Clin Oncol 1999;17(5):1558–67.

37. Lin P, Medeiros LJ. High-grade B-cell lymphoma/leukemia associated with t(14;18) and 8q24/MYC rearrangement: a neoplasm of germinal center immunophenotype with poor prognosis. Haematologica 2007;92(10):1297–301.

38. Relander T, Johnson NA, Farinha P, et al. Prognostic factors in follicular lymphoma. J Clin Oncol 2010; 28(17):2902–13.

39. Martinez-Climent JA, Alizadeh AA, Segraves R, et al. Transformation of follicular lymphoma to diffuse large cell lymphoma is associated with a heterogeneous set of DNA copy number and gene expression alterations. Blood 2003;101(8):3109–17.

40. Pasqualucci L, Khiabanian H, Fangazio M, et al. Genetics of follicular lymphoma transformation. Cell Rep 2014;6(1):130–40.

41. Morin RD, Mendez-Lago M, Mungall AJ, et al. Frequent mutation of histone-modifying genes in non-Hodgkin lymphoma. Nature 2011;476(7360): 298–303.

42. Morin RD, Mungall K, Pleasance E, et al. Mutational and structural analysis of diffuse large B-cell lymphoma using whole-genome sequencing. Blood 2013;122(7):1256–65.

43. Kiaii S, Clear AJ, Ramsay AG, et al. Follicular lymphoma cells induce changes in T-cell gene expression and function: potential impact on survival and risk of transformation. J Clin Oncol 2013;31(21): 2654–61.

44. Dighiero G, Hamblin TJ. Chronic lymphocytic leukaemia. Lancet 2008;371(9617):1017–29.

45. Hallek M, Cheson BD, Catovsky D, et al. Guidelines for the diagnosis and treatment of chronic lymphocytic leukemia: a report from the International Workshop on Chronic Lymphocytic Leukemia updating the National Cancer Institute-Working Group 1996 guidelines. Blood 2008;111(12):5446–56.

46. Dick FR, Maca RD. The lymph node in chronic lymphocytic leukemia. Cancer 1978;41(1):283–92.

47. Schmid C, Isaacson PG. Proliferation centres in B-cell malignant lymphoma, lymphocytic (B-CLL): an immunophenotypic study. Histopathology 1994; 24(5):445–51.

48. Ben-Ezra J, Burke JS, Swartz WG, et al. Small lymphocytic lymphoma: a clinicopathologic analysis of 268 cases. Blood 1989;73(2):579–87.

49. Hamblin TJ, Davis Z, Gardiner A, et al. Unmutated Ig V(H) genes are associated with a more aggressive form of chronic lymphocytic leukemia. Blood 1999; 94(6):1848–54.

50. Damle RN, Wasil T, Fais F, et al. Ig V gene mutation status and CD38 expression as novel prognostic indicators in chronic lymphocytic leukemia. Blood 1999;94(6):1840–7.

51. Crespo M, Bosch F, Villamor N, et al. ZAP-70 expression as a surrogate for immunoglobulin-variable-region mutations in chronic lymphocytic leukemia. N Engl J Med 2003;348(18):1764–75.

52. Richter MN. Generalized reticular cell sarcoma of lymph nodes associated with lymphatic leukemia. Am J Pathol 1928;4(4):285–292.7.

53. Tsimberidou AM, Keating MJ. Richter syndrome: biology, incidence, and therapeutic strategies. Cancer 2005;103(2):216–28.

54. Mao Z, Quintanilla-Martinez L, Raffeld M, et al. IgVH mutational status and clonality analysis of Richter's transformation: diffuse large B-cell lymphoma and Hodgkin lymphoma in association with B-cell chronic lymphocytic leukemia (B-CLL) represent 2 different pathways of disease evolution. Am J Surg Pathol 2007;31(10):1605–14.

55. Rossi D, Spina V, Deambrogi C, et al. The genetics of Richter syndrome reveals disease heterogeneity and predicts survival after transformation. Blood 2011;117(12):3391–401.

56. Tsimberidou AM, O'Brien S, Khouri I, et al. Clinical outcomes and prognostic factors in patients with Richter's syndrome treated with chemotherapy or chemoimmunotherapy with or without stem-cell transplantation. J Clin Oncol 2006;24(15):2343–51.

57. Rossi D, Cerri M, Capello D, et al. Biological and clinical risk factors of chronic lymphocytic leukaemia transformation to Richter syndrome. Br J Haematol 2008;142(2):202–15.

58. Chigrinova E, Rinaldi A, Kwee I, et al. Two main genetic pathways lead to the transformation of chronic lymphocytic leukemia to Richter syndrome. Blood 2013;122(15):2673–82.

59. Gine E, Martinez A, Villamor N, et al. Expanded and highly active proliferation centers identify a histological subtype of chronic lymphocytic leukemia ("accelerated" chronic lymphocytic leukemia) with aggressive clinical behavior. Haematologica 2010; 95(9):1526–33.

60. Melo JV, Wardle J, Chetty M, et al. The relationship between chronic lymphocytic leukaemia and prolymphocytic leukaemia. III. Evaluation of cell size by morphology and volume measurements. Br J Haematol 1986;64(3):469–78.

61. Tsimberidou AM, O'Brien S, Kantarjian HM, et al. Hodgkin transformation of chronic lymphocytic leukemia: the M. D. Anderson Cancer Center experience. Cancer 2006;107(6):1294–302.

62. Lee A, Skelly ME, Kingma DW, et al. B-cell chronic lymphocytic leukemia followed by high grade T-cell lymphoma. An unusual variant of Richter's syndrome. Am J Clin Pathol 1995;103(3):348–52.

63. Tadmor T, Shvidel L, Goldschmidt N, et al. Hodgkin's variant of Richter transformation in chronic lymphocytic leukemia; a retrospective study from the Israeli CLL study group. Anticancer Res 2014;34(2):785–90.

64. de Leval L, Vivario M, De Prijck B, et al. Distinct clonal origin in two cases of Hodgkin's lymphoma variant of Richter's syndrome associated With EBV infection. Am J Surg Pathol 2004;28(5):679–86.

65. Tsang WY, Chan JK, Sing C. The nature of Reed-Sternberg-like cells in chronic lymphocytic leukemia. Am J Clin Pathol 1993;99(3):317–23.

66. Rubin D, Hudnall SD, Aisenberg A, et al. Richter's transformation of chronic lymphocytic leukemia with Hodgkin's-like cells is associated with Epstein-Barr virus infection. Mod Pathol 1994;7(1):91–8.

Lymphoma Microenvironment and Immunotherapy

Mina L. Xu, MD[a], Yuri Fedoriw, MD[b]

KEYWORDS

- Immune surveillance • Tumor microenvironment • Immunomodulatory drugs • Immune checkpoint
- Tumor-associated macrophages

ABSTRACT

Understanding of the lymphoma tumor microenvironment is poised to expand in the era of next-generation sequencing studies of the tumor cells themselves. Successful therapies of the future will rely on deeper appreciation of the interactions between elements of the microenvironment. Although the phenotypic, cytogenetic, and molecular characterization of tumor cells in lymphomas has progressed faster than most other solid organ tumors, concrete advancements in understanding the lymphoma microenvironment have been fewer. This article explores the composition of the lymphoma tumor microenvironment; its role in immune surveillance, evasion, and drug resistance; and its potential role in the development of targeted therapies.

Key Features

- Understanding of the lymphoma tumor microenvironment is poised to expand in the era of next-generation sequencing studies of the tumor cells themselves.

- Successful therapies of the future will rely on deeper appreciation of the interactions between elements of the microenvironment.

OVERVIEW

Tumor microenvironment was initially addressed in the context of carcinoma metastases by Stephen Paget in 1889.[1] In examining the pattern of breast cancer metastases at autopsy, he found that some organs demonstrated a preponderance of metastases and generated the hypothesis that "seeds," or neoplastic cells, could only land and flourish in appropriate "soil," or microenvironment. Decades later, scientists discovered that lung-homing melanoma cells, when implanted in mice, selectively metastasize to lung and ectopically placed lung but not other tissues.[2]

Novel drugs targeting the tumor microenvironment in carcinomas have been primarily concentrated in the inhibition of tumor-related angiogenesis. Compounds include inhibitors of vascular endothelial growth factor (bevacizumab) and vascular endothelial growth factor receptor–2 tyrosine kinase (sorafenib and sunitinib). In patients with non–small cell lung cancer and colon cancer, bevacizumab, used in the conjunction with standard chemotherapy, demonstrated prolonged progression-free survival and overall survival.[3,4]

Although the phenotypic, cytogenetic, and molecular characterizations of tumor cells in lymphomas have progressed faster than for most other solid organ tumors, concrete advancements in understanding the lymphoma microenvironment have been fewer. This article explores the composition of the lymphoma tumor microenvironment; its role in immune surveillance, evasion, and drug resistance; and its potential role in the development of targeted therapies. In the context of morphologic and prognostic tumor evaluation, pathologists can provide insights critical for cutting-edge clinical care.

---

[a] Department of Pathology & Laboratory Medicine, Yale University School of Medicine, 310 Cedar Street, PO Box 208023, New Haven, CT 06520-8023, USA; [b] University of North Carolina School of Medicine, Department of Pathology and Laboratory Medicine, NC Cancer Hospital C3162-D, 101 Manning Drive, Chapel Hill, NC 27599, USA
E-mail address: mina.xu@yale.edu

Surgical Pathology 9 (2016) 93–100
http://dx.doi.org/10.1016/j.path.2015.10.001

TUMOR MICROENVIRONMENT IN LYMPHOMA

The key constituents of the lymphoma microenvironment and their pattern of distribution within tissue vary widely between tumors depending on the host inflammatory response as well as the genetics and proliferation rate of malignant cells (Box 1). For example, in tumors such as classic Hodgkin Lymphoma, polymorphic post-transplant lymphoproliferative disorders, and angioimmunoblastic T-cell lymphoma, the background non-neoplastic inflammatory components are prominent and often display typical morphologic features identifiable to the tumor type. In contrast, extranodal marginal zone lymphomas of mucosa-associated lymphoid tissues, follicular lymphomas, and some mantle cell lymphomas in the early stage retain or recapitulate normal lymphoid architecture. Further on the spectrum, many diffuse large B-cell lymphomas and virtually all Burkitt lymphomas show effacement of the underlying architecture. Often, the more aggressive lymphomas seem to demonstrate independence from the signals and supporting network provided by the microenvironment.

SIGNALS TO AND FROM THE TUMOR MICROENVIRONMENT

Lymphoma B cells have been shown to secrete CC-chemokine ligand 22 (CCL22), recruiting intratumoral regulatory T cells (Tregs) to suppress antitumor response. Substantially higher numbers of CD4[+] CD25[+] Tregs have been found in B-cell NHL biopsies than in non-neoplastic lymph nodes and normal peripheral blood mononuclear cells. These T cells have been shown to inhibit production of interferon γ and interleukin (IL)-4 by CD4[+] CD25[−] T cells.[5] In studying the attraction of Tregs for the tumor sites, it has been found that lymphoma B cells expressed significantly higher levels of CCL22. This chemokine may be responsible for chemotaxis and migration of intratumoral Tregs to sites of tumor.[6] In turn, the CD4[+] CD25[+] Tregs can directly down-regulate normal B-cell activation and humoral immune responses.[7,8]

Increased Tregs in B-cell lymphomas have been shown to be associated with down-regulation of T_H17 cells. T_H17 cells seem to abundantly secrete IL-17, a proinflammatory cytokine critical for host protection against a wide variety of pathogens. Although the exact mechanism for this process is not clear, costimulatory molecules CD70, CD80, and CD86 are involved in generation of Tregs; their blockade with targeted antibodies increases the number of IL-17–producing cells.[9]

EVASION FROM IMMUNE SYSTEM

In recent years, improved understanding of the tumor microenvironment highlighted the ways in which neoplastic cells escape from immune surveillance using its interactions with non-neoplastic neighboring cells.

A variety of lymphomas show decreased major histocompatibility complex (MHC) II expression, which may be a primary mode of evasion. In classic Hodgkin lymphoma and primary mediastinal (thymic) large B-cell lymphoma, genomic breaks in MHC class II transactivator CIITA are highly recurrent. These CIITA fusions lead to down-regulation of surface HLA class II expression as well as up-regulation of programmed cell death 1 ligands, CD274/PD-L1 and CD273/PD-L2.[10] Intriguing data also show homozygous deletions of HLA class II genes in testicular and central nervous system diffuse large B-cell lymphomas, likely contributing to the immune privilege of those sites.[11]

The function of PD-L1 and PD-L2 expression by malignant B cells is thought to cause T-cell exhaustion on contact with PD-1–bearing CD4[+] T cells. A subset of aggressive B-cell lymphomas and virus-associated and immunodeficiency-associated lymphoproliferative disorders have demonstrated overexpression of PD-L1 by tumor cells and infiltrating macrophages, identifying a group of tumors that could be rationally targeted with PD-1/PD-L1 therapies.[12] Primary non-Hodgkin lymphoma cells show increased numbers of functionally exhausted CD70[+] T cells that express PD-1 and Tim-3, a phenotype shown to be induced by transforming growth factor (TGF)-β.[13]

In addition, copy number analysis of classic Hodgkin lymphoma, nodular sclerosis subtype, and primary mediastinal (thymic) large B-cell lymphoma showed amplification at 9p24.1/PD-1 ligand as well as induction by JAK2. These findings suggest that consideration toward targeting PD-1 and JAK2 pathways may be warranted in these tumors.[14]

CHRONIC LYMPHOCYTIC LEUKEMIA

Chronic lymphocytic leukemia (CLL)/small lymphocytic leukemia cells disrupt the normal lymphoid architecture and show a distinctive morphology, often composed of pseudofollicles or proliferation centers that contain numerous prolymphocytes. This complete disruption of the normal microenvironment could explain the often associated immune deficiency and hypogammaglobulinemia seen in CLL patients.[15]

The tumor cells themselves express high levels of CXCR4 (the receptor for CXCL12) and tumor necrosis factor (TNF)-α to inhibit normal hematopoiesis.

Box 1
Components of the lymphoma tumor microenvironment

Tumor-associated macrophages

TAMs are cells from the macrophage/circulating monocyte lineage that are found in close proximity to tumor. TAMs seem to take on different roles depending on the tumor type. A high level of TAM infiltration has been correlated with poor prognosis in many neoplasms (including classic Hodgkin lymphoma) but better prognosis in other neoplasms.

Follicular dendritic cells

Follicular dendritic cells are $CD21^+$ $CD23^+$ $CD35^+$ cells found within B-cell follicles; they capture antigens and present them to other cells. They also help in development of germinal centers by participating in affinity maturation of B cells. They produce CXCL13, promoting B-cell migration into follicles.

Fibroblastic reticular cells

FRCs are stromal cells that regulate movement of dendritic cells, T cells, and B cells in secondary lymphoid tissue. They are primarily located in the T-cell zone. FRCs secrete chemokines CCL21 and CCL19, directing the movement of T cells and dendritic cells with CCR7 receptors.

Endothelial cells

Endothelial cells express adhesion molecules, CCL21, and peripheral lymph node addressin in blood endothelial cells. Specialized endothelial cells line the lymphatic vessels (lymphatic endothelial cells) and high endothelial venules (blood endothelial cells), permitting the trafficking of lymphocytes.

Follicular T helper cells

Tfh cells within tumor express PD-1, CXCR5, and BCL-6. They support B-cell activation and rescue malignant B cells from apoptosis. A higher proportion is found in follicular lymphoma than in diffuse large B-cell lymphoma or reactive lymph nodes.[19]

Regulatory T cells

Tregs are $CD4^+$ $CD25^+$, suppress autoimmune T-cell responses, and maintain peripheral tolerance. Under normal conditions, 5% to 10% of peripheral $CD4^+$ T cells in both mice and human. Forkhead/winged-helix transcription factor family member p3 (FOXP3) is a master regulator for the development and function of Tregs so the immunostain FOXP3 is now used to highlight Tregs. They are thought to suppress antitumor immunity by inhibiting intratumor $CD4^+$ and $CD8^+$ T cells.

Cytotoxic T cells

Cytotoxic T cells are $CD8^+$ T cells that kill cells displaying specific and recognizable antigen to the T cell. Once activated by an antigen presenting cell, cytotoxic T cells undergo clonal expansion with help from IL-2 and release cytotoxins, such as perforin and granzyme.

Natural killer cells

Natural killer cells are $CD16^+$ $CD56^+$ cytotoxic lymphocytes of the innate immune system that induce apoptosis even in the absence of antibodies and MHC.

Myeloid-derived suppressor cells

Myeloid-derived suppressor cells are myeloid lineage cells that seem to suppress immune surveillance, particularly in bone marrow. Myeloid-derived suppressor cells have been shown to form mature osteoclasts in response to receptor activator of nuclear factor κB ligand (RANKL), increasing bone resorption. They are thought to influence the ability of tumors to spread into the marrow niche.[23]

The elevated presence of nurse-like cells, currently understood to be of the myelomonocytic lineage, are associated with increased resistance to therapy and a shorter survival. The nurse-like cells secrete CXCL12, APRIL, and BAFF. APRIL, a proliferation-inducing ligand, seems to interact with trans-membrane activator and calcium modulator and cytophilin ligand interactor (TACI or CD267) and B-cell maturation antigen (BCMA or CD269). BAFF also interacts with TACI, which is associated with immunodeficiency.[16]

Studies have also began to elucidate the role of exosomes in the interaction between circulating tumor cells and the microenvironment. CLL-derived exosomes were shown to induce stromal cells to take on a cancer-associated fibroblast phenotype in vitro. The cancer-associated fibroblasts, in turn, support a niche that promotes CLL cell adhesion, survival, and growth in vivo.[17] Overview of the supporting cell types in the CLL microenvironment is provided through schematic in Fig. 1.

MICROENVIRONMENT-TARGETED IMMUNOTHERAPIES FOR CHRONIC LYMPHOCYTIC LEUKEMIA

- CXCR4 antagonists: blocks CLL cell trafficking and homing to marrow through interaction of CXCR4 with CXCL12 (eg, plerixafor [AMD3100] and T140 analogs)
- TACI decoy receptor: soluble TACI presumed to buffer APRIL and BAFF. Early studies in patients with refractory or relapsed CLL seem to suggest that the drug antagonizes the proliferation of CLL cells (eg, Atacicept).
- PI3K inhibitor: targets PI3K signaling in CLL, is thought to interfere with stromal cell interactions, releasing CLL tumor cells from protective microenvironments into blood. In circulation, they may be more sensitive to systemic chemotherapy (eg, Idelalisib).
- Bruton's tyrosine kinase inhibitor: disrupts B cell receptor (BCR) and nuclear factor κB signaling, causing tumor apoptosis, inhibition of proliferation, and prevention of tumor response to survival stimuli in the microenvironment. BTK inhibitor causes transient surge of tumor cells from lymph nodes into peripheral blood, likely due to disruption of homing mechanisms in tissue, causing lymphocytosis[18] (eg, ibrutinib).
- Thalidomide derivative: possibly works to inhibit Tregs and increase helper T-cell (T_H17) population (possible mechanism of action) (eg, lenalidomide)

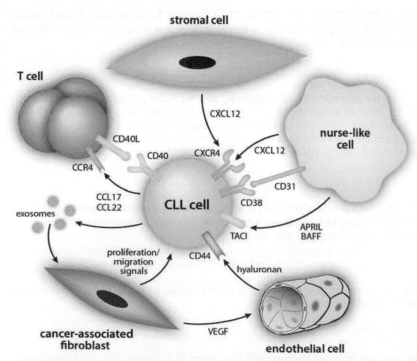

Fig. 1. The CLL tumor cells express CXCR4 at high levels, interacting with ligand CXCL12 from nurse-like cells as well as stromal cells. These signals induce CLL homing to the marrow. Expression of CD31 on nurse-like cells interact with CD38, helping to recruit monocytes and macrophages. Nurse-like cells also produce BAFF and APRIL, interacting with TACI on the surface of CLL cells. Crosstalk between T cells and CLL include CD40 stimulation, thereby allowing T cells to produce soluble factors, like IL-2, IL-4, and IL-10. CLL expression of CCL17 and CCl22 attract more CCR4+ T cells. Hyaluronan, on the basement membrane of high endothelial venules, interacts with CD44, likely promoting the production of matrix metalloproteinase 9. The latter has a possible role in CLL tumor cell migration into lymph nodes. CLL-derived exosomes seem to assist in the formation of cancer-associated fibroblasts, which work to promote the proliferation of CLL cells.

FOLLICULAR LYMPHOMA

Follicular lymphoma primarily occurs in lymph nodes, hijacking the normal follicle architecture. Compared with the normal lymph node, follicular lymphomas demonstrate increased Tregs and decreased effector T cells. Although earlier studies suggested that elevated numbers of Tregs predicted better survival in follicular lymphoma,[19] more recent studies have pointed to the importance of its localization. In a study using consistent treatment regimens, patients with predominantly follicular pattern Forkhead Box P3 (FOXP3) (which can highlight Tregs) demonstrated increased risk of transformation and shorter survival than those who had a diffuse pattern.[20] It also seems that the location of PD-1[+] T cells within follicles prolong the time to transformation.[21]

Helper T cells can be considered the opposite part of the equation from Tregs. Aside from T_H1, T_H2, and T follicular helper (Tfh) cells, T_H17 cells is another member of helper T cells, found to produce cytokines IL-17 and IL-22, thereby promoting inflammation. In follicular lymphoma, T_H17 cells were reduced when compared with other B-cell lymphomas and shown to be reduced by the neoplastic B cells themselves, in direct opposition to the up-regulation of Tregs by costimulatory molecules CD70, CD80 and CD86.[9] Thus, this skewing of the balance between T_H17 and Tregs could explain the lack of appropriate inflammatory response in follicular lymphoma. Tfh cells are increased in lymphoma samples. They express CXCR4 and CXCR5, which may help recruit neoplastic B cells into follicles. They interact with the tumor cells through CD40L/CD40 and secrete IL-4, thereby activating signal transducer and activator of transcription 6 (STAT6).[22]

Gene expression studies found that a monocyte/macrophage-related immune signature in follicular lymphomas predicted worse survival.[23] In tissue sections, increased CD68-positive lymphoma-associated macrophages was significantly correlated with poorer prognosis.[24] Tumor-associated macrophages (TAMs) are thought to promote angiogenesis by releasing suppressive cytokines, such as TGF-β, and expressing growth factors necessary for the tumor.[25] **Fig. 2** for a schematic of follicular lymphoma cell interaction with its microenvironment.

MICROENVIRONMENT-TARGETED IMMUNOTHERAPIES FOR FOLLICULAR LYMPHOMA

- PD-1 blocking antibody: disrupts interaction between immune checkpoint receptor PD-1 with its ligands PD-L1 and PD-L2, to prevent antitumor immunity (eg, nivolumab)
- Anti-CTLA4 antibody: CTLA4 signaling from T cells down-regulate T-cell activity and induces T-cell cycle arrest. Blocking CTLA4 promotes activation of infiltrating T cells within tumor (eg, ipilimumab).

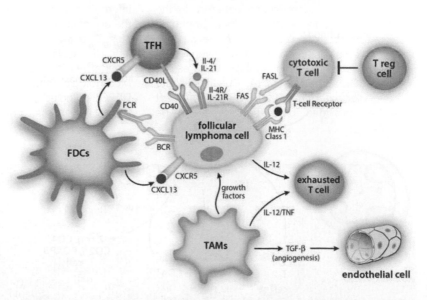

Fig. 2. Malignant B cells in follicular lymphoma have the power to induce important phenotypic changes in surrounding T cells. Conversely, the T cells can highly impact antitumor immunity. Tfh cells can assist in tumor cell growth and survival by secreting cytokines, such as IL-4 and IL-21, whereas stromal cells like follicular dendritic cells (FDCs) secrete CXCL13. BCR signaling can also take place through FDCs, which simultaneously supports the Tfh cells. Tregs act to inhibit the immune suppressive effects of cytotoxic T cells. TAMs secrete growth factors and also signals to induce angiogenesis.

- PI3K inhibitor: inhibits tumor cell migration, growth, angiogenesis (eg, idelalisib)
- Proteasome inhibitor: ubiquitin-proteasome pathway regulates cell trafficking, cell cycle progression, and apoptosis (eg, bortezomib).
- Immunomodulatory drugs: antiangiogenic activity, repair of T-cell defects in follicular lymphoma, and promotion of immune synapse function between host T cells and tumor cells (also direct toxic effects to tumor cells (eg, lenalidomide).

CLASSIC HODGKIN LYMPHOMA

Hodgkin Reed-Sternberg (HRS) cells of classic Hodgkin lymphoma seem to secrete and induce the secretion of a wide variety of chemokines and cytokines that maintain the polymorphous background cellularity richly composed of stromal cells, fibroblasts, plasma cells, numerous T cells, eosinophils, and neutrophils. For example, HRS cells secrete colony-stimulating factor 1 (CSF1) and CX3CL1, which may help recruit abundant macrophages. Recent findings that CSF1 receptor-enriched microenvironment appears associated with worse survival in a large cohort of Hodgkin lymphoma patients may lead to a

potential therapeutic target.[26] Macrophages, in turn, produce IL-8, a chemokine to enlist neutrophils into the tumor tissue whereas production of IL-5 by HRS cells attracts eosinophils.[27] HRS cells express CD30 abundantly, thus interacting with CD30 ligand on eosinophils and mast cells, leading to increased DNA synthesis in HRS cells.[28,29]

The production of TGF-β, IL-10, galectin-1, and prostaglandin E_2 by HRS cells, in addition to expression of PD-L1 by HRS cells, can all serve to induce T-cell anergy.[30] In EBV$^+$ cases of CHL, the latency type II pattern includes the expression of Latent Membrane Protein 1 (LMP1), LMP2, and Epstein-Barr nuclear antigen-1. Oncogene LMP1 mimics CD40 activation whereas LMP2 mimics BCR signaling.[31,32] CD40, in turn, interacts with the closely surrounding T cells expressing CD40 ligand, leading to prosurvival signaling.

There is evidence that the wide array of nonneoplastic cells is necessary for HRS cells to survive. HRS cells are rarely found in peripheral blood, do not persist in immunodeficient mice, and, even when metastatic to bone marrow, they are followed by the background cellularity. See **Fig. 3** for a schematic of HRS cell interaction with its microenvironment.

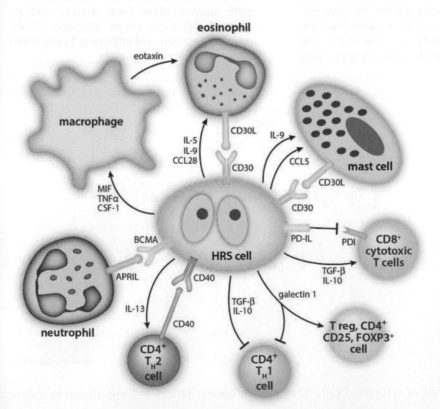

Fig. 3. In classic Hodgkin lymphoma, HRS cells produce abundant cytokines to support the cellular milieu that includes eosinophils and mast cells (IL-5 and IL-9). HRS cells also produce macrophage migration inhibitory factor (MIF), which support the infiltrate of M2 macrophages. Tregs are induced by galectin-1, secreted by HRS cells. CD4$^+$ T cells express high levels of CD40 ligand, which binds to CD40 on HRS cells, enhancing colony formation. Differentiation into T_H2 cells can be facilitated by IL-13, also secreted by HRS cells. PD-L1 expression by HRS cells may help the tumor escape immune responses by causing T-cell exhaustion.

MICROENVIRONMENT-TARGETED IMMUNOTHERAPIES FOR CLASSIC HODGKIN LYMPHOMA

- Histone deacetylace inhibitors: down-regulate PD-1 expression, stimulate antigen-specific memory T cells (eg, vorinostat and pabinostat)
- PD-1 blocking antibody: disrupts interaction between immune checkpoint receptor PD-1 with its ligands PD-L1 and PD-L2, to prevent antitumor immunity (eg, nivolumab)
- Anti-CTLA4 antibody: CTLA4 signaling from T cells down-regulate T-cell activity and induces T-cell cycle arrest. Blocking CTLA4 promotes activation of infiltrating T cells within tumor (eg, ipilimumab).
- Monoclonal antibodies targeting peritumor B cells (eg, rituximab), combined with gemcitabine, in combination with standard ABVD chemotherapy up front
- Anti-CD27: targets TNF stimulation by surrounding lymphocytes (eg, varlilumab)
- EBV antigen-specific cytotoxic T cells: requires ex vivo expansion of CTLs by antigen presenting cells[33]

SUMMARY

Understanding of the lymphoma tumor microenvironment is poised to expand in the era of next-generation sequencing studies of the tumor cells themselves. For example, in diffuse large B-cell lymphomas, loss-of-function mutations in B2M and CD58 as well as focal deletions in TNFSF9 have been demonstrated by RNA sequencing and exome sequencing.[34] B2M encodes a polypeptide β_2-microglobulin that helps form MHC class I. The latter functions to present antigens to cytotoxic T cells in immune surveillance activities. TNFSF9 is involved in antigen presentation while CD58 functions as a ligand to interact with T cells and natural killer cells. Targeting specific combinations of these escape strategies may lead to targeted reconstitution of antitumor immunity.

Novel therapeutics that take advantage of the tumor microenvironment include antiangiogenic drugs,[35] immune checkpoint blockade,[36] and mobilization of tumor cells away from their supportive niche.[37] A recent study used a combination of intratumoral CpG, which serves as an agonist for toll-like receptor 9, with systemic ibrutinib to activate surrounding natural killer cells and macrophages against the tumor. The investigators show that, in mice, the effectiveness of the therapy required an intact T-cell immune system.[38]

Successful therapies of the future will rely on deeper appreciation of the interactions between these elements of the microenvironment.

REFERENCES

1. Paget G. Remarks on a case of alternate partial anaesthesia. Br Med J 1889;1:1.
2. Kinsey DL. An experimental study of preferential metastasis. Cancer 1960;13:674.
3. Sandler A, Gray R, Perry MC, et al. Paclitaxel-carboplatin alone or with bevacizumab for non-small-cell lung cancer. N Engl J Med 2006;355:2542.
4. Hurwitz H, Fehrenbacher L, Novotny W, et al. Bevacizumab plus irinotecan, fluorouracil, and leucovorin for metastatic colorectal cancer. N Engl J Med 2004; 350:2335.
5. Sasada T, Kimura M, Yoshida Y, et al. CD4+CD25+ regulatory T cells in patients with gastrointestinal malignancies: possible involvement of regulatory T cells in disease progression. Cancer 2003;98:1089.
6. Yang ZZ, Novak AJ, Stenson MJ, et al. Intratumoral CD4+CD25+ regulatory T-cell-mediated suppression of infiltrating CD4+ T cells in B-cell non-Hodgkin lymphoma. Blood 2006;107:3639.
7. Bystry RS, Aluvihare V, Welch KA, et al. B cells and professional APCs recruit regulatory T cells via CCL4. Nat Immunol 2001;2:1126.
8. Lim HW, Hillsamer P, Banham AH, et al. Cutting edge: direct suppression of B cells by CD4+ CD25+ regulatory T cells. J Immunol 2005;175: 4180.
9. Yang ZZ, Novak AJ, Ziesmer SC, et al. Malignant B cells skew the balance of regulatory T cells and TH17 cells in B-cell non-Hodgkin's lymphoma. Cancer Res 2009;69:5522.
10. Steidl C, Shah SP, Woolcock BW, et al. MHC class II transactivator CIITA is a recurrent gene fusion partner in lymphoid cancers. Nature 2011;471:377.
11. Riemersma SA, Jordanova ES, Schop RF, et al. Extensive genetic alterations of the HLA region, including homozygous deletions of HLA class II genes in B-cell lymphomas arising in immune-privileged sites. Blood 2000;96:3569.
12. Chen BJ, Chapuy B, Ouyang J, et al. PD-L1 expression is characteristic of a subset of aggressive B-cell lymphomas and virus-associated malignancies. Clin Cancer Res 2013;19:3462.
13. Yang ZZ, Grote DM, Xiu B, et al. TGF-beta upregulates CD70 expression and induces exhaustion of effector memory T cells in B-cell non-Hodgkin's lymphoma. Leukemia 2014;28:1872.
14. Green MR, Monti S, Rodig SJ, et al. Integrative analysis reveals selective 9p24.1 amplification, increased PD-1 ligand expression, and further induction via JAK2 in nodular sclerosing Hodgkin

lymphoma and primary mediastinal large B-cell lymphoma. Blood 2010;116:3268.

15. Ravandi F, O'Brien S. Immune defects in patients with chronic lymphocytic leukemia. Cancer Immunol Immunother 2006;55:197.

16. Fecteau JF, Kipps TJ. Structure and function of the hematopoietic cancer niche: focus on chronic lymphocytic leukemia. Front Biosci (Schol Ed) 2012;4:61.

17. Paggetti J, Haderk F, Seiffert M, et al. Exosomes released by chronic lymphocytic leukemia cells induce the transition of stromal cells into cancer-associated fibroblasts. Blood 2015;126(9):1106–17.

18. Maffei R, Fiorcari S, Martinelli S, et al. Targeting neoplastic B cells and harnessing microenvironment: the "double face" of ibrutinib and idelalisib. J Hematol Oncol 2015;8:60.

19. Carreras J, Lopez-Guillermo A, Fox BC, et al. High numbers of tumor-infiltrating FOXP3-positive regulatory T cells are associated with improved overall survival in follicular lymphoma. Blood 2006;108:2957.

20. Tzankov A, Meier C, Hirschmann P, et al. Correlation of high numbers of intratumoral FOXP3+ regulatory T cells with improved survival in germinal center-like diffuse large B-cell lymphoma, follicular lymphoma and classical Hodgkin's lymphoma. Haematologica 2008;93:193.

21. Smeltzer JP, Jones JM, Ziesmer SC, et al. Pattern of CD14+ follicular dendritic cells and PD1+ T cells independently predicts time to transformation in follicular lymphoma. Clin Cancer Res 2014;20:2862.

22. Pangault C, Amé-Thomas P, Ruminy P, et al. Follicular lymphoma cell niche: identification of a preeminent IL-4-dependent T(FH)-B cell axis. Leukemia 2010;24:2080.

23. Dave SS, Wright G, Tan B, et al. Prediction of survival in follicular lymphoma based on molecular features of tumor-infiltrating immune cells. N Engl J Med 2004;351:2159.

24. Farinha P, Masoudi H, Skinnider BF, et al. Analysis of multiple biomarkers shows that lymphoma-associated macrophage (LAM) content is an independent predictor of survival in follicular lymphoma (FL). Blood 2005;106:2169.

25. Schmieder A, Michel J, Schonhaar K, et al. Differentiation and gene expression profile of tumor-associated macrophages. Semin Cancer Biol 2012;22:289.

26. Martin-Moreno AM, Roncador G, Maestre L, et al. CSF1R protein expression in reactive lymphoid tissues and lymphoma: its relevance in classical hodgkin lymphoma. PLoS One 2015;10:e0125203.

27. Scott DW, Gascoyne RD. The tumour microenvironment in B cell lymphomas. Nat Rev Cancer 2014;14:517.

28. Molin D, Fischer M, Xiang Z, et al. Mast cells express functional CD30 ligand and are the predominant CD30L-positive cells in Hodgkin's disease. Br J Haematol 2001;114:616.

29. Pinto A, Aldinucci D, Gloghini A, et al. Human eosinophils express functional CD30 ligand and stimulate proliferation of a Hodgkin's disease cell line. Blood 1996;88:3299.

30. Chemnitz JM, Eggle D, Driesen J, et al. RNA fingerprints provide direct evidence for the inhibitory role of TGFbeta and PD-1 on CD4+ T cells in Hodgkin lymphoma. Blood 2007;110:3226.

31. Kilger E, Kieser A, Baumann M, et al. Epstein-Barr virus-mediated B-cell proliferation is dependent upon latent membrane protein 1, which simulates an activated CD40 receptor. EMBO J 1998;17:1700.

32. Mancao C, Hammerschmidt W. Epstein-Barr virus latent membrane protein 2A is a B-cell receptor mimic and essential for B-cell survival. Blood 2007;110:3715.

33. Bollard CM, Gottschalk S, Leen AM, et al. Complete responses of relapsed lymphoma following genetic modification of tumor-antigen presenting cells and T-lymphocyte transfer. Blood 2007;110:2838.

34. Pasqualucci L, Trifonov V, Fabbri G, et al. Analysis of the coding genome of diffuse large B-cell lymphoma. Nat Genet 2011;43:830.

35. Stopeck AT, Unger JM, Rimsza LM, et al. A phase 2 trial of standard-dose cyclophosphamide, doxorubicin, vincristine, prednisone (CHOP) and rituximab plus bevacizumab for patients with newly diagnosed diffuse large B-cell non-Hodgkin lymphoma: SWOG 0515. Blood 2012;120:1210.

36. O'Mahony D, Morris JC, Quinn C, et al. A pilot study of CTLA-4 blockade after cancer vaccine failure in patients with advanced malignancy. Clin Cancer Res 2007;13:958.

37. Burger JA, Montserrat E. Coming full circle: 70 years of chronic lymphocytic leukemia cell redistribution, from glucocorticoids to inhibitors of B-cell receptor signaling. Blood 2013;121:1501.

38. Sagiv-Barfi I, Kohrt HE, Burckhardt L, et al. Ibrutinib enhances the antitumor immune response induced by intratumoral injection of a TLR9 ligand in mouse lymphoma. Blood 2015;125:2079.

Role of Flow Cytometry in the Diagnosis and Prognosis of Plasma Cell Myeloma

 CrossMark

Horatiu Olteanu, MD, PhD

KEYWORDS

- Flow cytometry • Myeloma • Plasma cells • MGUS • Minimal residual disease

ABSTRACT

This article provides an overview of the role of flow cytometry in the diagnosis and follow-up of plasma cell myeloma. A brief introduction to the general immunophenotypic features of normal and myeloma plasma cells is provided, followed by a discussion of technical issues as they relate to the application of flow cytometry in this entity. The prognostic and therapeutic utility of flow cytometric immunophenotyping in myeloma is also analyzed, with an emphasis on the growing role of minimal residual analysis as potential biomarker for evaluating treatment efficacy and for tailoring risk-adapted treatment, in prospective clinical trials.

Abbreviations

AL	Amyloid light chain
BMPC	Bone marrow plasma cell
CR	Complete response
CRAB	Hypercalcemia, renal insufficiency, anemia, bone lesions
FC	Flow cytometry
FS	Forward scatter
IMWG	International Myeloma Working Group
LPL	Lymphoplasmacytic lymphoma
MGUS	Monoclonal gammopathy of undetermined clinical significance
MM	Multiple myeloma
MRD	Minimal residual disease
MZL	Marginal zone lymphoma
NHL	Non-Hodgkin lymphoma
OS	Overall survival
PC	Plasma cell
PCM	Plasma cell myeloma
PFS	Progression-free survival
POEMS	Polyneuropathy, organomegaly, endocrinopathy, monoclonal plasma cell disorder, and skin changes
sFLCs	Serum free light chains
SMM	Smoldering multiple myeloma
SS	Side scatter
VGPR	Very good partial response
WHO	World Health Organization

Key Features

- During the past decade, a growing body of evidence has supported the role for flow cytometry (FC) in plasma cell myeloma (PCM), both at diagnosis and follow-up.

- Routine FC in myeloma requires careful consideration of several technical aspects related to plasma cell (PC) analysis.

- There are potential applications for FC in the differential diagnosis, prognosis, and treatment of PCM.

- Minimal residual disease (MRD) analysis by FC is a powerful predictor of outcome in myeloma in the clinical trial setting.

Disclosure Statement: The author has nothing to disclose.
Department of Pathology, Medical College of Wisconsin, 8701 Watertown Plank Road, Milwaukee, WI 53226, USA
E-mail address: holteanu@mcw.edu

Surgical Pathology 9 (2016) 101–116
http://dx.doi.org/10.1016/j.path.2015.09.009
1875-9181/16/$ – see front matter © 2016 Elsevier Inc. All rights reserved.

surgpath.theclinics.com

OVERVIEW

PCM or multiple myeloma (MM) is a common hematologic malignancy (10%–15% of hematopoietic neoplasms) and is defined by a triad of clinicopathologic criteria, including

1. The presence of a serum or urine monoclonal protein
2. The presence of a clonal PC population in the bone marrow (or plasmacytoma)
3. Disease-related end-organ or tissue impairment, usually summarized under the CRAB acronym:
   a. Hypercalcemia
   b. Renal insufficiency
   c. Anemia
   d. Bone lesions

and also including hyperviscosity, amyloidosis, or recurrent infections.

The current diagnostic criteria, as listed in the 2008 World Health Organization (WHO) classification of hematolymphoid neoplasms[1] and initially defined by the International Myeloma Working Group (IMWG) in 2003,[2] apply to symptomatic PCM (ie, requiring therapy) and have been used for the past decade in clinical practice and research trials.[3] The spectrum of PC neoplasms encompasses other entities, however, such as monoclonal gammopathy of undetermined clinical significance (MGUS); asymptomatic or smoldering MM (SMM); PC leukemia; solitary plasmacytoma; polyneuropathy, organomegaly, endocrinopathy, monoclonal plasma cell disorder, and skin changes (POEMS) syndrome; and systemic amyloid light chain amyloidosis.[1] From a clinical standpoint, it is postulated that PCM is almost always preceded by MGUS, which is present in 3% to 4% of the general population ages greater than 50 years[4,5] and has a rate of progression to PCM of approximately 1% per year.[6,7]

SMM is, by definition, an asymptomatic condition that constitutes an intermediate clinical phase between MGUS and PCM and has a higher risk of progression to myeloma (10% per year, during the first 5 years) compared with MGUS.[8]

Table 1 summarizes and compares the diagnostic criteria for PCM, SMM, and MGUS, as recently updated by the IMWG.[9,10] The rationale for updating these definitions is based on observations from several studies that a subset of patients with SMM showed a much higher progression risk to PCM, even in the absence of traditional CRAB features.[11–15] The introduction of these new myeloma-defining biomarkers (such as bone marrow plasma cells [BMPCs] ≥60%, involved:uninvolved serum free light chains [sFLCs] ratio ≥100, and MRI findings with more than 1 focal lesion) removes the need for documenting end-organ damage as an obligatory requirement for the definition of a neoplastic condition (PCM) and allows the identification of a cohort of SMM patients that may benefit from treatment initiation prior to the occurrence of irreversible end-organ damage. It is the recommendation of the IMWG that these criteria should be implemented in routine

---

Table 1
Revised International Myeloma Working Group diagnostic criteria for plasma cell myeloma, smoldering myeloma, and monoclonal gammopathy of undetermined clinical significance

Entity	Diagnostic Criteria	Progression Rate to Plasma Cell Myeloma

PCM	• Clonal bone marrow PCs ≥10% or biopsy-proved plasmacytoma
	• One or more myeloma-defining events:
	  ○ CRAB
	  ○ Clonal bone marrow PCs ≥60%
	  ○ Serum-free light chain ratio ≥100
	  ○ >1 Focal lesion on MRI scan
		N/A

MGUS (non-IgM)	Serum monoclonal protein <30 g/L Clonal bone marrow PCs <10% Absence of myeloma-defining events or amyloidosis	1% Per year
SMM	Serum monoclonal protein >30 g/L or Urine monoclonal protein ≥500 mg/24 h Clonal bone marrow PCs 10%–60% Absence of myeloma-defining events or amyloidosis	10% Per year (first 5 y)

Adapted from Rajkumar SV, Dimopoulos MA, Palumbo A, et al. International Myeloma Working Group updated criteria for the diagnosis of multiple myeloma. Lancet Oncol 2014;15:e541; and Rajkumar SV, Landgren O, Mateos MV. Smoldering multiple myeloma. Blood 2015;125:3070.

clinical practice and future trials.[9] Furthermore, it proposes the consideration of FC-based potential future biomarkers for the diagnosis of a PCM, such as high levels of circulating PC[16] and the presence of abnormal PC immunophenotype greater than or equal to 95% (in combination with immunoparesis).[17–19] With this background in mind, this review provides an overview of the diagnostic, prognostic, and therapeutic utility of flow cytometric immunophenotyping in PCM. In addition to discussing the rationale for the use of FC in this entity, a series of practical technical issue that may be encountered when analyzing normal and neoplastic PC is also covered.

DIAGNOSTIC UTILITY OF FLOW CYTOMETRY IN PLASMA CELL MYELOMA

FC is a powerful adjunct in the diagnostic work-up of hematologic malignancies and has a well-established role in the diagnosis and prognosis of leukemias and lymphomas. Although there are extensive literature data supporting the use of FC in PCM,[20–26] both at diagnosis and follow-up, its implementation in clinical practice may not be uniformly seen, due to several practical considerations.[27,28]

NORMAL VERSUS ABNORMAL PLASMA CELLS

When evaluating bone marrow specimens from patients with a clinical history or suspicion of PC dyscrasia, it is important to know the distinguishing immunophenotypic features between normal and clonal PCs. Unlike B-cell lymphoproliferative disorders, where evidence of clonality relies primarily on the demonstration of light chain restriction, for PCM and related disorders it is more important to detect an aberrant immunophenotype (in the presence or absence of distinct cytoplasmic light chain restriction), particularly in the MRD setting. By FC, PCs have been historically defined by their bright CD38 expression. Although normal PCs express CD38 at higher levels than any other normal nucleated marrow subsets, CD38 is not specific for PCs and is expressed by other maturing bone marrow elements (**Fig. 1**). Because myeloma cells tend to express CD38 at somewhat dimmer levels, CD138 has been recommended as a second antigen of PC identification.[22,24,29,30] This approach compensates for the relative nonspecificity of CD38 as a sole PC-defining marker, particularly in specimens that contain a low number of PCs. In addition to CD38 and CD138, a majority of normal PCs are positive for CD19 and CD45, are negative for

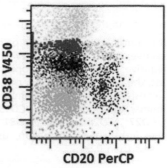

Fig. 1. CD38 expression on normal bone marrow subsets. PCs (*yellow*) show the brightest CD38 expression. Myeloblasts (*red*) and hematogones (*cyan*) also demonstrate uniform CD38 positivity, albeit at dimmer intensity compared with PCs. Additional populations that express CD38 (uniformly or on a subset of cells) include monocytes (*black*), T cells (*green*), or B lymphocytes (*blue*).

CD20 and CD56, and show polytypic cytoplasmic light chain expression, with a kappa:lambda immunoglobulin ratio ranging from 1 to 4. In addition, normal PCs express CD27 and CD81 and are predominantly lacking CD117, CD28, CD52, and CD200.[22,25,29,31–34] There are reports of minor subsets of normal PCs that are negative or dim for CD19, CD45, and CD27 and/or positive for CD20, CD28, CD56, and CD200,[24,29] which may potentially interfere with MRD analysis and the detection of very small populations of clonal and immunophenotypically aberrant PCs. The relative frequency of diagnostically useful antigen expression of myeloma cells is listed in **Table 2**.

Box 1 summarizes the most common features of normal and clonal PCs. Examples of common

Table 2
Frequency of immunophenotypic aberrancies in plasma cell myeloma. The list shows most relevant antigens and their most frequent expression patterns on myeloma cells

Antigen	Frequency of Expression
CD19[-]	~95%
CD20[+]	15%–20%
CD27[-]/dim positive	45%–65%
CD28[+]	15%–45%
CD45[-]	45%–80%
CD56[+]	75%
CD81[-]	45%–55%
CD117[+]	35%
CD200[+]	75%–80%

Box 1
Common immunophenotyptic features of normal and clonal plasma cells

The most common immunophenotype of normal PCs may be described as CD38 bright positive, CD138 bright positive, CD19⁺, CD20⁻, CD27 bright positive, CD28⁻, CD56⁻, CD81⁺, CD117⁻, CD200 predominantly negative, and polytypic cytoplasmic immunoglobulin.

In contrast, the typical immunophenotype of myeloma cells shows several deviations from the normal pattern, consisting of various combinations of immunophenotypic aberrancies, including CD38⁺ (often dimmer than normal PCs), CD138 bright positive, CD19⁻, CD20⁻ (may be positive in a subset of PCM), CD27⁻, CD28⁺, CD56⁺, CD81⁻, CD117⁻ (may be positive in a subset of PCM), CD200⁺, and monoclonal light chain expression, usually defined as a cytoplasmic kappa:lambda ratio greater than 5 or less than 0.5.

---

antigen expression patterns on normal and abnormal PCs are shown in **Fig. 2.**

Routine flow cytometric evaluation of PCM may be associated with several technical issues, which are described briefly. A separate set of technical aspects related to MRD analysis is discussed later.

GENERAL TECHNICAL ISSUES RELATED TO PLASMA CELL MYELOMA FLOW CYTOMETRY

It is well accepted that myeloma cells are generally under-represented in flow cytometric analyses compared with morphology-derived differential counts (**Box 2**).[20,24,35,36] The proportion of PCs

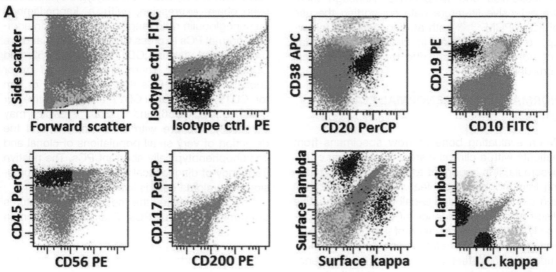

Fig. 2. Common antigen expression patterns in normal and abnormal PCs, shown in comparison with other bone marrow cell populations. (*A*) Normal PCs (*yellow*) are CD38 bright positive, CD19⁺, CD20⁻, CD45⁺, CD56⁻, CD117⁻, and CD200⁻; do not express surface immunoglobulin; and show polytypic intracytoplasmic (I.C.) light chain expression. Two other B-cell lineage populations are also illustrated: hematogones (*cyan*) and B-cell (*blue*). Hematogones express uniform and dimmer CD38 compared with PCs. An isotype control 2-D plot illustrates the high autofluorescence of PCs (shown for phycoerythrin [PE] and fluorescein isothiocyanate [FITC]), which may lead to overinterpretation of CD10 or CD56 expression on PCs in this case, if normal B cells were used as an internal negative control. (*B*) Myeloma cells (*red*) are CD38⁺, CD138⁺, CD19⁻, CD56⁻, CD45⁻, CD117⁺, CD200⁺, CD27⁻, and CD81⁻ and I.C. kappa light chain restricted. Normal B cells (*blue*) are also shown. (*C*) Coexistent normal (*yellow*) and abnormal (*red*) PC populations in a patient evaluated after autologous stem cell transplantation. There is also a significant population of hematogones (*cyan*) and normal B cells (*blue*) present in the bone marrow aspirate. Normal PCs that show brighter CD38 positivity compared with the neoplastic ones are CD19⁺, CD56⁻, CD45⁺, CD117⁻, CD81⁺, and CD27⁺; and express polytypic cytoplasmic light chains. The myeloma cells have an opposite immunophenotype and are I.C. kappa immunoglobulin restricted. Note the variable expression of CD138 on PCs (both normal and abnormal). Assessment of CD138 expression may be influenced by several technical issues, such as refrigeration, choice of lyse reagent, and bone marrow anticoagulant (heparin)—all these variables are known to lead to under-expression of this antigen on PCs by FC, as illustrated in this case. APC, allophycocyanin; ctrl, control; PerCP, peridinin chlorophyll protein.

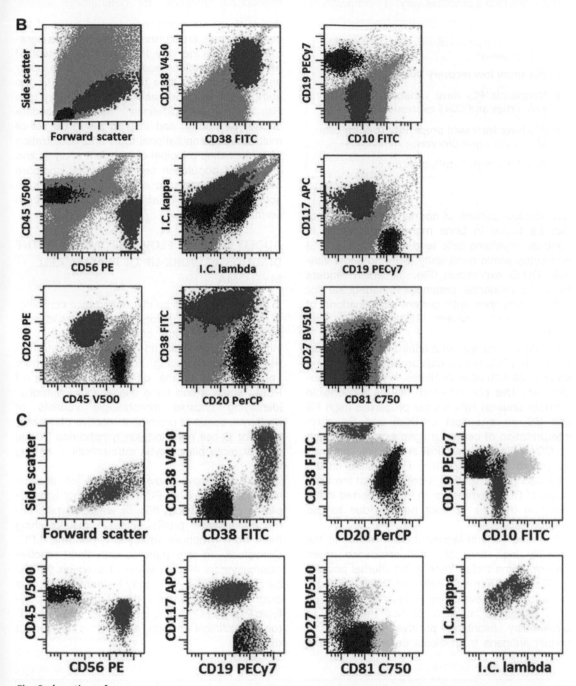

Fig. 2. (*continued*).

recovered by FC averages only one-third of those enumerated by morphology and may even be 1 order of magnitude lower. The factors responsible for this phenomenon are not entirely understood and possible causes are listed in **Box 3**.

Accurate quantification of BMPCs has prognostic value in the MRD setting, although there also are literature data on the prognostic value of flow cytometric enumeration of myeloma cells at

diagnosis compared with morphologic counts.[20] For practical purposes, however, the percentage of PCs used to establish a diagnosis of PCM is generated from morphology slides.

A second technical point relates to the variable light scatter and CD45 characteristics of PCs. In traditional FC data analysis, gating approaches using forward scatter (FS)/side scatter (SS) and CD45/SS 2-D plots offer a predictable and often

1. PCs show low recovery by FC

2. Neoplastic PCs have variable light scatter properties and CD45 expression.

3. PCs have increased propensity to form complexes with granulocytes.

4. PCs show high autofluorescence.

reproducible pattern of normal cell subsets that can be found in bone marrow specimens. In contrast, myeloma cells tend to vary in size (FS) and cytoplasmic complexity (SS) and show variable CD45 expression (**Fig. 3**), which renders these fluorescence parameters inadequate for gating compared with current combinations of recommended markers: CD38, CD138, and CD45.[24,29]

Related to this aspect is a third technical observation, that PCs have a high propensity to forming complexes with other cell types, in particular granulocytes. This phenomenon may be responsible for both unusual light scatter properties (high FS and SS on a subset of PCs) and for over-interpretation of certain antigen expression, such as CD45. From a practical standpoint, this may be evident when examining PC clusters on the CD45/SS plot (**Fig. 4**). It is possible that the wide range of CD45 expression in PCM reported in the literature may be at least partially due to this phenomenon.

The final general technical issue relates to the typically high level of autofluorescence noted with myeloma cells. When using internal populations, such as normal B cells and T cells, as negative controls for evaluating antigen expression on PCs, increased autofluorescence may lead to erroneously ascribing positive expression of certain antigens to myeloma cells. It is possible

that such an approach may explain some of the conflicting antigen expression data from the literature as well. One way to assess the extent of nonspecific autofluorescence in PCs is to apply an isotype control tube that includes CD38; the author uses this approach in the laboratory (see **Fig. 2A**). Current guidelines[24,29] do not mandate an isotype control and instead rely on a set of multivariate computational tools and visualization plots, including principal component analysis and automated population separators, that compare normal and neoplastic reference databases to achieve separation of aberrant populations from normal ones.[37,38]

ADDED VALUE OF FLOW CYTOMETRY IN THE DIAGNOSTIC WORK-UP OF PLASMA CELL MYELOMA

In general, PCM can be diagnosed by a combination of clinical, morphologic, radiologic, and laboratory criteria, and the contribution of FC in the initial evaluation is limited (**Box 4**). Flow cytometric immunophenotyping, however, plays a more important role in the differential diagnosis of PCM, where it can be a useful ancillary tool in identifying unusual morphologic variants of myeloma, cases of prominent reactive plasmacytosis, or B-cell non-Hodgkin lymphomas (NHLs) with extreme plasmacytic differentiation, among others.

As such, there may be cases of atypical morphology, such as PCM with distinct lymphoplasmacytoid cytology (**Fig. 5**), where a typical immunophenotypic profile helps in distinguishing them from lymphoplasmacytic lymphoma (LPL). Conversely, in rare patients with florid reactive plasmacytosis (**Fig. 6**) where, based on the PC percentage alone, PCM may be entertained as a diagnostic consideration, demonstration of polytypic PCs by FC, in conjunction with other laboratory and clinical findings, establishes the correct diagnosis.

1. Patchy, heterogeneous distribution of myeloma cells in the bone marrow

2. Relatively higher degree of hemodilution in the specimen processed for FC compared with the first-pull aspirate dedicated to morphology slides

3. Differential distribution of PCs in lipid-enriched particles in the morphology slides compared with the lipid-depleted liquid bone marrow aliquot analyzed by FC

4. Further loss during processing, staining, and acquisition on the flow cytometer, related to particular physical characteristics of myeloma cells, which render them potentially more susceptible to mechanical damage

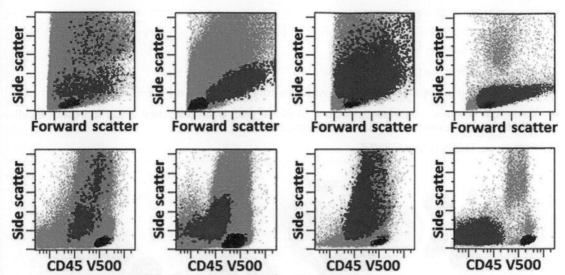

Fig. 3. Variable forward and SS characteristics (*top row*) and CD45 expression patterns (*bottom row*), corresponding cases, in myeloma PCs.

Perhaps more common is the situation of certain B-cell NHLs that may show extensive plasmacytic differentiation, usually seen with marginal zone lymphoma (MZL) and LPL. When the plasmacytic differentiation is as prominent as to raise the possibility of PCM, the distinction can be made by demonstrating 2 related clonal populations of B cells and PCs. FC is particularly adept at identifying even minor B cell clones that otherwise would be below the limit of detection of morphology or IHC. In addition to supporting a clonal relationship between the B-cell and PC components of NHLs with plasmacytic differentiation, FC offers immunophenotypic clues on the origin (PCM vs lymphoma) of the PCs. For practical purposes, positivity of CD19 in PCs was found the most helpful feature, because this antigen is expressed in only 5% of

PCM and 95% of NHL with plasmacytic differentiation[39–41] (**Fig. 7**).

A somewhat related issue may arise in the differential diagnosis of coexistent PC and B-cell populations with identical light chain expression detected in bone marrow specimens by morphology and FC. Although the most common situation is that of clonal relationship, as seen in NHL (LPL or MZL), there is also the possibility of a coincidental PCM or MGUS and an unrelated B-cell lymphoproliferative disorder. A recent study found that the identification of CD19[+], CD45[+] PCs in NHL and the presence of aneuploidy in PCM are the best discriminators in distinguishing B-cell NHLs with plasmacytic differentiation from PC neoplasms with an unrelated clonal B-cell process[42] (**Fig. 8**).

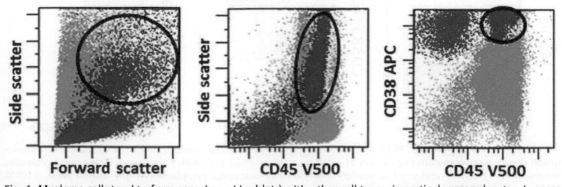

Fig. 4. Myeloma cells tend to form complexes (doublets) with other cell types, in particular granulocytes. In cases of distinct PC/granulocyte doublet formation, this particular subset may be readily discriminated from the main population of CD45[−] or dim positive myeloma cells (*circled areas*).

> **Box 4**
> **Applications of flow cytometry in the differential diagnosis of plasma cell dyscrasias**
>
> 1. Morphologic variants of PCM versus LPL
>
> 2. PCM versus florid reactive plasmacytosis
>
> 3. PCM versus low-grade B-cell lymphoma with extensive plasmacytic differentiation
>
> 4. Coexistent PCM and unrelated B-cell clone of similar light chain restriction versus low-grade B-cell lymphoma with extensive plasmacytic differentiation
>
> 5. PCM versus MGUS or SMM

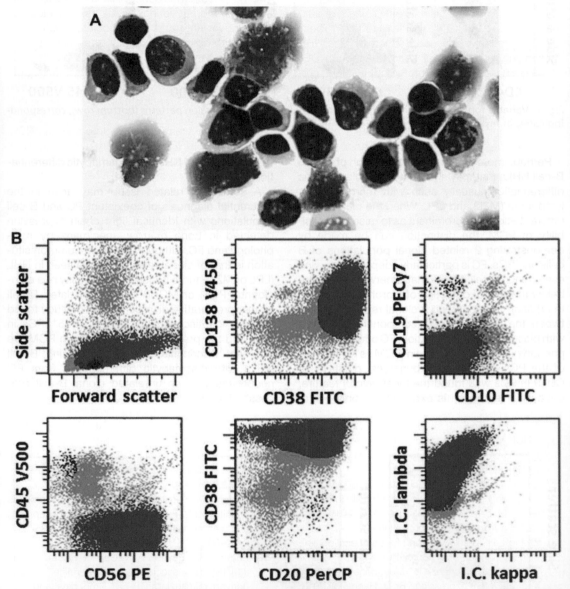

Fig. 5. Morphologic variant of PCM with distinct lymphoplasmacytoid cytology. (*A*) Flow cytospin microphotograph shows a predominant population of small to medium-sized cells with round nuclei, clumped chromatin, inconspicuous nucleoli, and small to moderate amounts of basophilic cytoplasm (Wright-Giemsa stain, ×1000). (*B*) Flow cytometric immunophenotyping showed an 83% population of aberrant PCs (*red*) that were CD38 bright positive, CD138+, CD19−, CD20 variably positive, CD45−, and CD56+ and intracytoplasmic lambda light chain restricted. Normal B cells (*blue*) are also shown. FITC, fluorescein isothiocyanate.

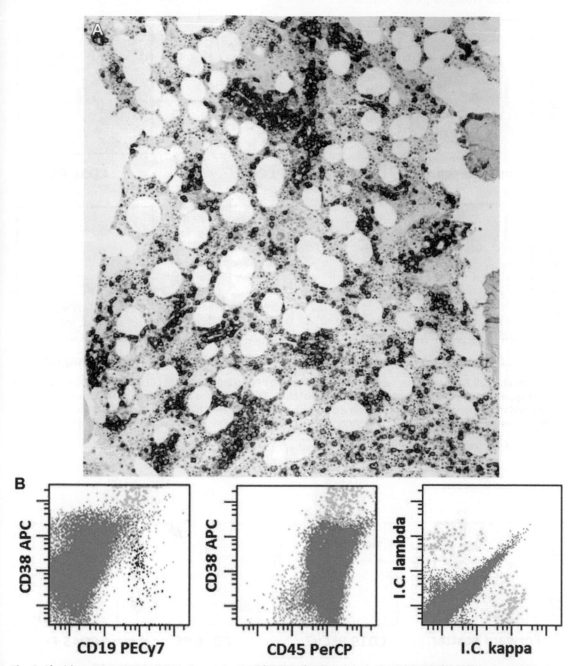

Fig. 6. Florid reactive plasmacytosis in a patient with HIV infection. (*A*) The core biopsy shows approximately 30% PCs by immunohistochemistry (CD138 immunohistochemistry, ×200). (*B*) FC demonstrates a population of normal PCs (*yellow*); B cells are shown in blue. APC, allophycocyanin; PECy7, phycoerythrin Cy7; PerCP, peridinin chlorophyll protein.

One area in which FC has generated interest is that of the differential diagnosis of MGUS and SMM versus PCM. Clonal PCs found in MGUS, SMM, and PCM are immunophenotypically aberrant and can be readily distinguished from normal ones, allowing their relative quantification by FC. As early as 1998, a study found the percentage of normal PCs, relative to total BMPCs, to be a significant parameter when trying to discriminate between MGUS and PCM.[43] That observation was based on greater than 3% normal PCs/BMPCs found in almost all MGUS cases but found in only less than 2% of PCMs. Later on, other investigators described a higher proportion of myelomas (14%) with greater than 5% normal PCs/BMPCs[44]; therefore, FC seems of limited practical

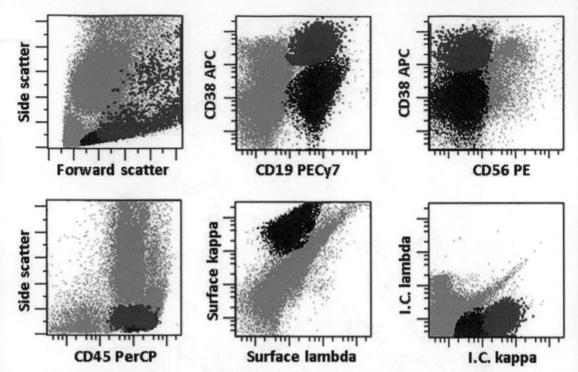

Fig. 7. Small B-cell NHL with plasmacytic differentiation. The PCs (*red*) are CD19⁺, CD45⁺, and CD56⁻ and show similar kappa light chain restriction to the clonal B cells (*blue*). The latter were also CD5⁻ and CD10⁻, and the patient had an IgM monoclonal protein, supporting a diagnosis of LPL. APC, allophycocyanin; FITC, fluorescein isothiocyanate; I.C., intracytoplasmic; PE, phycoerythrin; PECy7, phycoeytrhin Cyt; PerCP, peridinin chlorophyll protein.

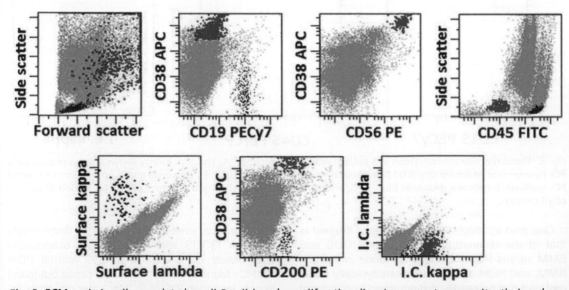

Fig. 8. PCM and clonally unrelated small B-cell lymphoproliferative disorder present concomitantly in a bone marrow biopsy. The PCs (*red*) are CD19⁻, CD56⁺, CD45⁻, and CD200⁺ and show the same kappa light chain restriction as the B cells (*blue*). The aberrant PC immunophenotype favors 2 unrelated processes, however, over an NHL with plasmacytic differentiation.

use in making a definite distinction between MGUS and PCM. The presence of a large (>95%) proportion of abnormal PCs/BMPCs, however, has been associated with a higher risk of progression of MGUS and SMM to PCM (discussed later).[17,19,45] From an immunophenotypic perspective, there is a similar prevalence of common antigen expression (CD19, CD56, CD20, CD45, and CD117) in clonal PCs from MGUS and PCM, with perhaps the exception of CD200, which in 1 study was found more frequently expressed in myeloma (73%) compared with MGUS (54%).[40]

Finally, several studies have looked at the predictive value of various immunophenotypic features for recurrent cytogenetic abnormalities in PCM. This is a topic of practical importance, because different genetic subgroups of myeloma are associated with different outcomes.[46–48] Investigators have reported associations of CD28 expression with t(14;16) and del(17p); lack of CD117 expression with t(4;14), del(13q), and nonhyperdiploid karyotype; and CD20 and CD23 expression with t(11;14), to name a few.[23,33,49–51] The clinical usefulness of these findings is limited, however, due to insufficient sensitivity and specificity.[24]

PROGNOSTIC UTILITY OF FLOW CYTOMETRY IN PLASMA CELL MYELOMA

Both qualitative and quantitative FC immunophenotypic features have been described relative to outcome in PCM (Box 5).

QUALITATIVE PROGNOSTIC PARAMETERS

In a large study of 685 newly diagnosed and uniformly treated patients, expression of CD19 and CD28 and lack of CD117 were associated with worse outcome (progression-free survival [PFS]

Box 5
Applications of flow cytometry in the prognosis of plasma cell dyscrasias

1. Qualitative prognostic markers
   a. CD19, CD28, CD45, CD56, CD81, CD117, and CD200
2. Quantitative prognostic markers
   a. Percentage of PCs (of total bone marrow cells)
   b. Percentage of clonal PCs (of bone marrow PCs)
   c. Normal circulating clonal PCs

---

and overall survival [OS]).[23] These findings allowed the separation of 3 distinct immunophenotypic risk groups: poor (CD28+/CD117−), intermediate (CD28+/CD117+ or CD28−/CD117−), and good (CD28−/CD117−), although the CD28/CD117 expression status lost its significance as an independent prognostic factor when cytogenetic information was added to multivariate analysis.

There are multiple reports on the prognostic significance of CD20, CD56, and CD45. Although some investigators have found that these markers carry no prognostic significance,[23] others have reported conflicting data with regard to CD45 and CD56. Specifically, lack of CD45 or CD56 expression in myeloma PCs has been demonstrated to be associated with a less favorable outcome.[52,53] Although the reasons for these discrepancies are not entirely clear, at least interpretation of CD45 data may be hampered by the broad range of CD45 expression in myeloma reported in the literature (20%–75%)[23,40,53–55]; this finding is likely the result of heterogeneous definitions and interpretations of positive antigen expression and variable gating approaches.

More recently, CD81 expression on PCs has been studied in PCM, MGUS, and SMM and was found to have both diagnostic and prognostic utility.[32,56,57] Dim to negative CD81 expression is found in approximately half of myeloma cases, and CD81 positivity has been identified as an independent prognostic factor for worse PFS and OS in a cohort of 230 patients.[32] Furthermore, because CD81 physiologically regulates CD19 expression in B cells, it is conceivable that CD81 expression is also linked in select cases to upregulation of CD19, which, in turn, has been identified as a prognostic marker associated with worse outcome in myeloma.[23]

The prognostic impact of CD200 expression in myeloma was the topic of several studies, and although there is no overall consensus, it seems that lack of CD200 was associated with a favorable outcome in most reports.[31,34,58]

QUANTITATIVE PROGNOSTIC PARAMETERS

The overall percentage of PCs (calculated as proportion of nucleated bone marrow cells) and the relative percentage of myeloma cells (reported as the proportion of BMPCs) were identified as quantitative FC parameters with prognostic significance. Despite the numerous variables implicated in the lower yield of PCs in flow cytometric analysis, 1 recent study found that the percentage of PCs generated by morphology and FC were both significant predictors of PFS and OS in univariate analysis, at cutoffs of 15% (by FC) and 30% (by morphology), respectively.[20] More surprisingly, only the FC enumeration of PCs maintained significance for OS in multivariate analysis, whereas the morphologic estimate was no longer significant.

Along the same lines, a relative higher proportion of normal PCs (>5% of BMPCs) at diagnosis has been associated with a better PFS and OS, in univariate analysis.[20] As discussed previously in this review, only a minority of PCMs (14% in this study[20]) show greater than 5% normal PCs, calculated as percentage of BMPCs, and typical diagnostic bone marrow biopsies from myeloma patients show few or no normal PCs.

In addition to the bone marrow compartment, there are data that the number of circulating PCs also have prognostic significance in PCM. Initial studies performed by immunofluorescent microscopy have identified a subset of patients with SMM and high levels of circulating PCs that had an elevated risk of progression within the first 2 to 3 years after diagnosis.[16] This approach was extended to flow cytometric quantitation of clonal circulating PCs and was able to stratify patients with newly diagnosed PCM in a higher risk group (with worse OS), based on a cutoff of greater than or equal to 400 clonal PCs.[59] Further data indicate that among patients with relapsing PCM, a higher number (≥100) of circulating clonal PCs may also predict for worse survival.[60]

MINIMAL RESIDUAL DISEASE ANALYSIS FLOW CYTOMETRY IN PLASMA CELL MYELOMA

In the near future, MRD analysis is the area where FC immunophenotyping is likely to exert the most impact in evaluating the effectiveness of new therapeutic drugs and in potentially identifying subsets of patients at risk for progression and in need of more intensive treatment.[27,29,61–65] PCM has well-defined and nuanced response criteria[3,66] (Table 3) and it is estimated that up to 33% of patients in complete response (CR) and 10% of those in near CR or very good partial response (VGPR) may be considered potentially cured (ie, relapse-free at 10-year follow-up).[67] These data prompt 2 observations. First, they imply that a better definition for CR is necessary, because 40% of patients with PCM in CR relapse, and 20% succumb to their disease within 4 years of initial treatment.[27] Second, accurate estimation of the depth of the response seems to correlate with better outcome in PCM, which supports the addition of MRD analysis to the definition of CR.[61,68]

MRD assessment in PCM can be performed by several methods, including FC, allele-specific oligonucleotide real-time quantitative polymerase chain reaction, next-generation sequencing, and PET/CT.[27] MRD monitoring by 4-color or 6-color FC was shown to be the most relevant prognostic factor when assessed in 2 large series of PCM patients.[21,61] The prognostic value of MRD assessment was demonstrated in those studies at different time points (preautologous and postautologous stem cell transplantation), and similar outcomes were noted outside the stem cell transplantation setting.[69] Furthermore, MRD status by FC maintained its prognostic value in patients with an unfavorable cytogenetic profile, and at least in 1 study showed benefit of more intensive treatment in MRD-positive patients.[21,63]

From a practical perspective, it is likely that clinical decision making should be based on the

---

Table 3
International Myeloma Working Group treatment response criteria in plasma cell myeloma

CR	<5% BMPCs Negative serum and urine immunofixation No soft tissue plasmacytomas
Stringent CR	CR criteria and the following: Normal sFLCs ratio No clonal BMPCs (documented by IHC or 2–4–color FC)
VGPR	Positive serum or urine immunofixation (but negative electrophoresis) ≥90% Reduction in serum monoclonal protein <100 mg/24-h urine monoclonal protein
Partial response	≥50% Reduction in serum monoclonal protein <200 mg/24-h urine monoclonal protein (or ≥90% reduction in urine 24-h monoclonal protein) ≥50% Reduction in sFLCs ratio (if serum or urine monoclonal protein is not measurable) ≥50% Reduction in BMPCs (if baseline BMPCs were ≥30%) ≥50% Reduction in the size of soft tissue plasmacytomas

Adapted from Refs.[3,56,66]

presence of MRD positivity (rather than the absence of MRD), because persistence of MRD has been shown to always be an adverse prognostic feature, even in PCM patients in CR. It is also envisioned that MRD may qualify as a biomarker to assess treatment efficacy at different stages (induction, transplantation, consolidation, and/or maintenance) and in the clinical trial setting, as a surrogate marker for OS. Currently, there are no guidelines that incorporate the use of MRD analysis in the routine clinical practice.

Because of its obvious potential benefits, there is a general and increased interest to advocate for the implementation of a standardized approach of performing MRD analysis by FC as a highly sensitive, cost-effective, and readily available technique.[27] From a clinical trial standpoint, the utilization of standardized FC MRD methods is more widespread in Europe than in the United States.[24,27–30,37,63] Some of the technical limitations related to routine FC analysis of PC also apply to MRD analysis, whereas others are specific to this particular technique.

For example, the clinically relevant threshold for MRD in PCM has been historically set at 0.01% (or 10^{-4}).[21,61] Because the level of sensitivity of published 4-color and 6-color FC assays was right at the required (10^{-4}) threshold for clinical relevance, many of the clinical studies evaluating this topic have typically reported results as either MRD positive or negative.[21,27,62] With the development of novel greater than or equal to 8-color antibody combinations, however, and the recognition of the prognostic value of MRD level reported as a continuous variable, current recommendations suggest a lower, clinically relevant threshold of 0.001% (or 10^{-5}).[27,29,61] For practical purposes, this requires transitioning from a conservative estimate of detecting a cluster of 20 abnormal PCs by collecting 200,000 events (for achieving a detection limit of 10^{-4}) to identifying populations of 30 to 50 myeloma cells in 3 to 5,000,000 events (for a lower limit of detection/limit of quantitation of 10^{-5}).

The choice of antibodies for MRD analysis has also been the subject of several consensus guidelines.[24,29,70] Current recommendations include CD38, CD138, CD45, CD19, and CD56 as surface markers to be simultaneously assessed, with CD117, CD27, and CD81 also described as the most useful in discriminating normal from abnormal PCs. Literature data provide evidence that these surface antibody combinations are effective in assessing MRD status in greater than 95% of cases, thus precluding the routine use of intracytoplasmic light chain analysis, although the latter may add value to select cases.

Finally, there is the issue of immunophenotypic variations occurring over time in myeloma cells and potentially compromising their detection, particularly in the MRD setting. Similar to other hematologic malignancies, PCs from patients with PCM have been shown to display immunophenotypic alterations when analyzed at different time points, including in antigens that are commonly assessed for MRD analysis (CD19, CD45, and CD56).[71] These variations in antigen expression were not dramatic, however, and thus less likely to compromise MRD analysis, particularly when using a reasonably flexible and robust approach.

UTILITY OF FLOW CYTOMETRY IN THERAPY-RELATED ISSUES IN PLASMA CELL MYELOMA

Immunotherapy holds great promise for the treatment of PCM as new therapeutic monoclonal antibodies have been developed against various surface PC molecules in recent years and are assessed in clinical trials.[72–75] These include antibodies recognizing CD38 and/or CD138, raising the possibility of interfering with the ability to detect PCs by FC. Several investigators have evaluated novel antibodies, such as CD54, CD229, CD307, and CD319, to assess their role in PC identification in the setting of specific immunotherapy.[70,73] Of these, CD229 seems the most promising in replacing CD38 as a potential marker for identifying PCs in patient treated with anti-CD38 monoclonal antibodies.

REFERENCES

1. McKenna RW, Kyle RA, Kuehl WM, et al. Plasma cell neoplasms. In: Swerdlow SH, Campo E, Harris NL, et al, editors. WHO classification of tumours of haematopoietic and lymphoid tissue. 4th edition. Lyon (France): IARC; 2008. p. 200–13.
2. International Myeloma Working Group. Criteria for the classification of monoclonal gammopathies, multiple myeloma and related disorders: a report of the International Myeloma Working Group. Br J Haematol 2003;121:749–57.
3. Kyle RA, Rajkumar SV. Criteria for diagnosis, staging, risk stratification and response assessment of multiple myeloma. Leukemia 2009;23:3–9.
4. Kyle RA, Therneau TM, Rajkumar SV, et al. Prevalence of monoclonal gammopathy of undetermined significance. N Engl J Med 2006;354:1362–9.
5. Dispenzieri A, Katzmann JA, Kyle RA, et al. Prevalence and risk of progression of light-chain monoclonal gammopathy of undetermined significance: a retrospective population-based cohort study. Lancet 2010;375:1721–8.

6. Kyle RA, Therneau TM, Rajkumar SV, et al. A long-term study of prognosis in monoclonal gammopathy of undetermined significance. N Engl J Med 2002; 346:564–9.

7. Turesson I, Kovalchik SA, Pfeiffer RM, et al. Monoclonal gammopathy of undetermined significance and risk of lymphoid and myeloid malignancies: 728 cases followed up to 30 years in Sweden. Blood 2014;123:338–45.

8. Kyle RA, Remstein ED, Therneau TM, et al. Clinical course and prognosis of smoldering (asymptomatic) multiple myeloma. N Engl J Med 2007;356:2582–90.

9. Rajkumar SV, Dimopoulos MA, Palumbo A, et al. International Myeloma Working Group updated criteria for the diagnosis of multiple myeloma. Lancet Oncol 2014;15:e538–48.

10. Rajkumar SV, Landgren O, Mateos MV. Smoldering multiple myeloma. Blood 2015;125:3069–75.

11. Rajkumar SV, Larson D, Kyle RA. Diagnosis of smoldering multiple myeloma. N Engl J Med 2011;365: 474–5.

12. Kastritis E, Terpos E, Moulopoulos L, et al. Extensive bone marrow infiltration and abnormal free light chain ratio identifies patients with asymptomatic myeloma at high risk for progression to symptomatic disease. Leukemia 2013;27:947–53.

13. Larsen JT, Kumar SK, Dispenzieri A, et al. Serum free light chain ratio as a biomarker for high-risk smoldering multiple myeloma. Leukemia 2013;27: 941–6.

14. Hillengass J, Fechtner K, Weber MA, et al. Prognostic significance of focal lesions in whole-body magnetic resonance imaging in patients with asymptomatic multiple myeloma. J Clin Oncol 2010;28:1606–10.

15. Kastritis E, Moulopoulos LA, Terpos E, et al. The prognostic importance of the presence of more than one focal lesion in spine MRI of patients with asymptomatic (smoldering) multiple myeloma. Leukemia 2014;28:2402–3.

16. Bianchi G, Kyle RA, Larson DR, et al. High levels of peripheral blood circulating plasma cells as a specific risk factor for progression of smoldering multiple myeloma. Leukemia 2013;27:680–5.

17. Perez-Persona E, Vidriales MB, Mateo G, et al. New criteria to identify risk of progression in monoclonal gammopathy of uncertain significance and smoldering multiple myeloma based on multiparameter flow cytometry analysis of bone marrow plasma cells. Blood 2007;110:2586–92.

18. Mateos MV, Hernandez MT, Giraldo P, et al. Lenalidomide plus dexamethasone for high-risk smoldering multiple myeloma. N Engl J Med 2013;369: 438–47.

19. Perez-Persona E, Mateo G, Garcia-Sanz R, et al. Risk of progression in smouldering myeloma and monoclonal gammopathies of unknown significance: comparative analysis of the evolution of monoclonal

20. Paiva B, Vidriales MB, Perez JJ, et al. Multiparameter flow cytometry quantification of bone marrow plasma cells at diagnosis provides more prognostic information than morphological assessment in myeloma patients. Haematologica 2009;94: 1599–602.

21. Paiva B, Vidriales MB, Cervero J, et al. Multiparameter flow cytometric remission is the most relevant prognostic factor for multiple myeloma patients who undergo autologous stem cell transplantation. Blood 2008;112:4017–23.

22. Paiva B, Almeida J, Perez-Andres M, et al. Utility of flow cytometry immunophenotyping in multiple myeloma and other clonal plasma cell-related disorders. Cytometry B Clin Cytom 2010;78:239–52.

23. Mateo G, Montalban MA, Vidriales MB, et al. Prognostic value of immunophenotyping in multiple myeloma: a study by the PETHEMA/GEM cooperative study groups on patients uniformly treated with high-dose therapy. J Clin Oncol 2008;26:2737–44.

24. Rawstron AC, Orfao A, Beksac M, et al. Report of the European Myeloma Network on multiparametric flow cytometry in multiple myeloma and related disorders. Haematologica 2008;93:431–8.

25. Raja KR, Kovarova L, Hajek R. Review of phenotypic markers used in flow cytometric analysis of MGUS and MM, and applicability of flow cytometry in other plasma cell disorders. Br J Haematol 2010;149: 334–51.

26. Frebet E, Abraham J, Genevieve F, et al. A GEIL flow cytometry consensus proposal for quantification of plasma cells: application to differential diagnosis between MGUS and myeloma. Cytometry B Clin Cytom 2011;80:176–85.

27. Paiva B, van Dongen JJ, Orfao A. New criteria for response assessment: role of minimal residual disease in multiple myeloma. Blood 2015;125:3059–68.

28. Keeney M, Halley JG, Rhoads DD, et al. Marked variability in reported minimal residual disease lower level of detection of 4 hematolymphoid neoplasms: a survey of participants in the College of American Pathologists flow cytometry proficiency testing program. Arch Pathol Lab Med 2015;139:1276–80.

29. Arroz M, Came N, Lin P, et al. Consensus guidelines on plasma cell myeloma minimal residual disease analysis and reporting. Cytometry B Clin Cytom 2015. [Epub ahead of print].

30. Stetler-Stevenson M, Paiva B, Stoolman L, et al. Consensus guidelines for myeloma minimal residual disease sample staining and data acquisition. Cytometry B Clin Cytom 2015. [Epub ahead of print].

31. Olteanu H, Harrington AM, Hari P, et al. CD200 expression in plasma cell myeloma. Br J Haematol 2011;153:408–11.

32. Paiva B, Gutierrez NC, Chen X, et al. Clinical significance of CD81 expression by clonal plasma cells in high-risk smoldering and symptomatic multiple myeloma patients. Leukemia 2012;26:1862–9.

33. Bataille R, Pellat-Deceunynck C, Robillard N, et al. CD117 (c-kit) is aberrantly expressed in a subset of MGUS and multiple myeloma with unexpectedly good prognosis. Leuk Res 2008;32:379–82.

34. Alapat D, Coviello-Malle J, Owens R, et al. Diagnostic usefulness and prognostic impact of CD200 expression in lymphoid malignancies and plasma cell myeloma. Am J Clin Pathol 2012;137:93–100.

35. Smock KJ, Perkins SL, Bahler DW. Quantitation of plasma cells in bone marrow aspirates by flow cytometric analysis compared with morphologic assessment. Arch Pathol Lab Med 2007;131:951–5.

36. Cogbill CH, Spears MD, vanTuinen P, et al. Morphologic and cytogenetic variables affect the flow cytometric recovery of plasma cell myeloma cells in bone marrow aspirates. Int J Lab Hematol 2015. [Epub ahead of print].

37. van Dongen JJ, Lhermitte L, Bottcher S, et al. EuroFlow antibody panels for standardized n-dimensional flow cytometric immunophenotyping of normal, reactive and malignant leukocytes. Leukemia 2012;26: 1908–75.

38. Costa ES, Pedreira CE, Barrena S, et al. Automated pattern-guided principal component analysis vs expert-based immunophenotypic classification of B-cell chronic lymphoproliferative disorders: a step forward in the standardization of clinical immunophenotyping. Leukemia 2010;24:1927–33.

39. Seegmiller AC, Xu Y, McKenna RW, et al. Immunophenotypic differentiation between neoplastic plasma cells in mature B-cell lymphoma vs plasma cell myeloma. Am J Clin Pathol 2007;127:176–81.

40. Olteanu H, Harrington AM, Kroft SH. CD200 expression in plasma cells of nonmyeloma immunoproliferative disorders: clinicopathologic features and comparison with plasma cell myeloma. Am J Clin Pathol 2012;138:867–76.

41. Morice WG, Chen D, Kurtin PJ, et al. Novel immunophenotypic features of marrow lymphoplasmacytic lymphoma and correlation with Waldenstrom's macroglobulinemia. Mod Pathol 2009;22:807–16.

42. Rosado FG, Morice WG, He R, et al. Immunophenotypic features by multiparameter flow cytometry can help distinguish low grade B-cell lymphomas with plasmacytic differentiation from plasma cell proliferative disorders with an unrelated clonal B-cell process. Br J Haematol 2015;169:368–76.

43. Ocqueteau M, Orfao A, Almeida J, et al. Immunophenotypic characterization of plasma cells from monoclonal gammopathy of undetermined significance patients. Implications for the differential diagnosis between MGUS and multiple myeloma. Am J Pathol 1998;152:1655–65.

44. Paiva B, Vidriales MB, Mateo G, et al. The persistence of immunophenotypically normal residual bone marrow plasma cells at diagnosis identifies a good prognostic subgroup of symptomatic multiple myeloma patients. Blood 2009;114:4369–72.

45. Olteanu H, Wang HY, Chen W, et al. Immunophenotypic studies of monoclonal gammopathy of undetermined significance. BMC Clin Pathol 2008;8:13.

46. Palumbo A, Avet-Loiseau H, Oliva S, et al. Revised international staging system for multiple myeloma: a report from International Myeloma Working Group. J Clin Oncol 2015;33(26):2863–9.

47. Fonseca R, Bergsagel PL, Drach J, et al. International Myeloma Working Group molecular classification of multiple myeloma: spotlight review. Leukemia 2009;23:2210–21.

48. Fonseca R, Barlogie B, Bataille R, et al. Genetics and cytogenetics of multiple myeloma: a workshop report. Cancer Res 2004;64:1546–58.

49. Mateo G, Castellanos M, Rasillo A, et al. Genetic abnormalities and patterns of antigenic expression in multiple myeloma. Clin Cancer Res 2005;11:3661–7.

50. Walters M, Olteanu H, Van Tuinen P, et al. CD23 expression in plasma cell myeloma is specific for abnormalities of chromosome 11, and is associated with primary plasma cell leukaemia in this cytogenetic sub-group. Br J Haematol 2010;149:292–3.

51. Buonaccorsi JN, Kroft SH, Harrington AM, et al. Clinicopathologic analysis of the impact of CD23 expression in plasma cell myeloma with t(11;14)(q13;q32). Ann Diagn Pathol 2011;15:385–8.

52. Sahara N, Takeshita A, Shigeno K, et al. Clinicopathological and prognostic characteristics of CD56-negative multiple myeloma. Br J Haematol 2002; 117:882–5.

53. Moreau P, Robillard N, Avet-Loiseau H, et al. Patients with CD45 negative multiple myeloma receiving high-dose therapy have a shorter survival than those with CD45 positive multiple myeloma. Haematologica 2004;89:547–51.

54. Morice WG, Hanson CA, Kumar S, et al. Novel multiparameter flow cytometry sensitively detects phenotypically distinct plasma cell subsets in plasma cell proliferative disorders. Leukemia 2007;21:2043–6.

55. Lin P, Owens R, Tricot G, et al. Flow cytometric immunophenotypic analysis of 306 cases of multiple myeloma. Am J Clin Pathol 2004;121:482–8.

56. Tembhare PR, Yuan CM, Venzon D, et al. Flow cytometric differentiation of abnormal and normal plasma cells in the bone marrow in patients with multiple myeloma and its precursor diseases. Leuk Res 2014;38:371–6.

57. Paiva B, Paino T, Sayagues JM, et al. Detailed characterization of multiple myeloma circulating tumor cells shows unique phenotypic, cytogenetic, functional, and circadian distribution profile. Blood 2013;122:3591–8.

58. Moreaux J, Hose D, Reme T, et al. CD200 is a new prognostic factor in multiple myeloma. Blood 2006; 108:4194–7.
59. Gonsalves WI, Rajkumar SV, Gupta V, et al. Quantification of clonal circulating plasma cells in newly diagnosed multiple myeloma: implications for redefining high-risk myeloma. Leukemia 2014;28:2060–5.
60. Gonsalves WI, Morice WG, Rajkumar V, et al. Quantification of clonal circulating plasma cells in relapsed multiple myeloma. Br J Haematol 2014; 167:500–5.
61. Rawstron AC, Gregory WM, de Tute RM, et al. Minimal residual disease in myeloma by flow cytometry: independent prediction of survival benefit per log reduction. Blood 2015;125:1932–5.
62. Paiva B, Puig N, Garcia-Sanz R, et al. Is this the time to introduce minimal residual disease in multiple myeloma clinical practice? Clin Cancer Res 2015; 21:2001–8.
63. Rawstron AC, Pavia B, Stetler-Stevenson M. Assessment of minimal residual disease in myeloma and the need for a consensus approach. Cytometry B Clin Cytom 2015. [Epub ahead of print].
64. Gormley NJ, Turley DM, Dickey JS, et al. Regulatory perspective on minimal residual disease flow cytometry testing in multiple myeloma. Cytometry B Clin Cytom 2015. [Epub ahead of print].
65. Paiva B, Chandia M, Puig N, et al. The prognostic value of multiparameter flow cytometry minimal residual disease assessment in relapsed multiple myeloma. Haematologica 2015;100:e53–5.
66. Durie BG, Harousseau JL, Miguel JS, et al. International uniform response criteria for multiple myeloma. Leukemia 2006;20:1467–73.
67. Martinez-Lopez J, Blade J, Mateos MV, et al. Long-term prognostic significance of response in multiple myeloma after stem cell transplantation. Blood 2011; 118:529–34.
68. Martinez-Lopez J, Lahuerta JJ, Pepin F, et al. Prognostic value of deep sequencing method for minimal residual disease detection in multiple myeloma. Blood 2014;123:3073–9.
69. Puig N, Sarasquete ME, Balanzategui A, et al. Critical evaluation of ASO RQ-PCR for minimal residual disease evaluation in multiple myeloma. A comparative analysis with flow cytometry. Leukemia 2014;28:391–7.
70. Flores-Montero J, de Tute R, Paiva B, et al. Immunophenotype of normal vs. myeloma plasma cells: toward antibody panel specifications for MRD detection in multiple myeloma. Cytometry B Clin Cytom 2015. [Epub ahead of print].
71. Spears MD, Olteanu H, Kroft SH, et al. The immunophenotypic stability of plasma cell myeloma by flow cytometry. Int J Lab Hematol 2011;33:483–91.
72. Raje N, Longo DL. Monoclonal antibodies in multiple myeloma come of age. N Engl J Med 2015;373(13): 1264–6.
73. Pojero F, Flores-Montero J, Sanoja L, et al. Utility of CD54, CD229, and CD319 for the identification of plasma cells in patients with clonal plasma cell diseases. Cytometry B Clin Cytom 2015. [Epub ahead of print].
74. Lokhorst HM, Plesner T, Laubach JP, et al. Targeting CD38 with Daratumumab monotherapy in multiple myeloma. N Engl J Med 2015;373(13):1207–19.
75. Lonial S, Dimopoulos M, Palumbo A, et al. Elotuzumab therapy for relapsed or refractory multiple myeloma. N Engl J Med 2015;373:621–31.

Immunoglobulin G4–Related Lymphadenopathy

Christine E. Bookhout, MD, Marian A. Rollins-Raval, MD, MPH*

KEYWORDS

- IgG4 • IgG4-related disease • Lymphadenopathy • Lymphoma • Immunohistochemistry

ABSTRACT

Immunoglobulin G4–related lymphadenopathy (IgG4-RLAD) occurs in the setting of extranodal IgG4-related disease (IgG4-RD), an immune-mediated process described in many organ systems characterized by lymphoplasmacytic infiltrates with abundant IgG4-positive plasma cells and fibrosis. Although the morphologic features in the lymph node sometimes resemble those seen at the extranodal sites, 5 microscopic patterns have been described, most of which resemble reactive lymphoid hyperplasia. This morphologic variability leads to unique diagnostic challenges and a broad differential diagnosis. As IgG4-RD may be exquisitely responsive to steroids or other immunotherapy, histologic recognition and inclusion of IgG4-RLAD in the differential diagnosis is vital.

Key Features

- Immunoglobulin G4–related lymphadenopathy (IgG4-RLAD), for which 5 main microscopic patterns have been described in association with increased IgG4-positive plasma cells, is seen before, concurrently with, and subsequent to a diagnosis of IgG4-related disease.

- The significance of reactive lymph nodes with increased IgG4-positive plasma cells is not clear, but the finding should be correlated with clinical features, serum IgG4 levels, and subsequent tissue evaluations.

- The differential diagnosis for this disease includes both reactive and neoplastic conditions, many of which have distinct prognoses and treatment courses, making it essential to exclude them when considering a lymph node with features of IgG4-RLAD.

OVERVIEW

Immunoglobulin G (IgG) comprises approximately 80% of total serum immunoglobulin, with 4 recognized subclasses related to variation in the γ heavy chain. The subclasses are named in order of prevalence, with IgG4 generally the least prevalent, accounting for less than 5% of total IgG in a healthy person.[1,2] IgG4-related disease (IgG4-RD) is a rapidly emerging pathologic entity that can lead to dysfunction of many organ systems, including the pancreas, biliary tree, salivary glands, periorbital tissues, lungs, kidneys, meninges, aorta, breast, prostate, thyroid, pericardium, and skin.[2]

IgG4-RD was first recognized in the context of extrapancreatic lesions and elevated IgG4 levels in patients with sclerosing autoimmune pancreatitis, also known as type 1 autoimmune pancreatitis, in the early 2000s.[3] Subsequently, several other disease entities have come under the umbrella of IgG4-RD. One is Mikulicz disease, characterized by submandibular, parotid, and lacrimal gland swelling, which was once considered a variant of Sjogren disease.[4] Other entities include Kuttner tumor (submandibular swelling), Reidel thyroiditis (fibrosing autoimmune thyroiditis), sclerosing aortitis, and inflammatory abdominal aortitis, retroperitoneal fibrosis, steroid-responsive

Disclosure Statement: The authors have nothing to disclose.
Department of Pathology and Laboratory Medicine, University of North Carolina, Campus Box 7525, Brinkhous-Bullitt Building, Chapel Hill, NC 27599-7525, USA
* Corresponding author.
E-mail address: Marian_Raval@med.unc.edu

Surgical Pathology 9 (2016) 117–129
http://dx.doi.org/10.1016/j.path.2015.09.005
1875-9181/16/$ – see front matter © 2016 Elsevier Inc. All rights reserved.

sclerosing cholangitis, orbital pseudotumor, and other inflammatory pseudotumors (including kidney, brain, lung, breast, and lymph nodes).[5,6]

IgG4-RD is a rare entity that most often occurs in older men. The estimated incidence in Japan for diagnosis of autoimmune pancreatitis is 0.28 to 1.08 per 100,000,[7] which likely underestimates the true incidence of all IgG4-RD. Incidence in other parts of the world is less well defined. However, because malignancy may be in the differential diagnosis for IgG4-RD, diagnostic accuracy is critical. IgG4-related lymphadenopathy (IgG4-RLAD) is lymphadenopathy that occurs in the setting of extranodal IgG4-RD.[8] In addition, an increasing number of case reports have been published associating IgG4-RD with hematologic malignancies, or showing elevated IgG4 expression in certain neoplasms, especially lymphoma.[9]

CLINICAL PRESENTATION AND GROSS FEATURES

The clinical presentation of IgG4-RLAD is variable. Incidentally involved regional lymph nodes may be noted in an excision specimen for extranodal IgG4-RD. Similarly, the patient may have extranodal disease, but simultaneously be found to have lymphadenopathy on clinical examination or imaging. Alternatively, a patient may present with extranodal disease and then develop lymphadenopathy after weeks to years. Finally, lymphadenopathy may present as the first manifestation of disease or in isolation.[8]

Symptoms of IgG4-RLAD generally result from mass effect of the enlarged nodes. Although individual nodes are typically no more than 1 to 3 cm in diameter, they can grow as large as 5 cm. Several groups of lymph nodes are usually involved, which may include the cervical, supraclavicular, mediastinal, hilar, intra-abdominal, axillary, and inguinal nodes.[10–12] The lymphadenopathy is usually nontender.

When excised, the lymph nodes generally show an intact capsule, although fibrotic thickening may occasionally be present.[13] The nodes are enlarged and the texture can range from rubbery to firm and fibrotic. The cut surface is tan-white and relatively homogeneous, generally without significant hemorrhage or necrosis, similar to a reactive lymph node. No gross features have been described for IgG4-RLAD, which specifically distinguishes it from reactive lymph nodes.

MICROSCOPIC FEATURES

In general, extranodal IgG4-RD shares similar histopathology. Usually, there are diffuse lymphoplasmacytic infiltrates with abundant IgG4-positive plasma cells, as well as tissue eosinophilia. Extensive fibrosis and sclerosis, often with a storiform pattern (whorling or "cartwheel" arrangement of cells), is commonly present. Obliterative phlebitis and arteritis are frequently identified, with narrowing or obliteration of the vessel lumen by a dense infiltrate of lymphocytes and plasma cells.[5,7,11,12,14,15]

Cheuk and Chan[8] describe 5 generally accepted microscopic patterns of IgG4-RLAD, all of which demonstrate increased IgG4 positivity. Many of these patterns show overlapping features, the common finding with all of these reactive-appearing patterns is increased plasma cells, often accompanied by increased eosinophils (**Fig. 1**).

The first is similar to multicentric, or plasma cell variant, Castleman disease, and demonstrates intact nodal architecture, including follicles, some hyperplastic as well as some regressed germinal centers with penetration by venules. Many plasma cells and increased endothelial venules may be present in the interfollicular zones, as well as possible scattered eosinophils. The second pattern is follicular hyperplasia, which is characterized by noncrowded follicles surrounded by discrete mantles containing germinal centers with a starry-sky appearance, characteristic of reactive follicles. Mature plasma cells are present in some germinal centers, as well as often increased in the interfollicular zones. Scattered eosinophils also may be present in the interfollicular areas. A third pattern is interfollicular expansion. In this group, follicles are less prominent, including some that may appear regressed with penetration of venules, with marked expansion of the interfollicular zone. A mixed cellular composition, with small lymphocytes, plasma cells, transformed cells (including immunoblasts), and eosinophils, is generally seen, as are numerous high-endothelial venules. The fourth subtype has an appearance of progressive transformation of germinal centers, notable for reactive follicles as well as larger "transformed" follicles with thickened, irregular mantles and distorted germinal centers. The interfollicular zone has a mixed cellular composition, including plasma cells and eosinophils. Last is the inflammatory pseudotumorlike pattern, involving replacement of lymph nodes by sclerotic tissue with variable infiltration of lymphocytes, plasma cells, and eosinophils. The collagen may show a storiform pattern similar to that seen in IgG4-RD of other organs.

Rare cases of IgG4-RLAD have been described with formation of perifollicular granulomas involving reactive follicles surrounded by a wreath

Fig. 1. The patterns of IgG4-related lymphadenopathy. (*A*) Type 1: Multicentric Castleman disease variant showing sheets of plasma cells in the interfollicular areas, regressed follicles with penetrating venules, but lacking the typical eosinophilia (hematoxylin-eosin [H&E], original magnification ×100). (*B*) Type 2: Follicular hyperplasia showing numerous reactive follicles with well-defined mantle zones (H&E, original magnification ×20). (*C, D*) Type 3: Interfollicular expansion showing increased numbers of transformed lymphocytes, plasma cells, eosinophils, and high-endothelial venules (H&E, original magnification ×40 and ×100, respectively).

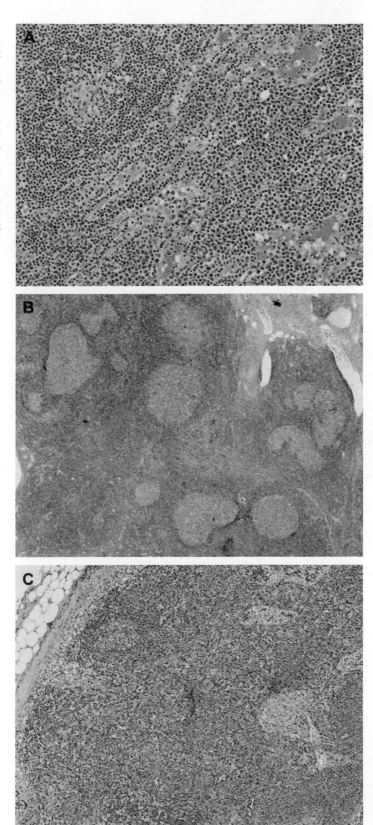

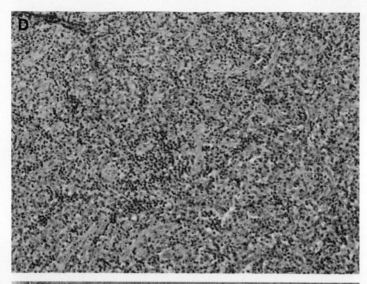

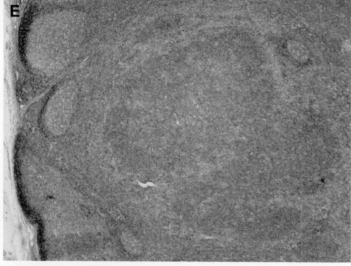

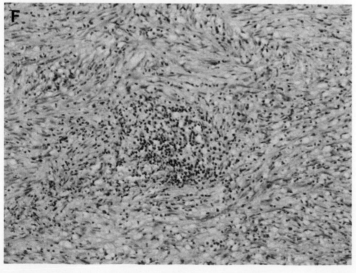

Fig. 1. (*continued*). (*E*) Type 4: Progressively transformed germinal centers (H&E, original magnification ×20). (*F*) Type 5: Inflammatory pseudotumor with spindled fibrosis, scattered plasma cells and small lymphoctyes (H&E, original magnification ×100).

of epithelioid histiocytes and multinucleated giant cells. Coagulative necrosis, epithelioid granulomas, and significant neutrophilic infiltration, however, are generally not features characteristic of IgG4-RLAD.[16] In general, the fibrosis and obliterative phlebitis characteristic of IgG4-RD at other sites are not prominent in lymph nodes.[10,15]

DIAGNOSIS

Serum IgG4 levels should be measured in patients in whom clinical or pathologic suspicion exists for IgG4-RD, and are often, but not always, elevated. This measurement is generally performed by automated nephelometry for total IgG and its subclasses. Normal levels of IgG4 are approximately 8 to 140 mg/dL. One study assessing the value of serum IgG4 in the diagnosis of autoimmune pancreatitis found that mild elevations can be seen in controls (less than twofold); however, higher elevations greater than twofold (>280 mg/dL) are quite specific for autoimmune pancreatitis (99%), but only 53% sensitive.[17] A more recent study assessed 190 patients with elevated IgG4 and 190 patients with normal levels, and found a sensitivity of 90% but a specificity of only 60% for IgG4-RD at a cutoff of 135 mg/dL. When the cutoff for IgG4 was doubled to 270 mg/dL, it improved specificity (91%), but greatly decreased sensitivity to 35%.[18] IgG4 concentrations can be normal in up to 40% to 50% of patients with biopsy-proven, active IgG4-RD.[15,19] Overall, an elevation in serum IgG4 can be helpful in assisting in making the diagnosis of IgG4-RD, but does not appear to have sufficient sensitivity or specificity to stand on its own as an independent diagnostic criterion.

Measurement of circulating plasmablast levels by flow cytometry, gating on CD19[low]CD38+CD20-CD27+ cells, shows promise for diagnosis of IgG4-RD. Marked elevations are noted in active IgG4-RD, even in those patients with normal serum IgG4 levels.[19–21]

The diagnosis for IgG4-RD is based primarily on tissue biopsy demonstrating the morphologic features described previously. For IgG4-RLAD, Cheuk and Chan[8] recommend testing for IgG4 by immunohistochemistry in reactive-appearing lymph nodes when IgG4-RD is a diagnostic consideration. An increase in IgG4-positive cells with an IgG4/total IgG ratio of greater than 40% has become an important diagnostic criterion for this disease. Recommendations for absolute number of IgG4-positive plasma cells for diagnosis vary by organ, with a recent consensus guideline considering more than 100 cells per high-power field (HPF) to be highly suggestive of IgG4-RLAD.[10,15] In isolation, however, neither increased

IgG4-positive cells nor increased serum IgG4 concentration is specific for the diagnosis, and correlation with specific histopathologic and clinical findings is essential.[22–24] Furthermore, other specific entities, such as Castleman disease and Rosai-Dorfman disease, should be considered and excluded before making a diagnosis of IgG4-RD (see Differential Diagnosis section later in this article).

Pathologic Key Features

Clinical

- Tumorlike enlargement of lymph nodes
- Usually nontender and involving multiple nodal groups
- May be associated with extranodal sclerosing disease

Gross

- Lymph node enlargement usually mild (1–3 cm), although can be up to 5 cm
- Texture ranges from rubbery to firm and fibrotic
- White-tan cut surface without hemorrhage or necrosis

Histologic

- IgG4-related lymphadenopathy (IgG4-RLAD) often lacks fibrosis and obliterative phlebitis seen in extranodal IgG4-related disease (IgG4-RD)
- Five patterns described in IgG4-RLAD
  1. Multicentric Castleman diseaselike
  2. Follicular hyperplasia
  3. Interfollicular expansion
  4. Progressive transformation of germinal centers
  5. Inflammatory pseudotumorlike
- Increase in IgG4-positive cells, with IgG4/total IgG ratio of greater than 40%, and greater than 100 IgG4-positive plasma cells per high-power field, is an important diagnostic criterion
- Coagulative necrosis, epithelioid granulomas, and significant neutrophilic infiltration are not expected

In a patient *with* known IgG4-RD, characteristic gross and microscopic findings as described previously in the lymph node, together with increased polytypic IgG4-positive plasma cells, can be diagnosed as IgG4-RLAD (Fig. 2). In a patient *without* IgG4-RD, a diagnosis can be made of reactive lymphoid hyperplasia with increased IgG4-positive cells (Fig. 3). These cases should include a comment stating that in a patient with systemic lymphadenopathy, these findings are more likely to represent IgG4-RLAD. In addition, correlation with the serologic IgG4 levels (as well as other emerging markers) and clinical follow-up, as some patients may develop subsequent extranodal involvement by IgG4-RD. However, at the current time the significance of these findings is unclear.[8,9]

Pitfalls

! Elevated serum IgG4 levels are not optimally sensitive or specific for IgG4-related disease

! On biopsy, increased IgG4/IgG ratios can be a nonspecific finding

! IgG4-related lymphadenopathy most often lacks the fibrosis and obliterative phlebitis characteristic of IgG4 disease at other sites

! Lymphomas can arise in association with IgG4-related disease or may express IgG4

DIFFERENTIAL DIAGNOSIS

Major differential diagnostic considerations for IgG4-RLAD include Castleman disease, Rosai-Dorfman syndrome, sarcoidosis, inflammatory pseudotumor, reactive lymphadenopathy, and malignancy, especially lymphoma.

The distinction between IgG4-RLAD and multicentric Castleman disease can be difficult due to overlapping histologic features. The former generally presents with mild to moderate lymph node enlargement and no constitutional symptoms, although anemia can be present, whereas the latter often is associated with malaise, fever, weight loss, skin rashes, and hepatosplenomegaly. IgG4-RD generally has increased serum IgG, IgE, and occasionally elevated erythrocyte sedimentation rate, but not IgA, IgM, interleukin-6, or C-reactive protein, all of which are commonly elevated in multicentric Castleman disease.[16,25,26] In Castleman disease, the germinal centers may be smaller and more regressive and lack eosinophil infiltration.[16,25] A significant increase in IgG4-positive plasma cells is also rare in multicentric Castleman disease, although it has been

reported.[26] Last, multicentric Castleman disease may have human herpesvirus-8–positive cells, especially in human immunodeficiency virus–associated cases. Making the correct diagnosis is imperative because IgG4-RD is generally steroid-responsive with a relatively benign clinical course, whereas multicentric Castleman disease is associated with significant mortality.[8,10,27]

Rosai-Dorfman disease, or sinus histiocytosis with massive lymphadenopathy, can show increased IgG4-positive plasma cells[28,29]; however, this disease predominantly affects younger patients rather than middle-aged or elderly patients. Additionally, biopsy findings of large, distinctive, S100-positive histiocytes are characteristic of this condition, and are not a feature of IgG4-RD.[30] Although some investigators have proposed that at least some cases of Rosai-Dorfman disease may represent part of the spectrum of IgG4-RD,[29] others feel that the 2 conditions are distinct, with Rosai-Dorfman disease having fewer IgG4-positive plasma cells and lower IgG4/IgG ratios.[28]

Although cases of IgG4-RD with generalized or hilar lymphadenopathy may resemble sarcoidosis by imaging and clinical evaluation, the biopsy findings of well-formed, non-necrotizing epithelioid granulomas expected in sarcoidosis are not characteristic of IgG4-RD. However, in rare cases of IgG4-RD with granulomatous inflammation, sarcoidosis may be a diagnostic consideration.[8] Serum angiotensin-converting enzyme levels are often elevated in sarcoidosis, whereas increases in serum IgG4 are often seen in IgG4-RD.

Inflammatory pseudotumor, or inflammatory myofibroblastic tumor, also may be in the differential for IgG4-RLAD, given that inflammatory pseudotumorlike pattern is one of the 5 described by Cheuk and Chan[8] and may show microscopic findings similar to the pattern seen in extranodal sites of IgG4-RD. However, inflammatory pseudotumor should show admixed anaplastic lymphoma kinase–positive cells. In addition, elevated IgG4 serum levels and IgG4-positive plasma cells have not been reported to be increased in inflammatory pseudotumor.

Reactive lymphadenopathy can show histologic patterns similar to several of those described in IgG4-RLAD, including follicular hyperplasia, interfollicular expansion, and progressive transformation of germinal centers. In most cases, neither increased IgG4-positive plasma cells (IgG4/total IgG ratio >40%) nor increased serum IgG4 concentration are present.[10] If a case of isolated lymphadenopathy is found to have increased IgG4-positive cells without other organ involvement characteristic of IgG4-RD, experts have

Fig. 2. IgG4-RLAD from a patient with known diagnosis of IgG4-RD. (*A*) Follicular hyperplasia (type 2) pattern (H&E, original magnification ×100). (*B*) Increased number of IgG-positive plasma cells (IgG immunohistochemistry [IHC], original magnification ×400). (*C*) IgG4-positive cells comprise greater than 40% of IgG-positive cells and greater than 100 cells per ×400 high-power field (IgG4 IHC, original magnification ×400).

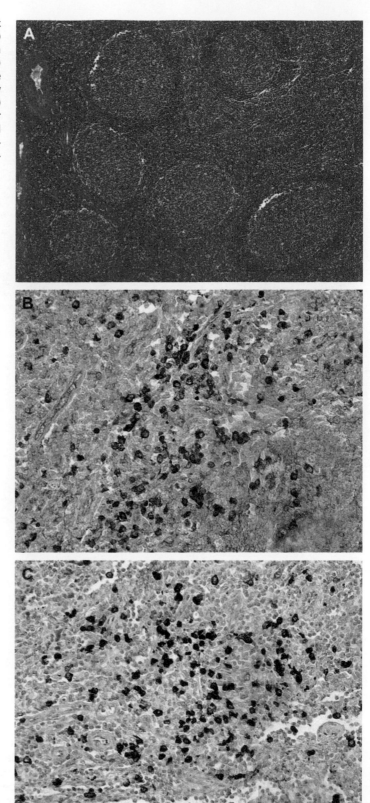

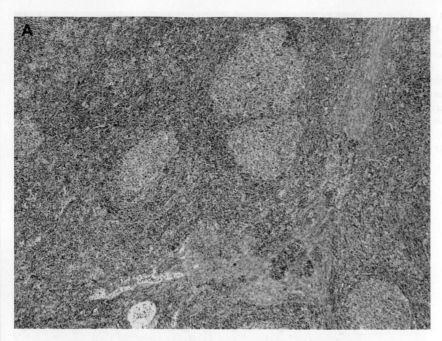

Fig. 3. (*A*) Patient 1 presented with cervical adenopathy that was biopsied and showed a reactive lymph node with follicular hyperplasia (H&E, original magnification ×40). (*B*) The lymph node from patient 1 shows focally increased IgG4-positive cells in germinal centers greater than 100 cells/HPF (IgG4 IHC, original magnification ×40).

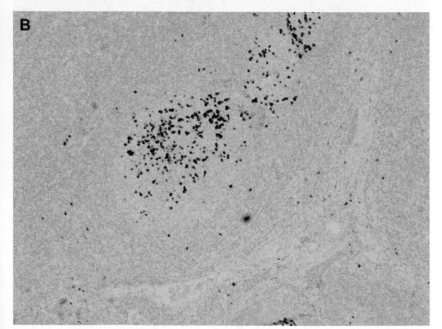

suggested giving a diagnosis only of reactive lymphoid hyperplasia with increased IgG4-positive cells along with a comment stating that the significance of this finding is unclear, but should be correlated with the clinical features and serologic studies.[8,9]

The distinction between IgG4-RLAD and lymphoma rests mostly on morphologic features and clonality studies, either by immunophenotyping or molecular studies. In general, effacement of the node by a monomorphic population of lymphoid cells and/or presence of a monotypic B or plasma cell population, by immunohistochemistry or molecular studies, should suggest lymphoma. Sato and colleagues[31] describe an IgG4-producing B-cell lymphoma with

Fig. 3. (*continued*). (*C*) Patient 2 presented with cervical adenopathy and showed atypical lymphoid hyperplasia with features of plasma cell variant Castleman disease (H&E, original magnification ×100). (*D*) Patient 2 showed numerous IgG4-positive plasma cells greater than 100/HPF (IgG4 IHC, original magnification ×40). Neither patient had a diagnosis of IgG4-RD, so for both a diagnosis of a lymph node with reactive features including increased IgG4-positive cells was rendered.

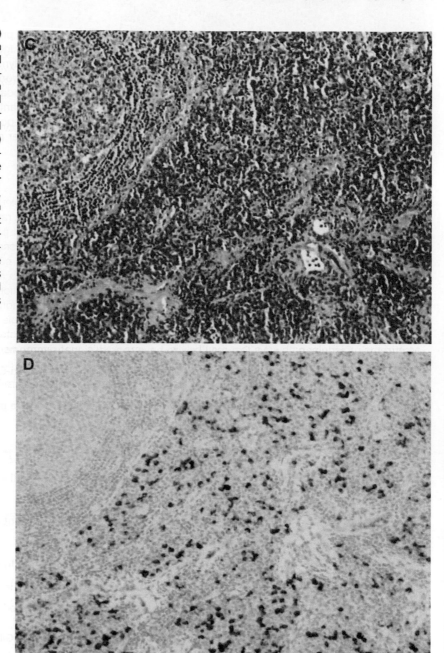

plasmacytic differentiation in a 72-year-old man with retroperitoneal lymphadenopathy; however, typically most lymphocytes in IgG4-RD are T cells rather than B cells. This latter observation highlights another potential diagnostic challenge between the interfollicular expansion pattern of IgG4-RLAD and angioimmunoblastic T-cell lymphoma, both of which can show architectural distortion, increased vascularity, and a mixed cellular population. In angioimmunoblastic T-cell lymphoma, clonal CD10-positive atypical T cells with irregular nuclei, scattered Epstein-Barr virus–positive lymphoid cells, as well as expanded CD21-positive follicular dendritic cell meshworks should be present, without a marked increase in IgG4/IgG ratio.[16,25]

Increasing numbers of case reports are appearing in the literature showing IgG4-positive lymphomas. Many are mucosa-associated lymphoid tissue lymphoma arising in the background of IgG4-RD of the head and neck.[32–35] A case of mantle cell lymphoma has been described in association with Mikulicz syndrome.[36] In addition, a significant percentage of dural marginal zone lymphomas and cutaneous marginal zone lymphomas have been shown to produce IgG4 without a known association with IgG4-RD.[37,38] The association of IgG4-RD and lymphoma, as well as the significance of IgG4 production by lymphomas, both nodal and extranodal, will require additional and larger studies for clarification.[39,40] In the presence of increased IgG4-positive cells, the possibility of lymphoma or other malignancy needs to be excluded.

△△	*Differential Diagnosis*
IgG4-Related Lymphadenopathy vs:	**Helpful Distinguishing Features**
Multicentric Castleman disease (MCD)	• MCD more likely to have constitutional symptoms • Elevated immunoglobulin (Ig)A, IgM, interleukin-6, and C-reactive protein (versus IgG and IgE in IgG4-related disease) • Rare to have significant increase in IgG4-positive plasma cells • May have human herpesvirus-8–positive cells • Less steroid responsive with higher mortality
Rosai-Dorfman syndrome	• Predominantly young patients rather than middle-aged to elderly • Distinctive S100-positive histiocytes on biopsy • May have increased IgG4-positive plasma cells but generally lower IgG4/IgG ratios
Sarcoidosis	• Well-formed, non-necrotizing epithelioid granulomas are characteristic • Elevated serum angiotensin-converting enzyme levels • No increase in IgG4-positive plasma cells expected
Inflammatory pseudotumor	• May appear similar to microscopic findings in IgG4-related disease (IgG4-RD) • Anaplastic lymphoma kinase positive • No increase in IgG4-positive plasma cells or serum IgG4
Reactive lymphadenopathy	• May show similar histologic patterns (follicular hyperplasia, interfollicular expansion, progressive transformation of germinal centers) • No increase in IgG4-positive plasma cells or serum IgG4 expected
Malignancy	• Effacement of node by monomorphic lymphoid population • Monoclonal population present (versus polyclonal plasma cells in IgG4-related lymphadenopathy) • Often B cells (versus IgG4-RD mostly T cells)

PROGNOSIS

IgG4-RD is generally steroid responsive, and initial therapy consists of glucocorticoids, such as prednisone. Most patients respond within several weeks, with reduced size of the tumorlike swelling of affected organs, improvements in organ functions, and decreases in serum levels of IgG4. There are patients who respond more slowly, requiring months of therapy, or those who have little to no response. It is possible that some of these patients may have more pronounced fibrosis and sclerosis that has become irreversible.[41]

Treatment should be initiated in patients who are symptomatic from disease; however, in those with mild lymphadenopathy or incidentally detected organ involvement without symptoms, no immediate treatment may be required. Therapy is generally initiated at a higher steroid dose, then tapered with the goal of very low-dose maintenance steroid therapy or eventual discontinuation of therapy.[12,41]

In patients who do not respond to steroids sufficiently or who do not remain in remission after dose tapering, rituximab, a monoclonal antibody against CD20, may be used for B-cell depletion. In small case series, this therapy has led to a rapid decline in serum IgG4 concentrations, with often striking clinical improvement within a few weeks.[42–44] Rituximab therapy has proven to be effective even in patients not being treated with glucocorticoids, with a 97% response rate in one study of 30 patients.[44] Serum IgG4 concentrations decrease with relative preservation of other immunoglobulin subclasses, suggesting that rituximab therapy depletes the B-lymphocytes responsible for replenishing the short-lived IgG4-secreting plasma cells.[42]

The often swift and marked response to treatment in IgG4-RD, if therapy is initiated before dense fibrosis and sclerosis develop, is characteristic and can prove diagnostically helpful. It also suggests that long-term prognosis is likely to be relatively favorable, although most patients experience chronic disease with relapses and variable rates of progression. Because the recognition of IgG4-RD as a distinct entity occurred relatively recently, long-term studies of prognosis are not

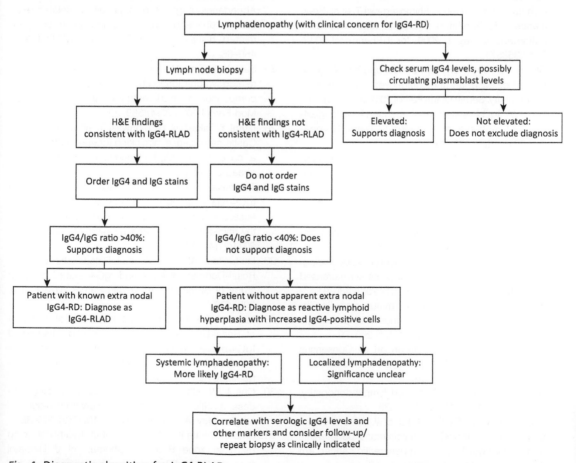

Fig. 4. Diagnostic algorithm for IgG4-RLAD.

yet available. Although further study is indicated, treatment and prognosis of the cases of malignancies associated with IgG4-RD likely mirror similar cases that are not associated with IgG4 (Fig. 4).

REFERENCES

1. Sigal LH. Basic science for the clinician 58: IgG subclasses. J Clin Rheumatol 2012;18(6):316–8.
2. Stone JH, Zen Y, Deshpande V. IgG4-related disease. N Engl J Med 2012;366(6):539–51.
3. Okazaki K, Uchida K, Miyoshi H, et al. Recent concepts of autoimmune pancreatitis and IgG4-related disease. Clin Rev Allergy Immunol 2011;41(2):126–38.
4. Takahashi H, Yamamoto M, Tabeya T, et al. The immunobiology and clinical characteristics of IgG4 related diseases. J Autoimmun 2012;39(1–2):93–6.
5. Khosroshahi A, Deshpande V, Stone JH. The clinical and pathological features of IgG(4)-related disease. Curr Rheumatol Rep 2011;13(6):473–81.
6. Furukawa S, Moriyama M, Kawano S, et al. Clinical relevance of Kuttner tumour and IgG4-related dacryoadenitis and sialoadenitis. Oral Dis 2015;21(2): 257–62.
7. Uchida K, Masamune A, Shimosegawa T, et al. Prevalence of IgG4-related disease in Japan based on nationwide survey in 2009. Int J Rheumatol 2012; 2012:358371.
8. Cheuk W, Chan JK. Lymphadenopathy of IgG4-related disease: an underdiagnosed and overdiagnosed entity. Semin Diagn Pathol 2012;29(4):226–34.
9. Ferry JA. IgG4-related lymphadenopathy and IgG4-related lymphoma: moving targets. Diagn Histopathol 2013;19(4):128–39.
10. Cheuk W, Yuen HK, Chu SY, et al. Lymphadenopathy of IgG4-related sclerosing disease. Am J Surg Pathol 2008;32(5):671–81.
11. Mahajan VS, Mattoo H, Deshpande V, et al. IgG4-related disease. Annu Rev Pathol 2014;9:315–47.
12. Kamisawa T, Zen Y, Pillai S, et al. IgG4-related disease. Lancet 2015;385(9976):1460–71.
13. Grimm KE, Barry TS, Chizhevsky V, et al. Histopathological findings in 29 lymph node biopsies with increased IgG4 plasma cells. Mod Pathol 2012;25(3):480–91.
14. Inoue D, Zen Y, Abo H, et al. Immunoglobulin G4-related lung disease: CT findings with pathologic correlations. Radiology 2009;251(1):260–70.
15. Deshpande V, Zen Y, Chan JK, et al. Consensus statement on the pathology of IgG4-related disease. Mod Pathol 2012;25(9):1181–92.
16. Sato Y, Yoshino T. IgG4-related lymphadenopathy. Int J Rheumatol 2012;2012:572539.
17. Ghazale A, Chari ST, Smyrk TC, et al. Value of serum IgG4 in the diagnosis of autoimmune pancreatitis and in distinguishing it from pancreatic cancer. Am J Gastroenterol 2007;102(8):1646–53.
18. Carruthers MN, Khosroshahi A, Augustin T, et al. The diagnostic utility of serum IgG4 concentrations in IgG4-related disease. Ann Rheum Dis 2015;74(1): 14–8.
19. Wallace ZS, Deshpande V, Mattoo H, et al. IgG4-related disease: clinical and laboratory features in 125 patients. Arthritis Rheum 2015;67(9): 2466–75.
20. Mattoo H, Mahajan VS, Della-Torre E, et al. De novo oligoclonal expansions of circulating plasmablasts in active and relapsing IgG4-related disease. J Allergy Clin Immunol 2014;134(3):679–87.
21. Wallace ZS, Mattoo H, Carruthers M, et al. Plasmablasts as a biomarker for IgG4-related disease, independent of serum IgG4 concentrations. Ann Rheum Dis 2015;74(1):190–5.
22. Rollins-Raval MA, Felgar RE, Krasinskas AM, et al. Increased numbers of IgG4-positive plasma cells may rarely be seen in lymph nodes of patients without IgG4-related sclerosing disease. Int J Surg Pathol 2012;20(1):47–53.
23. Cotta CV, Hsi ED. IgG4+ plasma cells in isolated reactive lymphadenopathy. Am J Clin Pathol 2014; 142(4):432–4.
24. Martinez LL, Friedlander E, van der Laak JA, et al. Abundance of IgG4+ plasma cells in isolated reactive lymphadenopathy is no indication of IgG4-related disease. Am J Clin Pathol 2014;142(4): 459–66.
25. Sato Y, Kojima M, Takata K, et al. Systemic IgG4-related lymphadenopathy: a clinical and pathologic comparison to multicentric Castleman's disease. Mod Pathol 2009;22(4):589–99.
26. Izumi Y, Takeshita H, Moriwaki Y, et al. Multicentric Castleman disease mimicking IgG4-related disease: a case report. Mod Rheumatol 2014;1–4 [Epub ahead of print].
27. Takenaka K, Takada K, Kobayashi D, et al. A case of IgG4-related disease with features of Mikulicz's disease, and retroperitoneal fibrosis and lymphadenopathy mimicking Castleman's disease. Mod Rheumatol 2011;21(4):410–4.
28. Liu L, Perry AM, Cao W, et al. Relationship between Rosai-Dorfman disease and IgG4-related disease: study of 32 cases. Am J Clin Pathol 2013;140(3): 395–402.
29. Menon MP, Evbuomwan MO, Rosai J, et al. A subset of Rosai-Dorfman disease cases show increased IgG4-positive plasma cells: another red herring or a true association with IgG4-related disease? Histopathology 2014;64(3):455–9.
30. Cheuk W, Chan JK. IgG4-related sclerosing disease: a critical appraisal of an evolving clinicopathologic entity. Adv Anat Pathol 2010;17(5):303–32.
31. Sato Y, Takata K, Ichimura K, et al. IgG4-producing marginal zone B-cell lymphoma. Int J Hematol 2008;88(4):428–33.

32. Sato Y, Ohshima K, Ichimura K, et al. Ocular adnexal IgG4-related disease has uniform clinicopathology. Pathol Int 2008;58(8):465–70.

33. Sato Y, Ohshima K, Takata K, et al. Ocular adnexal IgG4-producing mucosa-associated lymphoid tissue lymphoma mimicking IgG4-related disease. J Clin Exp Hematop 2012;52(1):51–5.

34. Mulay K, Aggarwal E. IgG4-related dacryoadenitis evolving into an extra-nodal, marginal zone B-cell lymphoma (EMZL): a tale of two lacrimal glands. Pathology 2014;46(5):464–6.

35. Cheuk W, Yuen HK, Chan AC, et al. Ocular adnexal lymphoma associated with IgG4+ chronic sclerosing dacryoadenitis: a previously undescribed complication of IgG4-related sclerosing disease. Am J Surg Pathol 2008;32(8):1159–67.

36. Krishnamurthy A, Shah A, Ganesan P, et al. Mantle cell lymphoma presenting as Mikulicz syndrome. J Cancer Res Ther 2011;7(3):372–5.

37. Venkataraman G, Rizzo KA, Chavez JJ, et al. Marginal zone lymphomas involving meningeal dura: possible link to IgG4-related diseases. Mod Pathol 2011;24(3):355–66.

38. Brenner I, Roth S, Puppe B, et al. Primary cutaneous marginal zone lymphomas with plasmacytic differentiation show frequent IgG4 expression. Mod Pathol 2013;26(12):1568–76.

39. Ferry JA, Deshpande V. IgG4-related disease in the head and neck. Semin Diagn Pathol 2012;29(4): 235–44.

40. Stone JH, Khosroshahi A, Deshpande V, et al. Recommendations for the nomenclature of IgG4-related disease and its individual organ system manifestations. Arthritis Rheum 2012;64(10):3061–7.

41. Khosroshahi A, Stone JH. Treatment approaches to IgG4-related systemic disease. Curr Opin Rheumatol 2011;23(1):67–71.

42. Khosroshahi A, Bloch DB, Deshpande V, et al. Rituximab therapy leads to rapid decline of serum IgG4 levels and prompt clinical improvement in IgG4-related systemic disease. Arthritis Rheum 2010; 62(6):1755–62.

43. Khosroshahi A, Carruthers MN, Deshpande V, et al. Rituximab for the treatment of IgG4-related disease: lessons from 10 consecutive patients. Medicine 2012;91(1):57–66.

44. Carruthers MN, Topazian MD, Khosroshahi A, et al. Rituximab for IgG4-related disease: a prospective, open-label trial. Ann Rheum Dis 2015;74(6): 1171–7.

T-cell Lymphomas
Updates in Biology and Diagnosis

Sarah L. Ondrejka, DO, Eric D. Hsi, MD*

KEYWORDS

- T-cell lymphoma • Non-Hodgkin lymphoma • T-cell lymphoma subtypes
- Pathobiology • Anaplastic large cell lymphoma • Peripheral T-cell lymphoma
- Angioimmunoblastic T-cell lymphoma • Nodal • T-follicular helper cells

ABSTRACT

Nodal-based peripheral T-cell lymphomas are heterogeneous malignancies with overlapping morphology and clinical features. However, the current World Health Organization classification scheme separates these tumors into prognostically relevant categories. Since its publication, efforts to uncover the gene expression profiles and molecular alterations have subdivided these categories further, and distinct subgroups are emerging with specific profiles that reflect the cell of origin for these tumors and their microenvironment. Identification of the perturbed biologic pathways may prove useful in selecting patients for specific therapies and associating biomarkers with survival and relapse.

Key Features

- Peripheral T-cell lymphomas comprise a diverse group of neoplasms that can present a diagnostic dilemma to clinicians and pathologists.

- Accurate diagnosis usually requires knowledge of clinical data, laboratory test results and an adequate tissue biopsy for routine and ancillary tests.

- The classification scheme for T-cell lymphomas will continue to be updated alongside emerging information about cell(s) of origin, genetic alterations and oncogenesis.

- Many types of peripheral T-cell lymphoma have a poor prognosis and aggressive course, and additional studies are underway to identify the best treatment options.

OVERVIEW AND PRACTICAL CONSIDERATIONS

T-cell lymphomas represent 5% to 10% of non-Hodgkin lymphomas in Western countries and 15% to 20% in the Asian continent, yet are classified in numerous distinct clinicopathologic entities that reflect etiologic factors, morphology, cell of origin, and behavior. Our understanding of the biology and diversity of these tumors has grown progressively in the past several decades, and the classification schemes are continually modified to reflect new information.[1,2] Most types are aggressive neoplasms that demonstrate a poor response to conventional therapies. The T-cell lymphoma subtypes vary in frequency by geographic region, with natural killer (NK)/T-cell lymphoma and adult T-cell leukemia/lymphoma most common in Asia, and peripheral T-cell lymphoma, unspecified (PTCL-NOS), as the most common subtype in both North America and Europe.[1]

The diagnosis of these tumors can be difficult because they are rare and lack certain histologic features that are specific to subtypes of B-cell lymphomas. Most importantly, clinical context is extremely important in classifying T-cell neoplasia and/or generating a differential diagnosis and must be considered in every case. Core needle biopsies are generally suboptimal for diagnosis and

The authors have no commercial or financial conflicts of interest to disclose.
Department of Laboratory Medicine, Robert J. Tomsich Pathology and Laboratory Medicine Institute, Cleveland Clinic, 9500 Euclid Avenue, L-30, Cleveland, OH 44195, USA
* Corresponding author.
E-mail address: hsie@ccf.org

Surgical Pathology 9 (2016) 131–141
http://dx.doi.org/10.1016/j.path.2015.11.002

are typically useful to heighten suspicion for lymphoma and thereby elicit subsequent procedures. Ideally, tissue samples are excisional biopsies with ample fresh tissue for ancillary diagnostics, including flow cytometry and molecular tests. Immune profiling by immunohistochemistry is helpful but there is much overlap in phenotype among the various entities. Polymerase chain reaction (PCR) studies of T-cell receptor gene rearrangements are often performed to document clonality in T-cell proliferations and aid in separating reactive from neoplastic causes. Even with ample pathologic material, accurate diagnosis is difficult and lacks 100% consensus agreement even by experts in the field. The International Peripheral T-cell and NK/T-cell Lymphoma Study reported an overall agreement of 81%,[1] whereas consistent use of a specified algorithm may improve consensus agreement to 92%.[3] In a comparison of diagnoses made by referring institutions versus central review for patients with T-cell lymphoma in the National Comprehensive Cancer Network, 44% (57/131) had concordant results, 24% were discordant, and 32% were assigned a provisional diagnosis.[4]

Although advanced molecular modalities, such as gene expression profiling and/or genomic sequencing technologies are not currently being used in routine diagnosis of T-cell lymphomas, the information gained from these studies is helping to flesh out the classification of these entities and uncover useful biomarkers that represent important biologic pathways and provide opportunities for tailored treatment regimens.

The current review will discuss the most common nodal types of peripheral T-cell lymphoma, including key features for recognition, immunohistochemistry, and molecular modalities to assist in diagnosis and differential diagnosis, and recent biomarkers and genetic alterations that provide clues to prognosis or classification.

ANAPLASTIC LARGE CELL LYMPHOMA, OVERVIEW

Anaplastic large cell lymphoma (ALCL) is currently classified as being anaplastic lymphoma kinase (ALK) positive, ALK negative, or primary cutaneous, according to the World Health Organization (WHO) 2008 classification.[5] There is also a site-specific form not yet incorporated into this classification scheme; that is, ALCL associated with breast implants, an indolent form when strictly confined to the breast capsule.[6,7] This discussion is limited to the nodal types of ALCL, which represent 3% of non-Hodgkin lymphomas in adults and 30% of childhood non-Hodgkin lymphoma. There is a biphasic age distribution with medians centering on the second and seventh decade, and ALK-positive ALCL is more often seen in the younger age group with a male predominance.[1,5]

ANAPLASTIC LARGE CELL LYMPHOMA, ANAPLASTIC LYMPHOMA KINASE POSITIVE

ALK protein expression defines this specific clinicopathologic entity, and the tumor cells express an ALK fusion protein derived from a rearrangement at the *ALK* 2p23 locus.[8] Both ALK-positive and ALK-negative ALCLs are neoplasms of large CD30-positive cells with pleomorphic, horseshoe-shaped nuclei, a prominent Golgi zone, and eosinophilic cytoplasm. All cases contain the so-called "hallmark cells." Staining for CD30 is strong and diffuse; the quality can be membranous and Golgi, and/or cytoplasmic.[5]

ALK-positive ALCL often presents with B symptoms, peripheral adenopathy, and variable involvement of extranodal sites, including skin, soft tissue, liver, lung, and bone.[9,10] The bone marrow is sometimes involved, and the detection rate is increased with a CD30 immunostain.[11] Rarely, circulating ALCL cells are present in peripheral blood and associated with the small cell variant.[12] The normal counterpart is thought to be a CD4-positive T cell with similarities to the T-helper 17 subset, although not all cases express CD4.[13] ALK-positive ALCL has a favorable prognosis compared with ALK-negative ALCL and many other types of peripheral T-cell lymphoma. The 5-year overall survival rates are in the 70% to 80% range.[14,15]

Lymph node involvement can be sinusoidal or diffuse, and in extranodal sites, ALCL grows in a sheetlike pattern. In addition to the common pattern, there are several histologic variants described in the WHO classification, including lymphohistiocytic, small-cell, and Hodgkinlike. A composite pattern may be seen in few cases.[5] Some cases have rather unusual features and do not fit as one of the recognized variants. These have been described as sarcomatoid, myxoid, round cell, or neutrophil rich.[16] In addition to ALK and CD30 expression, the immunophenotype might include loss of multiple T-cell antigens, with CD2 and CD4 often preserved. Cytotoxic markers (perforin, TIA-1, and granzyme B) are frequently expressed and can be helpful,[17] and sometimes epithelial membrane antigen (EMA) or clusterin is positive. The pattern of ALK staining gives clues to the partner gene, as the *NPM-ALK* fusion (t[2;5] [p23;q35]) protein is distributed in both the nucleus and the cytoplasm, whereas many other partners are restricted to the cytoplasm.[18]

ANAPLASTIC LARGE CELL LYMPHOMA, ANAPLASTIC LYMPHOMA KINASE NEGATIVE

ALCL, ALK negative, is a provisional category in the WHO 2008 classification scheme that has recently been an area of focused research efforts. It is morphologically indistinguishable from ALCL, ALK positive, and bears the same immunophenotype, but lacks detection of ALK. Although differences in survival exist, ALK-positive and ALK-negative lymphomas share some similarities in their genetic profile,[19] distinctive from PTCL-NOS. However, it is important to separate ALK-negative ALCL from PTCL-NOS because the former is associated with a better survival.[19] Some cases are difficult to separate based on morphology and immunohistochemistry. An International T-cell Lymphoma Project Study of 331 cases of PTCL-NOS found that 32% of cases had CD30 expression in some cells, and 15 cases had CD30 expression in 80% of cells.[15] Some researchers have turned toward other technologies to make this distinction. For example, the European T-cell lymphoma study group applied quantitative reverse transcriptase PCR to formalin-fixed and frozen tumors and validated a 3-gene model (*TNFRSF8*, *BATF3*, and *TMOD1*) that could accurately separate ALCL, ALK negative, from PTCL-NOS.[20] However, this has not been translated to clinical settings. ALCL, ALK negative, must also be distinguished from primary cutaneous ALCL and this can be accomplished by correlation with clinical findings and radiographic studies.

In the past several years, great strides have been made toward the task of uncovering the molecular genetics of ALK-negative ALCL. This began with discovery of a novel t(6;7) (p25.3q32.3) by massively parallel genomic sequencing,[21] reported in approximately 10% of cases. Next generation sequencing analysis revealed the translocation involves *DUSP22* at 6p25.[21] This was also seen in primary cutaneous ALCL (25%) and in rare cases of lymphomatoid papulosis.[22] DUSP22 is a dual-specificity phosphatase that is thought to dephosphorylate *MAPK* gene products and may play a role in regulating T-cell receptor signaling. The translocation appears to result in decreased expression of *DUSP22* and it is questioned whether *DUSP22* might normally function as a tumor suppressor.[9] A separate recurrent translocation was identified by genome-wide analysis that was found to inhibit p53-related genes. These novel *TP63* rearrangements were identified in a subset of PTCLs, mutually exclusive of ALK rearrangements, and associated with an inferior survival.[23]

To put these discoveries into practical context and query a cohort of cases for incidence of these genetic events, a large study commenced to determine whether combined biomarker testing for *TP63* and *DUSP22* rearrangements would be useful in diagnosis and risk stratification. Of 73 ALK-ALCLs, 30% were DUSP22 translocated and 8% were *TP63* translocated. The *DUSP22*-rearranged cases demonstrated favorable outcomes similar to ALK-positive ALCLs, whereas the other genetic subtypes were associated with inferior outcomes. The findings will need to be validated in future cohorts, but the ease of fluorescence in situ hybridization (FISH) testing to identify these rearrangements should allow for analysis in subsequent studies.[24]

A histopathologic analysis of ALK-negative ALCL blinded to translocation status identified some morphologic features that were specific to those lymphomas with *DUSP22* translocations. This study found that *DUSP22* rearranged cases were significantly more likely to have a common growth pattern, with "doughnut cells," and a monomorphic population of smaller hallmark cells imparting a mini-doughnut appearance (**Fig. 1**). There was also an inverse association with TIA-1 expression.[25]

Other differential diagnostic considerations for ALCL, ALK negative, include CD30+ diffuse large B-cell lymphoma with a sinusoidal growth pattern, and using 2 B-cell markers to effectively exclude a B-cell phenotype will help in that regard. Classic Hodgkin lymphoma is an important consideration, and CD15 is not enough to discriminate the two.[26] The phenotype of Hodgkin lymphoma must be fulfilled, and, rarely, ALCL can express CD15. Finally, metastatic carcinoma should be excluded, as both ALCL and carcinoma can show cohesive growth of tumor cells.

ANGIOIMMUNOBLASTIC T-CELL LYMPHOMA

Angioimmunoblastic T-cell lymphoma (AITL) is a primarily nodal-based mature T-cell neoplasm with an often dramatic systemic presentation in the form of generalized lymphadenopathy, hepatosplenomegaly, B-symptoms, and occasionally a skin rash. There is laboratory evidence of immune abnormalities in many patients who exhibit polyclonal hypergammaglobulinemia and/or hemolytic anemia with a positive Coombs test. It is a common type of peripheral T-cell lymphoma and is the most common type in Europe, presenting in middle-aged to elderly adults with an equal male-to-female distribution.[27]

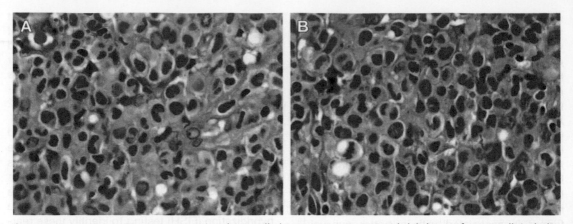

Fig. 1. ALK-negative ALCL case representing the so-called "common pattern," with (*A*) sheets of tumor cells including numerous hallmark cells, some of which are deeply invaginated (hematoxylin-eosin [H&E], ×1000). (*B*) Several "doughnut" cells (H&E, ×1000). FISH analysis identified a *DUSP22* rearrangement. (*Courtesy of* James R. Cook, MD, PhD, Cleveland Clinic, Cleveland, Ohio.)

The microscopic findings are characteristic, with a nodal architecture that typically is completely effaced by medium-sized T cells with abundant cytoplasm, mixed inflammatory cells, aggregates of follicular dendritic cells, and abundant arborizing high endothelial venules (**Fig. 2**). At low power, this constellation imparts a hypocellular depleted appearance. The subcapsular sinus may be open, but the infiltrate often extends into perinodal adipose tissue. Germinal centers are variably present, and form the basis for designating AITLs as histologic pattern I (hyperplastic follicles), pattern II (loss of architecture with regressed follicles), or pattern III (complete effacement with absent follicles). Of note, a mixture of patterns can occur at presentation or patients may relapse with a different pattern.[28] The characteristic immunophenotype is CD3+/CD4+ cells with occasional aberrant loss of pan T-cell antigens. By flow cytometry, a subset of cells may lack CD3 and/or coexpress CD10. AITL cells express markers related to T-follicular helper cells (T$_{FH}$) (CXCL13, PD1, BCL6, ICOS, SAP) indicative of their derivation from this T-helper subset, and are used in hematopathology practice to reinforce the diagnosis. It has been suggested that positivity for 3 markers is ideal to establish this relationship, as the presence of only a single marker may reflect a partial conversion of effector T-helper cells.[29] Epstein-Barr virus (EBV) is detectable in most AITL cases and infects bystander B-cells, potentially transforming them into overt B-cell proliferations that may complicate the presentation with underlying T-cell lymphoma.[30] AITL patients experience a moderately aggressive clinical course with a median survival of less than 2 years, but some can spontaneously remit or show partial responsiveness to corticosteroids.[27]

The differential diagnosis includes a reactive lymphadenopathy related to human immunodeficiency virus infection (patterns B and C), other immune reactions, or certain medications. Similarly,

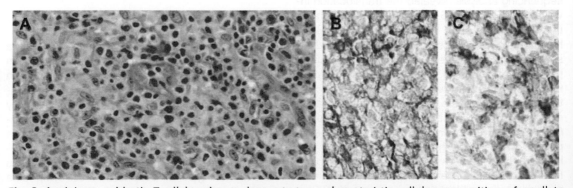

Fig. 2. Angioimmunoblastic T-cell lymphoma demonstrates a characteristic cellular composition of small to medium-sized atypical lymphocytes and other inflammatory cells. (*A*) This case has prominent follicular dendritic cells and few scattered immunoblasts (H&E, ×500). The neoplastic T cells are positive for (*B*) CD3 and (*C*) CXCL13, a chemokine that is highly upregulated in the germinal center T-helper cell subset (×500).

early stages can be missed or masked by treatment with steroids. An early morphologic stage with hyperplastic germinal centers, poorly developed mantles, an increase in vascularity, and slight architectural distortion may be overlooked. Expansion of the CD21-positive follicular dendritic cell meshworks is a helpful feature, as is observation of CD4+ T-cells expressing CD10 that hug depleted follicles.[31] Identifying a clonal population by flow cytometry or PCR for T-cell receptor gene rearrangements is a supportive adjunct when present. When the diagnosis of a T-cell lymphoma is unmistakable, other differential diagnostic possibilities include PTCL-NOS, particularly one that may express T_{FH} markers and fall into a "gray zone" category between AITL and PTCL-NOS.[32] Rare cases of T-cell lymphoma have features intermediate between AITL and PTCL-NOS and might show a nondescript diffuse growth pattern with some AITL characteristics, but these cannot be better classified even by experts. The TFH phenotype is not completely specific to AITL because it is found in rare cases of peripheral T-cell lymphoma, particularly those cases with a follicular growth pattern,[33] as well as the WHO provisional category of primary cutaneous small/medium CD4-positive T-cell lymphoma. EBV-positive diffuse large B-cell lymphomas are also in the differential diagnosis of AITL, but clues to detect an AITL in these cases include proliferated follicular dendritic cell meshworks, positive T-cell receptor gene rearrangement studies (although not foolproof logic), and the clinical systemic presentation of AITL. PTCL-NOS also can be EBV positive, and either type of T-cell lymphoma may contain Reed-Sternberg–like B-cells associated with EBV infection, potentially contributing to diagnostic confusion.[34]

Gene expression profiling (GEP) has defined diagnostic signatures for peripheral T-cell lymphoma subtypes and can define unique molecular signatures that either better refine classification or bridge entities with commonalities. This has yielded important contributions to AITL in particular, in which GEP established the putative link between AITL and its microenvironment, its cell of origin from T_{FH} cells, and the upregulation of genes related to B-cells and vasculogenesis.[35,36] Yet, although the gene expression signature of AITL is characteristic, it is not exclusive, as a few cases of PTCL-NOS were found to have a profile similar to AITL in GEP studies.[35] Some of these cases had focal follicular dendritic cell expansion or a few EBV-positive large cells, but fell short of a diagnosis of AITL during slide review. This suggests that the spectrum of AITL might be broader than suspected or initially thought. Regardless, in most cases, AITL and PTCL-NOS have distinct molecular features, and a gene set containing functional categories of cell adhesion, vascular biology, extracellular matrix, and B-cell/plasma cell–related genes was able to significantly separate AITL from PTCL-NOS.[35]

Additional discoveries related to the genetic basis for AITL have come about in the past several years, thanks to studies using high-throughput genomic sequencing technologies (Table 1). Mutations in the epigenetic regulators TET2, DNMT3A, and IDH2 frequently occur in AITL, but are not specific to this disease and can be found in PTCL-NOS at a lower frequency.[37–39] Many of the myeloid malignancies share these mutations, although IDH2 mutations in AITL are confined to the R172 position.[39] Unlike in acute myeloid leukemia, these recurring mutations are not mutually exclusive. The patterns of mutation overlap have yielded some interesting findings, such that TET2 is present in almost 80% of AITL, and that most tumors with DNMT3A mutations or IDH2 R172 mutations also have TET2 mutations.[40] Most specific to AITL was the recent discovery of a point mutation in the Ras homolog gene family, member A (RHOA G17V) in almost 70% of AITL samples, resulting in a dominant negative form of RHOA GTPase and disruption of RHOA signaling. This was present in PTCL-NOS at a much lower frequency and positive cases were enriched in those that showed a T_{FH}-immunophenotype.[41,42] Interestingly, these studies proposed that these mutations may be acquired in a multistep manner, because all the RHOA-mutated samples were TET2 mutated, and the smaller percentage of IDH2-mutated tumors harbored both TET2 and RHOA mutations. Sakata-Yanagimoto and colleagues[42] proposed that TET2 mutations might be a prerequisite for subsequent RHOA G17V and development of an angioimmunoblastic T-cell lymphoma. Consequences of the G17V alteration on RHOA function have been studied in vitro, and the functional effects include inability to bind guanosine triphosphate (GTP), resulting in increased cell proliferation and migration via increases in AKT phosphorylation.[43] Indeed, more than a decade earlier, mouse models provided evidence that disruption of RHOA signaling can lead to neoplastic transformation of T cells in mice.[44]

Analysis of mutation-specific subgroups in AITL has been a recent focus. A recent comparison of clinical and pathologic features between RHOA G17V and wild-type groups identified significantly higher mean vessel density and a greater number of T_{FH} markers by immunohistochemistry than wild-type cases.[45] A study of the IDH2 R172

Table 1
A summary of recurrent mutations identified in nodal peripheral T-cell lymphomas

Gene	AITL, %	PTCL-NOS, %	PTCL-NOS with T_{FH} Phenotype, %	ALCL, ALK+, %	ALCL, ALK−, %
RHOA	67[41] 71[42] 72[46] 53[43] 63[45]	18[41] 0[42] 26[46]	62[42]	—	—
TET2	33[37] 73[41] 83[42] 76[40] 47[47] 82[46]	20[37] 24[47] 29[41] 49[42] 46[46]	58[47]	0[41]	0[37] 0[47] 50[41] (n = 2) 33[46]
IDH1	0[42]	0[42]	—	—	—
IDH2 R172	13[41] 30[42] 20[40] 25[39] 32[46]	0[42] 0[39] <1[46]	—	—	—
DNMT3A	23[41] 26[42] 33[40] 38[46]	27[42] 36[46]	—	—	16[46]

Abbreviations: ALCL, anaplastic large cell lymphoma; ALK, anaplastic lymphoma kinase; PTCL-NOS, peripheral T-cell lymphoma not otherwise specified.

subgroup of AITLs showed that the TET/IDH2-mutated cases have a distinct gene expression profile compared with other AITLs, with upregulation of T_{FH} genes and downregulation of genes associated with other T-helper subsets. The consequence of this mutational alteration was biochemical evidence of histone demethylase inhibition, and the investigators use this rationale to consider the use of hypomethylating agents in AITL.[46] A common theme seems to be emerging, as TET2 mutations were also shown to correlate with T_{FH}-features, building on the premise that this phenotype might be the consequence of several specific mutations working in concert to execute a final disease-specific pathway.[47]

PERIPHERAL T-CELL LYMPHOMA, NOT OTHERWISE SPECIFIED

PTCL-NOS was introduced in the Revised European American Lymphoma (REAL) classification in 1994 and has subsequently been a unique category in the WHO 2001 and 2008 classifications. It encompasses a heterogeneous group of mature T-cell neoplasms that lack specific features of any of the other subtypes of peripheral T-cell lymphomas. Its unfortunate reputation as a "wastebasket" category and diagnosis of exclusion holds promise for the future, as new discoveries using novel approaches such as next-generation sequencing and gene expression arrays are helping to define subsets within this broad group. PTCL-NOS tends to affect older adults with a median age of onset of 60 years, with a male predominance. Patients often present with generalized disease and occasionally extranodal presentations, and sometimes demonstrate peripheral blood eosinophilia, pruritis, or hemophagocytic syndrome.

PTCL-NOS is typically composed of a pleomorphic or monomorphic infiltrate of variably sized cells with or without an inflammatory background. The pattern causes diffuse effacement of the lymph node without sparing of the marginal sinus, as in AITL. Provisional cytologic grades were found to have no definite prognostic significance, so grading is not typically done.[48] The WHO 2008 classification describes 3 less common morphologic variants: T-zone, lymphoepithelioid ("Lennert's lymphoma"), and the more recently recognized follicular variant. Although rare, it is important to be aware of the variant patterns to avoid confusing PTCL-NOS with another type of lymphoma or with a reactive process. The T-zone pattern is predominantly interfollicular and the neoplastic infiltrate spares the reactive follicles. The lymphoepithelioid variant shows effacement of the architecture by lymphoma with abundant collections of epithelioid histiocytes imparting a granulomatous appearance, and occasionally contains admixed Hodgkin/Reed-Sternberg-like cells.[49] The follicular variant was first recognized as those cases that can truly be mistaken for follicular lymphoma on routine sections[50] (Fig. 3), but subsequent studies expanded the morphologies of this variant to those resembling lymphocyte-predominant Hodgkin lymphoma or marginal zone lymphoma.[51] The follicular variant of PTCL-NOS was found to bear a novel t(5;9) (q33;q22) ITK-SYK translocation in a subset of cases,[52] and is thought to lack certain features of AITL, despite having a T_{FH} immunophenotype. It is characterized clinically as having a lower stage and lacking typical AITL

symptomatology, and pathologically as lacking hyperplastic high endothelial venules or follicular dendritic cell meshwork proliferation.[32] The ITK-SYK translocation juxtaposes the interleukin-2–inducible T-cell kinase (ITK) gene on chromosome 5 and the spleen tyrosine kinase (SYK) gene on chromosome 9, and the resultant fusion protein was shown to be a catalytically active tyrosine kinase capable of inducing T-cell lymphoproliferation.[52,53] However, this fusion may not be entirely specific to PTCL, as it was recently detected in a case of AITL, and may argue against separating peripheral T-cell lymphoma, follicular variant (PTCL-F) from AITL.[54]

The immunophenotype of PTCL-NOS is as varied as its histologic appearance. It typically shows expression of pan T-cell antigens (CD3, CD2, CD5, CD7), with loss of one or more antigens in up to 80% of cases. This is helpful in distinguishing a

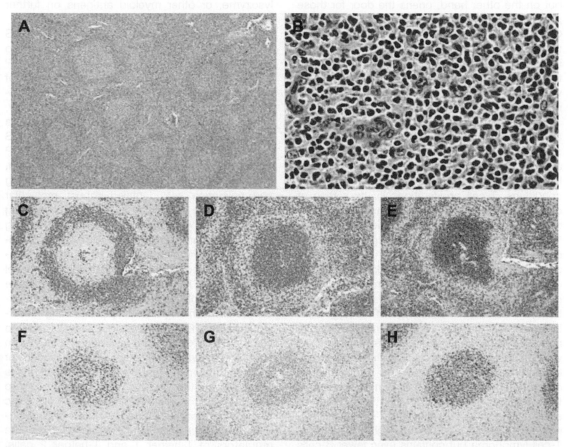

Fig. 3. Microscopic images from a case of PTCL-NOS, follicular variant, mimicking a follicular lymphoma on routine histologic sections. (A) At low magnification, the follicle density is increased and the germinal centers contain mantles, but are not polarized (H&E, ×20). (B) High magnification inside a follicle. There is a proliferation of atypical, intermediately sized lymphocytes with irregular nuclei (H&E, ×400). (C–H) Immunostains highlight the lymphoma cells, which are localized in the follicle centers and in the interfollicular areas, sparing the mantles (×100). The lymphoma cells are negative for CD20 (C), and positive for CD3 (D), positive for CD4 (E), positive for CD57 (F), and positive for the T_{FH} markers BCL6 (G) and CD10 (H).

T-cell proliferation from an inflammatory lesion. Most cases are positive for CD4, and less often CD8, and even fewer are double positive for CD4 and CD8. Skewing of the CD4 to CD8 ratio, although often observed, cannot be used as a surrogate of clonality. Positivity for EBV may be associated with an adverse prognosis, and Ki-67 labeling index was also found to be prognostically relevant.[55] Some tumors are negative for both CD4 and CD8, and may be associated with a worse prognosis. Expression of cytotoxic molecules trends with a CD8+ phenotype, and these PTCL-NOS derived from CD8+ cytotoxic T cells have been associated with clinical findings indicative of a poor prognosis.[56] The neoplastic cells express TCRαβ in most PTCL-NOS, while fewer are of gamma-delta T-cell receptor derivation.[57] Many cases of PTCL-NOS present with CD30 expression, possibly up to half.[55,58] This makes the differential diagnosis with ALCL ALK more challenging but on the other hand, opens the door for those patients to the possibility of benefit from anti-CD30 therapy. Helpful immunostains to differentiate CD30+ PTCL-NOS from ALCL, ALK negative, include CD3, which is more frequently present in the former, and cytotoxic molecules and EMA, which are more often positive in ALCL, ALK negative.[15]

The differential diagnosis of PTCL-NOS includes an abnormal immune response or atypical hyperplasia. Loss of pan T-cell antigens and monoclonality are useful characteristics that favor a T-cell lymphoma, but can rarely be present in reactive conditions. T-cell proliferations in the setting of certain medications such as phenytoin or carbamazepine can closely mimic a peripheral T-cell lymphoma, and therefore knowledge of the medication record and patient history is necessary in pathologic evaluation. Classic Hodgkin lymphoma can be difficult to distinguish from a T-cell lymphoma with Hodgkin/Reed-Sternberg cells, because the immunophenotype of the large cells is remarkably similar.[59] In addition, EBV-positive and EBV-negative variants of T-cell lymphoma with HRS-like cells do exist.[60] In these cases, the background architecture and inflammatory composition as well as a solid understanding of the subtypes of classic Hodgkin lymphoma will assist in this difficult distinction. T-cell/histiocyte-rich large B-cell lymphoma might resemble a T-cell lymphoma but contains even fewer B-cells than a T-cell lymphoma (particularly almost no small B cells) and the small T cells are not neoplastic. Nodal involvement by other, rare types of T-cell lymphoma that are distinct entities must be recognized (for example, adult T-cell leukemia/lymphoma, mycosis fungoides, or T-prolymphocytic leukemia [T-PLL]). This is another circumstance in which knowledge of peripheral blood findings, infectious exposures, or skin lesions is critical. TCL1 is a helpful immunohistochemical stain that identifies 77% of cases of T-PLL,[61] but a specific tissue biomarker is not available for most of these other T-cell lymphoma types that can take up residence in the lymph node. A process of elimination is often required to arrive at the diagnosis of PTCL-NOS, and sometimes a recommendation to check for human T-lymphotropic virus (HTLV) serologies, review a peripheral blood smear, and/or to consider a cutaneous T-cell lymphoma history is included in the comment section of the pathology report. Finally, a myeloid sarcoma could theoretically be mistaken for a T-cell lymphoma if a restrictive immunohistochemistry screening panel is used, as it might express CD43 but no other T-cell markers, and may variably express myeloperoxidase, lysozyme, or other myeloid antigens on further immunophenotyping.

GEP has provided insights into PTCL-NOS biology and has been suggested as a way to improve the diagnosis of PTCL-NOS. The GEP signatures reflect the inherent characteristics of the neoplastic cells themselves, as well as a contribution from their microenvironment. Certainly, studies using GEP have reassigned lymphoma types; for example, 14% to 20% of PTCL-NOS cases were reclassified as AITL using a GEP signature.[62,63] A different study of formalin-fixed, paraffin-embedded tissue that used a training and validation set identified robust molecular classifiers that were fairly accurate in separating ALK-negative ALCL from PTCL-NOS, including cases that were CD30 positive.[19] After molecularly reclassifying cases into other WHO categories, diagnostic signatures for 2 novel subgroups of PTCL were identified: the first, a GATA3 high subgroup with enrichment of cell-cycle/proliferation signatures (upregulating MYC-induced and PI3K-induced pathways), and the second, a TBX21 subgroup (enriching interferon and NF-κβ pathways). A statistically significant survival difference was identified between these groups, with the GATA3 high signature group demonstrating worse overall survival. A cytotoxic group was also associated with a worse prognosis.[63] Given that TBX21 and GATA3 are regulators of T-helper 1 and T-helper 2 cells, respectively, this connection between cell of origin and the contribution of polarizing cytokines within the microenvironment helps to understand lymphomagenesis and reinforces using GEP as a tool in this effort. A study of GATA3 protein expression confirmed that it is expressed in a subset of PTCL-NOS cases (45%) and is associated with a poor outcome, using a cutoff of greater than 10% considered as positive by immunohistochemistry.[64]

SUMMARY

Peripheral T-cell non-Hodgkin lymphomas are a generally aggressive group of neoplasms that are sometimes difficult to diagnose and frequently complicated by persistent disease or tumor relapse. Entities within this larger category have been identified based on differences in etiology, pathogenesis, tumor cell of origin and genetic and microenvironmental information. It is sometimes difficult to apply all that is known about T-cell lymphomas in routine practice, but an understanding of the pathobiology of these disease subtypes can lead to a better diagnosis and perhaps optimized therapy for each patient.

REFERENCES

1. Vose J, Armitage J, Weisenburger D, International T-Cell Lymphoma Project. International peripheral T-cell and natural killer/T-cell lymphoma study: pathology findings and clinical outcomes. J Clin Oncol 2008;26(25):4124–30.
2. Jaffe E, Harris N, Stein H, et al. Introduction and overview of the classification of lymphoid neoplasms. In: Swerdlow, editor. WHO classification of tumours of the haematopoietic and lymphoid tissues. 4th edition. Lyon (France): International Agency for Research on Cancer; 2008. p. 161–6.
3. Hsi ED, Said J, Macon WR, et al. Diagnostic accuracy of a defined immunophenotypic and molecular genetic approach for peripheral T/NK-cell lymphomas. A North American PTCL study group project. Am J Surg Pathol 2014;38(6):768–75.
4. Herrera AF, Crosby-Thompson A, Friedberg JW, et al. Comparison of referring and final pathology for patients with T-cell lymphoma in the national comprehensive cancer network. Cancer 2014; 120(13):1993–9.
5. Swerdlow S, Campo E, Harris N, et al, editors. WHO classification of the haematopoietic and lymphoid tissues. 4th edition. Lyon (France): IARC; 2008.
6. Aladily TN, Medeiros LJ, Amin MB, et al. Anaplastic large cell lymphoma associated with breast implants: a report of 13 cases. Am J Surg Pathol 2012;36(7):1000–8.
7. de Jong D, Vasmel WL, de Boer JP, et al. Anaplastic large-cell lymphoma in women with breast implants. JAMA 2008;300(17):2030–5.
8. Morris SW, Kirstein MN, Valentine MB, et al. Fusion of a kinase gene, ALK, to a nucleolar protein gene, NPM, in non-Hodgkin's lymphoma. Science 1994; 263(5151):1281–4.
9. Xing X, Feldman AL. Anaplastic large cell lymphomas: ALK positive, ALK negative, and primary cutaneous. Adv Anat Pathol 2015;22(1):29–49.
10. Sandlund JT, Pui CH, Roberts WM, et al. Clinicopathologic features and treatment outcome of children with large-cell lymphoma and the t(2;5)(p23;q35). Blood 1994;84(8):2467–71.
11. Fraga M, Brousset P, Schlaifer D, et al. Bone marrow involvement in anaplastic large cell lymphoma. Immunohistochemical detection of minimal disease and its prognostic significance. Am J Clin Pathol 1995;103(1):82–9.
12. Bayle C, Charpentier A, Duchayne E, et al. Leukaemic presentation of small cell variant anaplastic large cell lymphoma: report of four cases. Br J Haematol 1999;104(4):680–8.
13. Matsuyama H, Suzuki HI, Nishimori H, et al. miR-135b mediates NPM-ALK-driven oncogenicity and renders IL-17-producing immunophenotype to anaplastic large cell lymphoma. Blood 2011; 118(26):6881–92.
14. Gascoyne RD, Aoun P, Wu D, et al. Prognostic significance of anaplastic lymphoma kinase (ALK) protein expression in adults with anaplastic large cell lymphoma. Blood 1999;93(11):3913–21.
15. Savage KJ, Harris NL, Vose JM, et al. ALK-anaplastic large-cell lymphoma is clinically and immunophenotypically different from both ALK+ ALCL and peripheral T-cell lymphoma, not otherwise specified: report from the international peripheral T-cell lymphoma project. Blood 2008;111(12): 5496–504.
16. Benharroch D, Meguerian-Bedoyan Z, Lamant L, et al. ALK-positive lymphoma: a single disease with a broad spectrum of morphology. Blood 1998; 91(6):2076–84.
17. Foss HD, Anagnostopoulos I, Araujo I, et al. Anaplastic large-cell lymphomas of T-cell and null-cell phenotype express cytotoxic molecules. Blood 1996;88(10):4005–11.
18. Falini B, Nicoletti I, Bolli N, et al. Translocations and mutations involving the nucleophosmin (NPM1) gene in lymphomas and leukemias. Haematologica 2007;92(4):519–32.
19. Piccaluga PP, Fuligni F, De Leo A, et al. Molecular profiling improves classification and prognostication of nodal peripheral T-cell lymphomas: results of a phase III diagnostic accuracy study. J Clin Oncol 2013;31(24):3019–25.
20. Agnelli L, Mereu E, Pellegrino E, et al. Identification of a 3-gene model as a powerful diagnostic tool for the recognition of ALK-negative anaplastic large-cell lymphoma. Blood 2012;120(6):1274–81.
21. Feldman AL, Dogan A, Smith DI, et al. Discovery of recurrent t(6;7)(p25.3;q32.3) translocations in

ALK-negative anaplastic large cell lymphomas by massively parallel genomic sequencing. Blood 2011;117(3):915–9.

22. Karai LJ, Kadin ME, Hsi ED, et al. Chromosomal re-arrangements of 6p25.3 define a new subtype of lymphomatoid papulosis. Am J Surg Pathol 2013; 37(8):1173–81.

23. Vasmatzis G, Johnson SH, Knudson RA, et al. Genome-wide analysis reveals recurrent structural abnormalities of TP63 and other p53-related genes in peripheral T-cell lymphomas. Blood 2012; 120(11):2280–9.

24. Parrilla Castellar ER, Jaffe ES, Said JW, et al. ALK-negative anaplastic large cell lymphoma is a genet-ically heterogeneous disease with widely disparate clinical outcomes. Blood 2014;124(9):1473–80.

25. King RL, Dao LN, McPhail ED, et al. Morphologic features of ALK-negative anaplastic large cell lymphomas with DUSP22 rearrangements. Am J Surg Pathol 2015;40(1):36–43.

26. Rosso R, Paulli M, Magrini U, et al. Anaplastic large cell lymphoma, CD30/ki-1 positive, expressing the CD15/leu-M1 antigen. immunohistochemical and morphological relationships to Hodgkin's disease. Virchows Arch A Pathol Anat Histopathol 1990; 416(3):229–35.

27. Federico M, Rudiger T, Bellei M, et al. Clinicopatho-logic characteristics of angioimmunoblastic T-cell lymphoma: analysis of the international peripheral T-cell lymphoma project. J Clin Oncol 2013;31(2): 240–6.

28. Attygalle AD, Kyriakou C, Dupuis J, et al. Histologic evolution of angioimmunoblastic T-cell lymphoma in consecutive biopsies: clinical correlation and in-sights into natural history and disease progression. Am J Surg Pathol 2007;31(7):1077–88.

29. Laurent C, Fazilleau N, Brousset P. A novel subset of T-helper cells: follicular T-helper cells and their markers. Haematologica 2010;95(3):356–8.

30. Dunleavy K, Wilson WH, Jaffe ES. Angioimmuno-blastic T cell lymphoma: pathobiological insights and clinical implications. Curr Opin Hematol 2007; 14(4):348–53.

31. Attygalle A, Al-Jehani R, Diss TC, et al. Neoplastic T cells in angioimmunoblastic T-cell lymphoma ex-press CD10. Blood 2002;99(2):627–33.

32. Huang Y, Moreau A, Dupuis J, et al. Peripheral T-cell lymphomas with a follicular growth pattern are derived from follicular helper T cells (TFH) and may show overlapping features with angioimmunoblastic T-cell lymphomas. Am J Surg Pathol 2009;33(5): 682–90.

33. Rodriguez-Pinilla SM, Atienza L, Murillo C, et al. Peripheral T-cell lymphoma with follicular T-cell markers. Am J Surg Pathol 2008;32(12):1787–99.

34. Quintanilla-Martinez L, Fend F, Moguel LR, et al. Peripheral T-cell lymphoma with Reed-Sternberg-like cells of B-cell phenotype and genotype associ-ated with Epstein-Barr virus infection. Am J Surg Pathol 1999;23(10):1233–40.

35. de Leval L, Rickman DS, Thielen C, et al. The gene expression profile of nodal peripheral T-cell lym-phoma demonstrates a molecular link between an-gioimmunoblastic T-cell lymphoma (AITL) and follicular helper T (TFH) cells. Blood 2007;109(11): 4952–63.

36. Piccaluga PP, Agostinelli C, Califano A, et al. Gene expression analysis of angioimmunoblastic lym-phoma indicates derivation from T follicular helper cells and vascular endothelial growth factor dereg-ulation. Cancer Res 2007;67(22):10703–10.

37. Quivoron C, Couronne L, Della Valle V, et al. TET2 inac-tivation results in pleiotropic hematopoietic abnormal-ities in mouse and is a recurrent event during human lymphomagenesis. Cancer Cell 2011;20(1):25–38.

38. Couronne L, Bastard C, Bernard OA. TET2 and DNMT3A mutations in human T-cell lymphoma. N Engl J Med 2012;366(1):95–6.

39. Cairns RA, Iqbal J, Lemonnier F, et al. IDH2 muta-tions are frequent in angioimmunoblastic T-cell lymphoma. Blood 2012;119(8):1901–3.

40. Odejide O, Weigert O, Lane AA, et al. A targeted mutational landscape of angioimmunoblastic T-cell lymphoma. Blood 2014;123(9):1293–6.

41. Palomero T, Couronne L, Khiabanian H, et al. Recur-rent mutations in epigenetic regulators, RHOA and FYN kinase in peripheral T cell lymphomas. Nat Genet 2014;46(2):166–70.

42. Sakata-Yanagimoto M, Enami T, Yoshida K, et al. Somatic RHOA mutation in angioimmunoblastic T cell lymphoma. Nat Genet 2014;46(2):171–5.

43. Yoo HY, Sung MK, Lee SH, et al. A recurrent inactivat-ing mutation in RHOA GTPase in angioimmunoblastic T cell lymphoma. Nat Genet 2014;46(4):371–5.

44. Cleverley SC, Costello PS, Henning SW, et al. Loss of rho function in the thymus is accompanied by the development of thymic lymphoma. Oncogene 2000;19(1):13–20.

45. Ondrejka SL, Grzywacz B, Bodo J, et al. Angioim-munoblastic T-cell lymphomas with the RHOA p.Gly17Val mutation have classic clinical and patho-logic features. Am J Surg Pathol 2015. [Epub ahead of print].

46. Wang C, McKeithan TW, Gong Q, et al. IDH2R172 mutations define a unique subgroup of patients with angioimmunoblastic T-cell lymphoma. Blood 2015;126(15):1741–52.

47. Lemonnier F, Couronne L, Parrens M, et al. Recur-rent TET2 mutations in peripheral T-cell lymphomas correlate with TFH-like features and adverse clinical parameters. Blood 2012;120(7):1466–9.

48. Gisselbrecht C, Gaulard P, Lepage E, et al. Prog-nostic significance of T-cell phenotype in aggressive non-Hodgkin's lymphomas. groupe d'etudes des

lymphomes de l'adulte (GELA). Blood 1998;92(1): 76–82.

49. Suchi T, Lennert K, Tu LY, et al. Histopathology and immunohistochemistry of peripheral T cell lymphomas: a proposal for their classification. J Clin Pathol 1987;40(9):995–1015.

50. de Leval L, Savilo E, Longtine J, et al. Peripheral T-cell lymphoma with follicular involvement and a CD4+/bcl-6+ phenotype. Am J Surg Pathol 2001; 25(3):395–400.

51. Hu S, Young KH, Konoplev SN, et al. Follicular T-cell lymphoma: a member of an emerging family of follicular helper T-cell derived T-cell lymphomas. Hum Pathol 2012;43(11):1789–98.

52. Streubel B, Vinatzer U, Willheim M, et al. Novel t(5;9)(q33;q22) fuses ITK to SYK in unspecified peripheral T-cell lymphoma. Leukemia 2006;20(2):313–8.

53. Dierks C, Adrian F, Fisch P, et al. The ITK-SYK fusion oncogene induces a T-cell lymphoproliferative disease in mice mimicking human disease. Cancer Res 2010;70(15):6193–204.

54. Attygalle AD, Feldman AL, Dogan A. ITK/SYK translocation in angioimmunoblastic T-cell lymphoma. Am J Surg Pathol 2013;37(9):1456–7.

55. Went P, Agostinelli C, Gallamini A, et al. Marker expression in peripheral T-cell lymphoma: a proposed clinical-pathologic prognostic score. J Clin Oncol 2006;24(16):2472–9.

56. Asano N, Suzuki R, Kagami Y, et al. Clinicopathologic and prognostic significance of cytotoxic molecule expression in nodal peripheral T-cell lymphoma, unspecified. Am J Surg Pathol 2005;29(10):1284–93.

57. Gaulard P, Bourquelot P, Kanavaros P, et al. Expression of the alpha/beta and gamma/delta T-cell receptors in 57 cases of peripheral T-cell lymphomas. Identification of a subset of gamma/delta T-cell lymphomas. Am J Pathol 1990;137(3): 617–28.

58. Sabattini E, Pizzi M, Tabanelli V, et al. CD30 expression in peripheral T-cell lymphomas. Haematologica 2013;98(8):e81–2.

59. Moroch J, Copie-Bergman C, de Leval L, et al. Follicular peripheral T-cell lymphoma expands the spectrum of classical Hodgkin lymphoma mimics. Am J Surg Pathol 2012;36(11):1636–46.

60. Nicolae A, Pittaluga S, Venkataraman G, et al. Peripheral T-cell lymphomas of follicular T-helper cell derivation with Hodgkin/Reed-Sternberg cells of B-cell lineage: both EBV-positive and EBV-negative variants exist. Am J Surg Pathol 2013; 37(6):816–26.

61. Herling M, Patel KA, Teitell MA, et al. High TCL1 expression and intact T-cell receptor signaling define a hyperproliferative subset of T-cell prolymphocytic leukemia. Blood 2008;111(1):328–37.

62. Iqbal J, Weisenburger DD, Greiner TC, et al. Molecular signatures to improve diagnosis in peripheral T-cell lymphoma and prognostication in angioimmunoblastic T-cell lymphoma. Blood 2010;115(5): 1026–36.

63. Iqbal J, Wright G, Wang C, et al. Gene expression signatures delineate biological and prognostic subgroups in peripheral T-cell lymphoma. Blood 2014; 123(19):2915–23.

64. Wang T, Feldman AL, Wada DA, et al. GATA-3 expression identifies a high-risk subset of PTCL, NOS with distinct molecular and clinical features. Blood 2014;123(19):3007–15.

Genetic Testing in Acute Myeloid Leukemia and Myelodysplastic Syndromes

Valentina Nardi, MD, Robert P. Hasserjian, MD*

KEYWORDS

- Myelodysplastic syndrome • Acute myeloid leukemia • Mutations • Translocations • Cytogenetics
- Molecular genetic analysis

ABSTRACT

Cytogenetic analysis of acute myeloid leukemia (AML) and myelodysplastic syndrome (MDS) is essential for disease diagnosis, classification, prognostic stratification, and treatment guidance. Molecular genetic analysis of *CEBPA*, *NPM1*, and *FLT3* is already standard of care in patients with AML, and mutations in several additional genes are assuming increasing importance. Mutational analysis of certain genes, such as *SF3B1*, is also becoming an important tool to distinguish subsets of MDS that have different biologic behaviors. It is still uncertain how to optimally combine karyotype with mutation data in diagnosis and risk-stratification of AML and MDS, particularly in cases with multiple mutations and/ or several mutationally distinct subclones.

OVERVIEW

Myelodysplastic syndromes (MDSs) are clonal hematopoietic stem cell neoplasms characterized by morphologic dysplasia, ineffective hematopoiesis resulting in peripheral blood cytopenias, and risk of progression to acute myeloid leukemia (AML). AML is a clonal hematopoietic neoplasm with increased myeloblasts, usually comprising at least 20% of leukocytes in the bone marrow and/or blood. Both MDS and AML are heterogeneous diseases with variable morphologic, immunophenotypic, and genetic features; a range of clinical aggressiveness; and multiple treatment options.

Key Features

- Conventional karyotyping of bone marrow provides critical information regarding risk stratification of both MDS and AML and should be obtained in all cases.

- Mutational analysis of AML routinely includes *FLT3*, *NPM1* and *CEBPA*, but is moving towards including an additional small group of genes (*IDH1*, *IDH2*, *RUNX1*, *MLL*, *DENMT3A*, and others) that have been shown to have prognostic and/or therapeutic relevance in large-scale genomic studies.

- Mutational analysis of a limited set of genes in MDS is also becoming a useful tool for the purposes of prognosis (with *TP53*, *EZH2*, *ASXL1*, and *RUNX1* among genes conferring a poor prognosis independently of other factors); however, the finding of gene mutations alone in a cytopenic patient is currently considered insufficient to establish a primary diagnosis of MDS in the absence of required diagnostic criteria.

- While there is still a role for single gene testing in some contexts, the field is moving towards testing multiple genes (from 10 to over 100) at once in dedicated panels, often using next generation sequencing technology.

In the World Health Organization's (WHO) 4th edition *Classification of Tumors of Haematopoietic and Lymphoid Tissues* published in 2008,[1] several

---

Disclosure: Both authors have no relevant financial interests or funding sources to disclose.
Department of Pathology, Massachusetts General Hospital, Harvard Medical School, 55 Fruit Street, Boston, MA 02114, USA
* Corresponding author.
E-mail address: rhasserjian@partners.org

recurrent genetic abnormalities were formally incorporated in the diagnostic algorithms of AML and MDS, given their major impact on the prognosis[2,3] and clinical management of these diseases. Regarding the diagnosis of MDS and AML, certain specific cytogenetic abnormalities are considered as presumptive evidence for MDS when they are detected in a patient with unexplained cytopenias.[1] Similarly, a diagnosis of AML can be made with less than 20% myeloblasts when the specific AML-defining chromosomal abnormalities t(8;21)(q22;q22), inv(16)(p13.1q22), t(16;16)(p13.1;q22), or t(15;17)(q22;q12) are detected. With regard to disease classification, genetic abnormalities have been incorporated into the definitions of certain AML and MDS disease categories. These are generally cytogenetic abnormalities, but mutations in *NPM1* and *CEBPA* genes were used to define two new provisional AML subtypes.

Since the publication of the 2008 WHO classification, the advent of high-throughput next generation sequencing (NGS) technologies has revealed the complexity of the genomic landscape of MDS and AML.[4–8] These technologies have led to the discovery of numerous recurrent mutations in genes and cellular pathways not previously implicated in these neoplasms (or previously missed by older, less sensitive methods of analysis), several of which have been shown to have diagnostic, prognostic, and/or therapeutic implications. Although conventional karyotyping to detect numerical chromosomal abnormalities and translocations remains a cornerstone in the diagnosis, classification, and management of AML and MDS, our review focuses mainly on the recently unraveled molecular genetic abnormalities in these diseases. These newly discovered genetic markers are refining existing prognostic schemes for AML and MDS and may help dictate targeted therapies.

CYTOGENETIC TESTING IN MYELODYSPLASTIC SYNDROME AND ACUTE MYELOID LEUKEMIA

Cytogenetic abnormalities are present in approximately 50% to 60% of MDS and AML cases at diagnosis. The cytogenetic findings provide critical diagnostic and prognostic information for both MDS and AML, and a conventional karyotype should always be performed on bone marrow taken at the time of primary diagnosis. Targeted fluorescent in situ hybridization (FISH) studies that interrogate for gains or losses of specific loci or translocations may miss abnormalities that are not included in the panel. FISH analysis for common abnormalities in MDS may be helpful if the karyotype fails or is insufficient (less than 20 metaphases),[9] but probably does not add information if the karyotype is successful.[10,11]

The most common recurring clonal cytogenetic aberrations in MDS are shown in **Table 1**.[12–15] Most of the genetic abnormalities in MDS are chromosomal gains or losses, such as –7, del(5q), –5, and +8. Translocations are less frequent in MDS and, if present, are often unbalanced. According to the 2008 WHO classification, the presence of any of the MDS-defining cytogenetic abnormalities listed in **Table 1** (with the exception of +8, del20q, and –Y), is sufficient to confirm a diagnosis of MDS in a cytopenic patient, even if significant morphologic dysplasia is lacking.[16–18] A recent study suggests that +15, often accompanied by –Y, is another cytogenetic abnormality that does not necessarily indicate MDS.[19] The only genetic abnormality that currently defines a specific MDS subtype is an isolated del(5q), reflecting the strong association of this abnormality with a particular disease phenotype (**Fig. 1**A), response to a specific therapy (lenalidomide), and favorable prognosis. A central role of the del(5q) in the pathogenesis of this MDS subtype has been recently validated by its identification in the most primitive MDS stem cells and its occurrence as an apparent founding event before the acquisition of any other mutations.[20] A number of genes in the commonly deleted region have been hypothesized to contribute to the disease pathogenesis. Haploinsufficiency of the RPS14 ribosomal structural protein,[21] as well as the microRNAs miR-145 and miR-146a in the deleted region, are thought to influence the characteristic megakaryocyte abnormalities and anemia,[22] whereas casein kinase 1A1 (*CSNK1A1*) haploinsufficiency that dysregulates the WNT/beta-catenin pathway has been implicated in proliferation of the del(5q) clone.[23] Beyond the del(5q), it is well established that specific cytogenetic abnormalities strongly influence the prognosis of MDS, and thus the karyotype findings represent a critical aspect of MDS risk-stratification schemes, such as the revised International Prognostic Scoring System (IPSS-R).[3]

Although chromosomal gains and losses are also common in AML, recurring translocations that activate oncogenes are a hallmark of many types of AML. A listing of the common cytogenetic aberrations in AML is shown in **Table 2**. As with MDS, cytogenetics is very important in AML risk stratification. Karyotype abnormalities are strongly correlated with clinical behavior in AML and certain abnormalities define specific AML disease subtypes that often have distinctive morphologies. Examples of these genetic-morphologic correlations in AML

Table 1
Cytogenetic abnormalities in myelodysplastic syndromes: significance in the WHO classification and prognostic risk grouping according to the revised International Prognostic Scoring System (IPSS-R) scheme

Cytogenetic Abnormality and IPSS-R risk group	Genes Involved	Significance in WHO Classification
Very good risk group		
−Y	Unknown	Not sufficient to diagnose MDS in the absence of significant dysplasia
del(11q)	Unknown	Sufficient to diagnose MDS in a cytopenic patient, even in the absence of dysplasia
Good-risk group		
Normal karyotype	NA	None
del(5q) (isolated or with one other abnormality)	*RPS14* haploinsufficiency	Sufficient to diagnose MDS in a cytopenic patient, even in the absence of dysplasia; defines a specific MDS subtype, provided other criteria for MDS with isolated del(5q) are fulfilled
del(12p)	Unknown	Sufficient to diagnose MDS in a cytopenic patient, even in the absence of dysplasia
del(20q)	Unknown	Not sufficient to diagnose MDS in the absence of significant dysplasia
Intermediate-risk group		
del(7q)	Unknown	Sufficient to diagnose MDS in a cytopenic patient, even in the absence of dysplasia
iso(17q)	*TP53*	Sufficient to diagnose MDS in a cytopenic patient, even in the absence of dysplasia
+8	Unknown	Not sufficient to diagnose MDS in the absence of significant dysplasia
1 or 2 other abnormalities	Unknown	None; some abnormalities are considered sufficient to diagnose MDS even in the absence of significant dysplasia
Poor-risk group		
−7 (isolated or with 1 or 2 other abnormalities)	Unknown	Sufficient to diagnose MDS in a cytopenic patient, even in the absence of dysplasia; common in therapy-related MDS
del(7q) (with 1 or 2 other abnormalities)	Unknown	Sufficient to diagnose MDS in a cytopenic patient, even in the absence of dysplasia; common in therapy-related MDS
inv(3), translocations of 3q, deletion 3q	*RPN1-EVI1* or other abnormalities of *RPN1* or *EVI1*	Sufficient to diagnose MDS in a cytopenic patient, even in the absence of dysplasia
3 abnormalities	Unknown	Sufficient to diagnose MDS in a cytopenic patient, even in the absence of dysplasia
Very poor risk group		
>3 abnormalities	Unknown	Sufficient to diagnose MDS in a cytopenic patient, even in the absence of dysplasia

Abbreviations: MDS, myelodysplastic syndrome; NA, not applicable; WHO, World Health Organization.

Data from Swerdlow S, Campo E, Harris NL, et al. WHO Classification of Tumours of Haematopoietic and Lymphoid Tissues. Lyon (France): International Agency for Research on Cancer (IARC); 2008; and Greenberg PL, Tuechler H, Schanz J, et al. Revised international prognostic scoring system for myelodysplastic syndromes. Blood 2012;120:2454–65.

are shown in **Fig.** 1B–D. Identification of a t(15;17) *PML-RARA* rearrangement to confirm a diagnosis of acute promyelocytic leukemia (APML) is especially critical, as this unique AML subtype requires specific up-front therapy. Institution of inappropriate therapy may precipitate fulminant disseminated intravascular coagulation, which is a major cause of death in patients with APML. This clinical

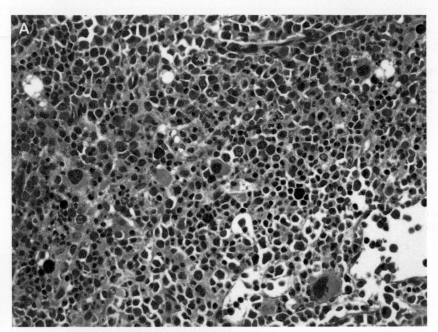

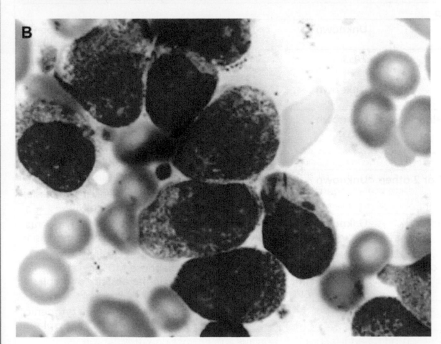

Fig. 1. Morphologic correlations of cytogenetic abnormalities in MDS and AML. (*A*) MDS with isolated del(5q), showing numerous megakaryocytes with rounded, unilobated nuclei (hematoxylin-eosin [H&E], bone marrow biopsy, original magnification ×20). (*B*) APML with t(15;17) (q22;q12); *PML-RARA.* Blasts and promyelocytes contain azurophilic granules and one has multiple Auer rods (Wright-Giemsa, bone marrow aspirate smear, original magnification ×100).

association mandates that *PML-RARA* rearrangement be investigated in all new acute leukemias in which APML is a diagnostic consideration. The *PML-RARA* rearrangement can be rapidly demonstrated (in <24 hours) by a direct harvest karyotype, targeted FISH, reverse transcriptase-polymerase chain reaction (RT-PCR), or immunofluorescent staining showing aberrant PML nuclear staining pattern; the latter technique is the fastest way to confirm the *PML-RARA*, but it is not widely available.[24–26] In addition to the role of karyotype in the WHO classification of AML, most clinical risk-stratification schemes use karyotype findings to predict prognosis and help direct risk-adjusted therapy for patients with AML. These include the United Kingdom Medical Research Council (most recently updated in 2010),[27] Southwest Oncology Group/ Eastern Cooperative Oncology Group,[28] and the

Fig. 1. (continued). (*C*) AML with t(8;21) (q22;q22); *RUNX1-RUNX1T1*. Blasts have relatively abundant pink cytoplasm (Wright-Giemsa, bone marrow aspirate smear, original magnification ×100). (*D*) AML with inv(16) (p13.1q22); *BCFB-MYH11*. Blasts have monocytic features, with folded and bilobed nuclei, and there is prominent background eosinophilia (H&E, bone marrow biopsy, original magnification ×100).

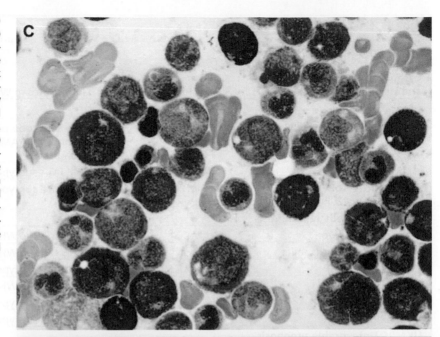

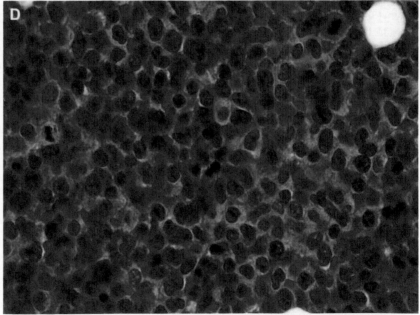

Cancer and Leukemia Group B AML cytogenetic classifications.[29]

MOLECULAR GENETIC RISK-STRATIFICATION IN MYELODYSPLASTIC SYNDROME AND ACUTE MYELOID LEUKEMIA

As mentioned previously, the most widely used risk-stratification scheme for MDS, the IPSS-R,[3]

incorporates 5 cytogenetic risk groups (**Table 1**). However, this scheme does not take into account the influence of gene mutations on prognosis, which is substantial. Although the effect of karyotype on prognosis has been studied for decades in studies that have collectively examined thousands of patients with long follow-up, data on mutations in MDS are still relatively immature, given the relatively recent availability of robust mutation testing. One recent study found that mutations in

Table 2
Cytogenetic abnormalities in AML: significance in the WHO classification and prognostic risk grouping according to the UKMRC scheme

Cytogenetic Abnormality and UKMRC Risk Grouping	Genes Involved	Significance in WHO Classification
UKMRC Favorable prognosis		
t(15;17)(q22;q21)[a]	PML-RARA	AML-RGA subtype; treated differently from other AML, necessitating rapid diagnosis
t(8;21)(q22;q21)[a]	RUNX1T1-RUNX1	AML-RGA subtype
inv(16)(p13.1q22)/ t(16;16)(p13.1;q22)[a]	CBFB-MYH11	AML-RGA subtype
UKMRC Intermediate prognosis		
Normal karyotype	NA	Not a specific WHO subtype
+8, +21, other trisomies	Unknown	Not a specific WHO subtype
t(9;11)(p22;q23)	MLLT3-MLL	AML-RGA subtype
t(11;19)(q23;p13)	MLL-ELL or MLL-MLLT1	Not a specific WHO subtype
t(6;9)(p23;q34)	DEK-NUP214	AML-RGA subtype
t(1;22)(p13;q13)	RBM15-MKL1	AML-RGA subtype
UKMRC Unfavorable prognosis		
inv(3)(q21q26)/t(3;3)(q21;q26)	RPN1-EVI1	AML-RGA subtype
t(3;21)(q26.2;q22.1)	RUNX1-EVI1	AML-MRC defining
t(1;3)(p36.3;q21.1)	PRDM16-RPN1	AML-MRC defining
t(3;5)(q25;q34)	MLF1-NPM1	AML-MRC defining
-5, del(5q), -7, del(7q)	Unknown	AML-MRC defining
Abnormal 17p (translocation or deletion), including i(17q)	TP53	AML-MRC defining
-17	TP53	Not a specific WHO subtype
Complex (≥4 unrelated abnormalities)	Variable	AML-MRC defining
Other t(11q23) excluding t(9;11) and t(11;19)	MLL	Not a specific WHO subtype; some MLL rearrangements are AML-MRC defining
t(9;22)(q34;q11)	BCR-ABL1	Not a specific WHO subtype

Abbreviations: AML-MRC, acute myeloid leukemia with myelodysplasia-related changes; AML-RGA, acute myeloid leukemia with recurrent genetic abnormalities; NA, not applicable; UKMRC, United Kingdom Medical Research Council; WHO, World Health Organization.

[a] Cases are still classified as AML-RGA and considered to have favorable UKMRC karyotype even if other cytogenetic abnormalities are present; these abnormalities are AML-defining even if blasts are less than 20%.

Data from Grimwade D, Hills RK, Moorman AV, et al. Refinement of cytogenetic classification in acute myeloid leukemia: determination of prognostic significance of rare recurring chromosomal abnormalities among 5876 younger adult patients treated in the United Kingdom Medical Research Council trials. Blood 2010;116:354–65; and Arber DA, Brunning RD, Orazi A, et al. Acute myeloid leukaemia with myelodysplasia-related changes. In: Swerdlow SH, Campo E, Harris NL, et al, editors. WHO Classification of Tumours of Haematopoietic and Lymphoid Tissues. 4th edition. Lyon (France): International Agency for Research on Cancer (IARC); 2008. p. 124–6.

any of 5 genes (*TP53, EZH2, ETV6, RUNX1*, and *ASXL1*, each discussed separately later in this article) had a significant adverse impact on prognosis in MDS that was independent of age and the IPSS grouping[30]; in effect, the presence of any one of these mutations predicted significantly worse outcome than would have been expected from the existing IPSS grouping. Another study used a prognostic model with the mutation status of 14 genes to create 4 prognostic groups with significantly different outcomes.[31] It is still uncertain how to apply these schemes in clinical practice, and much more data are required to fully understand the implication of mutations on current MDS treatment algorithms. The level of complexity is increased by the frequent presence of multiple mutations in combination, diverse subclones with different mutation profiles in a single patient, and varying levels of mutant allele fraction in different cases.

In AML, the mutation status of 3 genes (*NPM1*, *FLT3*, and *CEBPA*) has been used (since at least 2008) in combination with the cytogenetic risk group to guide treatment. Evidence has shown that patients with AML with intermediate-risk karyotype and *NPM1* or dual *CEBPA* mutations and lacking *FLT3*-ITD (internal tandem duplications) have a favorable prognosis and may not require treatment with stem cell transplantation. Since 2008, as with MDS, large amounts of data have been accumulating concerning the effect of other mutations on AML outcome. A listing of the recurrently mutated genes in AML is shown in **Table 3**. One study found that in intermediate-risk karyotype AML, *NPM1* in combination with *IDH1* and *IDH2* and no FLT3-ITD conferred a prognosis

similar to the favorable-risk karyotype group, whereas mutations in *TET2*, *MLL*, *ASXL1*, *PHF6*, or combination of *FLT3*-ITD with *DNMT3A* mutation or trisomy 8 conferred a prognosis similar to the unfavorable-risk karyotype group.[32] Another scheme proposed by the European LeukemiaNet developed 5 AML risk groups based on a combination of karyotype and mutation status of *NPM1*, *FLT3*, *CEBPA*, *DNMT3A*, *MLL*, and *TP53*.[33] The optimal way to combine karyotype with mutation data (particularly in cases with multiple mutations and/or several mutationally distinct subclones) to guide treatment decisions is still under active investigation. Importantly, targeted therapies have been developed against several pathways or proteins that are affected by mutations in AML, making it critically important to better understand mutation hierarchies and how these should dictate the use of targeted therapies in conjunction with standard cytotoxic therapies.

Table 3
Recurrently mutated genes in AML and MDSs

Gene	Estimated Incidence in MDS	Estimated Incidence in AML	References
Transcription factors			
CEBPA	1%–4%	8%–15%	44–46
ETV6	3%	2%	54,55
RUNX1	9%	6%–9%	58–61
Signal transducers			
FLT3	2%–6%	20%–30%	66,67
NPM1	4%	30%	67,124,125
TP53	10%–15% (40% t-AML/MDS)	10%–15%, (40% in t-AML/MDS)	72–74
KIT	<1%	<5% (20%–30% in core-binding factor AML)	66,79,80
Splicing factors	43%–85% overall	7% overall (27% of t-AML)	7,83–85
SF3B1	28%	—	7,86
U2AF1	7%–9%	—	7,86
SRSF2	12%–15%	—	7,86
ZRSR2	3%–11%	—	7,86
Cohesin complex genes	8%–17%	8%–20%	91
DNA methylation			
DNMT3A	2%–8%	22%	5,96
TET2	10%–25%	7%–23%	98,99
IDH1/2	5%–10%	15%–25%	101,126
Chromatin modifiers			
ASXL1	10%	17%	77
MLL	3%	3%–8%	58,118
EZH2	6%	2%	121–123,127

Abbreviations: AML, acute myeloid leukemia; MDS, myelodysplastic syndrome; t-AML, therapy-related AML; t-MDS, therapy-related MDS.

METHODS OF DETECTING GENETIC ABERRATIONS IN MYELODYSPLASTIC SYNDROME AND ACUTE MYELOID LEUKEMIA

DETECTION OF TRANSLOCATIONS

Translocations between genes (gene rearrangements) are detected most commonly by conventional karyotyping, FISH, and RT-PCR, and, more recently, by NGS assays.

Conventional karyotyping has the advantage of being a genome-wide assay and is therefore capable of detecting both known and novel gene rearrangements. It requires fresh, viable tissue, has a limit of detection of approximately 5 Mb, and will miss cryptic rearrangements, including some (such as PML-RARA and MLL rearrangements) that occur in AML. Because only 20 metaphases are typically examined (and a minimum of 2 metaphases showing the same aberration need to be detected), cytogenetics has a sensitivity of only approximately 10%.

FISH, in which fluorescent probes are used to locate genes or sequences of interest on one or more chromosomes, is also routinely used in cytogenetics and molecular diagnostic laboratories to detect translocations. The assay can be performed on metaphase preparations from growing cells (metaphase FISH, requiring fresh tissue) or on nondividing cells (interphase FISH, which is applicable to fixed, paraffin-embedded tissue). The assay sensitivity depends on laboratory cutoffs established during the validation of the assay, on the number of cells scored, and on whether the assay is performed on whole nuclei or thin [5 μm] sections; typically, the sensitivity ranges from 1-15%. The disadvantage of FISH is that one needs to know which translocations to look for and it may not detect all possible rearrangements due in part to its limit of detection of 50Kb to 1Mb (depending on the size of the probes).

RT-PCR is widely available in most molecular laboratories and a very sensitive assay, down to 0.01-0.001%, making it an ideal assay to use for minimal residual disease monitoring during treatment. Similar to FISH, one needs to know which translocation to look for, including both 5′ and 3′ translocated genes, when designing the primers and probes for the assay; this is a disadvantage compared with FISH assays that can usually detect rearrangements even when only one fusion partner is known by using "break-apart" probes. Furthermore, RT-PCR can be used only to detect gene fusions, whereas it cannot generally detect gene rearrangements in which a gene is translocated to promoter or enhancer elements of another gene.

NGS also can be used to detect recurrent gene rearrangements. Whole-genome sequencing (WGS) allows unbiased genome-wide detection of any structural rearrangements, both known and novel, but is not generally in clinical use. Targeted DNA or RNA sequencing assays are increasingly being used to detect gene rearrangements. As with RT-PCR or FISH, these targeted assays will detect only rearrangements specifically dictated by the assay design. Recently, targeted RNA sequencing assays have been developed that require knowing only one of the genes involved in a rearrangement and can thus be used to detect rearrangements with not only known but also novel fusion partners.[34]

DETECTION OF COPY NUMBER ABNORMALITIES

Conventional karyotyping is routinely used to detect chromosomal copy number abnormalities at the level of chromosomes or chromosome arms, often seen in patients with MDS and particularly important for the disease-defining del(5q).

Chromosomal microarray platforms are based on measuring the difference in fluorescence intensity between co-hybridized sample and control DNA, which is fluorescently labeled. For hematological neoplasms, some laboratories have been successfully using arrays with oligonucleotide probes for single nucleotide polymorphisms (SNP-arrays) that provide copy number information with superior resolution compared with conventional karyotyping and also allow the detection of acquired copy-neutral loss of heterozygosity.[35] The analysis of candidate genes in regions of copy-neutral loss of heterozygosity and in microdeletions identified by these SNP-array platforms has led to the discovery of several genes recurrently mutated in MDS and AML, such as the TET2 gene.[36]

NGS assays also are successfully used to detect copy number abnormalities. WGS is the ideal platform to detect all types of structural variants, including translocations. It provides coverage across the genome, including intragenic, intronic, and exonic regions, but is not routinely used for clinical testing. Restricting NGS analysis to certain regions of the genome (whole-exome sequencing [WES], whole transcriptome sequencing, or targeted gene panels) will not capture the full complexity of all structural variation in a tumor, which often involves intronic and intragenic regions, but is more cost-effective and clinically implementable. The use of both tumor and normal tissue from the same patient for SNP-arrays and NGS assays can be very useful in correctly distinguishing somatically acquired, cancer-specific lesions from patient-specific inherited copy number variations.

DETECTION OF POINT MUTATIONS AND INSERTION/DELETIONS

Recent studies have demonstrated that a relatively small core of genes (fewer than 30) is recurrently mutated in the vast majority of patients with MDS and AML,[37,38] thus routine WGS or WES is not considered necessary for uncovering recurrent genetic mutations in most cases. Although WGS allows a comprehensive and unbiased overview of a tumor genome and identifies translocations and copy number alterations (discussed previously) in addition to gene mutations, sequencing 6 billion bases is associated with high costs, complex analysis, slow turnaround time, and relatively low sensitivity for variant detection; at this point in time, WGS is still considered largely a research tool. WES typically analyzes approximately 1.5% of the genome, being restricted to exonic regions of the approximately 25,000 protein-coding genes where most of the known pathogenic mutations occur. Although WES is not currently routinely performed in clinical practice, it may be considered for selected patients, such as those in whom a mutation cannot not be identified with routine testing or in the setting of clinical trials. Most molecular laboratories currently use multiplex targeted genotyping panels that are based on NGS sequencing technologies.

Single gene testing may occasionally be used for disease monitoring of a known genetic abnormality. Sanger sequencing technology uses primers that hybridize to PCR products and are extended using 4 deoxynucleotides (dNTPs), and 4 fluorescently labeled dideoxynucleotides (ddNTPs); products are analyzed by capillary electrophoresis. The technique is labor intensive, not amenable to multiplexing, and has low sensitivity (20%–25%), but it is relatively cheap and it is still widely used for single gene mutational analysis. Allele-specific PCR assays are also still widely used in most molecular laboratories for both gene mutation panels and single gene testing. The assay relies on primers or probes hybridizing to the wild type or to the alternative nucleotide. Allele-specific PCR is cheap, fast, and sensitive (typically 0.1%–1%), but is useful only for mutational hotspots; it cannot easily be used for interrogating genes where pathogenic mutations occur at multiple sites.

Targeted NGS assays require target enrichment strategies that usually are either hybrid capture based (in which DNA fragments are hybridized in solution to sequence-specific capture probes corresponding to target regions of the genome)[39] or amplicon capture based (in which targeted multiplex PCR amplifies regions of interest). These targeted NGS assays provide high throughput and can be very sensitive. Some NGS methods like anchored multiplex assay technologies,[34] hybrid capture–based assays, or the use of molecular barcodes[40] allow accurate quantification of mutated allele burden. Knowledge of the mutated allele burden can help reveal oncogenic subclones and thus elucidate the clonal hierarchy, which may have important prognostic and therapeutic implications.

Although molecular genetic testing is already the standard of care in patients with AML (at least with regard to NPM1, FLT3, and CEBPA mutations), it is still not common practice for patients with MDS, despite several recent studies demonstrating prognostic and therapeutic advantages derived from detection of specific mutations. An important note of caution is that mutations in MDS-related genes may be detected in healthy individuals,[41,42] particularly in elderly individuals, and therefore in the absence of cytopenias and morphologic dysplasia, the presence of mutations alone should not be used to diagnose MDS.[42]

RELEVANCE OF SPECIFIC MUTATIONS IN MYELODYSPLASTIC SYNDROME AND ACUTE MYELOID LEUKEMIA

MYELOID TRANSCRIPTION FACTORS

CCAAT/Enhancer Binding Protein Alpha

The CCAAT/enhancer binding protein alpha (CEBPA) gene is a single-exon intronless gene encoding a member of the basic region leucine zipper family of transcription factors, composed of 2 transactivation domains in the N-terminal part, a leucine zipper region (for homo- or hetero-dimerization with other CEBP family members) and a DNA-binding domain in the C-terminal part. CEBPA function is crucial for granulocytic differentiation and proliferation.[43] Various mechanisms contribute to its dysregulation in patients with AML. The most well-characterized consist of mutations at the N-terminus and at the C-terminus of the gene, either in combination on separate alleles (ie, in trans) or as a sole mutation. CEBPA mutations affect 8% to 15% of patients with AML, particularly those with normal karyotype and are only rarely seen in patients with MDS.[44–46] The mutations occurring in the N-terminus are usually frameshift insertion/deletions (indels) resulting in translation of a truncated protein form that lacks the transactivation domains and exerts a dominant-negative effect over the full-length protein form. Conversely, mutations in the C-terminus are generally in-frame indels that affect the leucine zipper region and disrupt DNA binding and homo- or heterodimerization with other CEBP family members.[47] Double, but not single, *CEBPA* mutations in AML are associated with a favorable prognosis with regard to increased remission duration and overall survival, in the absence of adverse cytogenetic abnormalities or *FLT3* internal tandem duplications (*FLT3-ITD*).[48–50] Of note, germline *CEBPA* mutations, particularly in the N-terminal domain, have been detected in familial AML. In these patients, a second somatic mutation (usually in the C-terminal domain) is detected in the leukemic blasts.[51] In the 2008 WHO classification, AML with mutated *CEBPA* is recognized as a provisional subtype of AML with recurrent genetic abnormalities (AML-RGA). *CEBPA* mutation testing is currently recommended by the National Comprehensive Cancer Network guidelines and other cooperative groups in de novo AML that lacks other defining genetic features.

Ets Variant 6 Gene (ETV6)

The Ets variant 6 gene (*ETV6*), previously known as *TEL* (translocation, ETS, leukemia) encodes an ETS family transcription factor required for hematopoiesis and maintenance of the developing vascular network. This gene is dysregulated through a variety of mechanisms in hematological malignancies, including gene fusions with a variety of partners[52] and gene deletions[53] that are mostly found in acute lymphoblastic leukemia. ETV6 point mutations are found in a small subset of MDS and appear to independently predict poorer survival.[54,55]

Runt-related Transcription Factor 1 (RUNX1)

RUNX1 (Runt-related transcription factor 1), formerly known as *AML1* (acute myeloid leukemia 1) or *CBFA2* (core-binding factor subunit alpha-2) encodes the alpha subunit of the core-binding factor protein, a transcription factor that regulates the differentiation of hematopoietic stem cells into mature blood cells.[56]

RUNX1 was first identified at the translocation site t(8;21) in AML.[57] In addition to this and other translocations, mutations of *RUNX1* are detected in approximately 6% to 9% of AML[58–60] and 9%

of MDS.[55,60,61] Leukemia-associated *RUNX1* point mutations are commonly clustered within the functionally important Runt domain, but they can be distributed throughout the full length of the gene. Most mutations are predicted to cause a loss of normal RUNX1 trans-activating activity due to disruption of DNA binding and/or heterodimerization capabilities (haploinsufficiency), with some also exerting a dominant-negative effect. *RUNX1* mutations are more commonly seen in older patients with normal karyotype AML with undifferentiated (FAB M0) morphology as well as in therapy-related or MDS-associated AML. *RUNX1* mutations are positively associated with *MLL-PTD* and *IDH* mutations, whereas they do not usually occur together with *NPM1* or *CEBPA* mutations.

Mutations of *RUNX1* detected in patients with MDS and AML are distributed throughout the full length of the protein. N-terminal mutations are exclusively within the Runt homology domain (RHD). Nearly half are missense mutations that replace amino acid residues in direct contact with DNA, and most of the other mutations are frameshift or nonsense mutations that abolish the function of the RHD. On the other hand, the bulk of the C-terminal mutations result in frameshifts, with a few missense mutations. The consequences of C-terminal mutations are unusual: typically, frameshift mutations result in truncation of the authentic protein followed by a relatively short additional stretch of amino acid residues originating from the wrong reading frame or from intronic sequences. However, in nearly half of the C-terminal *RUNX1* mutations, the stretches of additional amino acids resulting from the wrong reading frame are relatively long (approximately 200–350 residues in length). The mutated *RUNX1* proteins in these cases are even longer than wild-type *RUNX1*, resembling fusion proteins rather than truncations.

In AML, *RUNX1* mutations are associated with thrombocytopenia and predict resistance to chemotherapy and shorter overall survival, but allogeneic stem cell transplantation seems to improve the prognosis.[55,62,63] Of note, germline mutations of *RUNX1* have been identified as a cause of an autosomal familial platelet dysfunction with predisposition to AMLs (OMIM 601399).[64]

SIGNAL TRANSDUCTION

FMS Like Tyrosine Kinase 3 (FLT3)

The FMS like tyrosine kinase 3 (FLT3) is a receptor tyrosine kinase expressed on hematopoietic precursor cells that plays a key role in stem cell differentiation and proliferation.[65] Mutations in *FLT3* are detected in 20% to 30% of AML[66] and in only 2%

to 6% of MDS cases.[67] In AML, these mutations are often associated with high white blood count and "cup-shaped" blasts (Fig. 2A).[68] Two main mutations occur, both of which result in dysregulated kinase activity: internal tandem duplications (*FLT3*-ITD) in the juxtamembrane domain, varying in size between 5 and 400 nucleotides, and, in a smaller proportion of patients, missense point mutations in the tyrosine kinase domain (TKD), most frequently at codon 835 or 836. In AML, *FLT3*-

ITD mutations predict increased frequency of relapse and shorter overall survival, but their prognostic impact is influenced by cooperating mutations, such as *NPM1* and *DNMT3A*. The presence of only mutated *FLT3*-ITD sequences with absence of wild-type *FLT3* portends an even more dismal prognosis.[69] Patients with AML with *FLT3*-ITD mutation appear to benefit from allogeneic stem cell transplantation.[70] The prognostic role for the *FLT3*-TKD mutations

Fig. 2. Morphologic and immunohistochemical correlations of mutations in MDS and AML. (*A*) AML with *FLT3*-ITD. Blasts have irregular or lobulated nuclei and some have cup-shaped nuclear invaginations (Wright-Giemsa, peripheral blood smear, original magnification ×100). (*B*) AML with mutated *NPM1*. Blasts show abnormal cytoplasmic staining for NPM1, in addition to the expected nuclear staining (NPM1 immunohistochemistry, bone marrow biopsy, original magnification ×100).

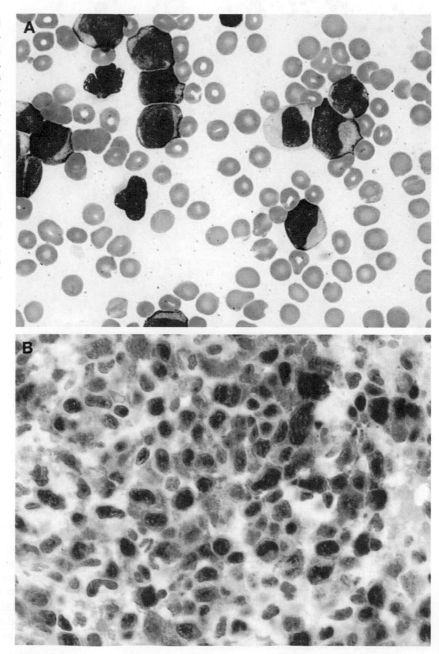

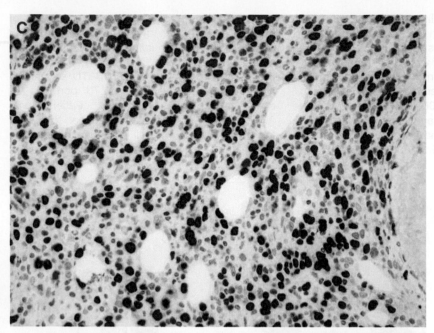

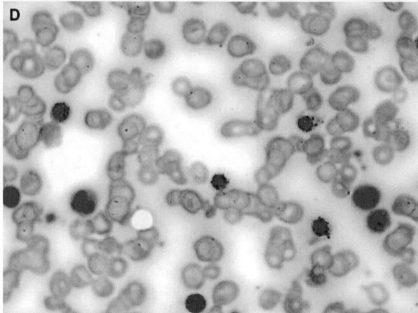

Fig. 2. (continued). (*C*) MDS with *TP53* mutation. Many cells (mostly blasts and early erythroids) show strong nuclear immunoreactivity for TP53 (TP53 immunohistochemistry, bone marrow biopsy, original magnification ×20). (*D*) MDS with ring sideroblasts and *SF3B1* mutation. Ring sideroblasts are erythroid elements with iron granules surrounding the nucleus (iron stain, bone marrow aspirate smear, original magnification ×100).

remains controversial. In MDS, *FLT3* mutations are mainly restricted to higher-risk subtypes, are associated with complex karyotype, and often rapidly progress to AML.[67] Small molecule multikinase inhibitors with activity against FLT3 have been evaluated in patients with *FLT3*-mutated AML, both as single agents as well as in combination with chemotherapy, with generally limited and short-lasting effects due to acquired resistance.[71]

Nucleophosmin 1 (NPM1)

The Nucleophosmin 1 (*NPM1*) gene is mutated in approximately 30% of all AML and it is the most frequently mutated gene in normal karyotype AML, being found in up to 85% of such cases. NPM1 is a shuttle protein, predominantly localized in the nucleolus and involved in many cellular functions, particularly in ribosomal biogenesis, chromatin remodeling, control of DNA replication and repair, cell cycle progression, and cell survival. Mutations in *NPM1* are usually small insertions (mostly 4 bp in size, but sometimes up to 11 bp) in exon 12 resulting in loss of 2 tryptophan residues (Trp-288 and Trp-290) in the C-terminus. The mutation introduces a nuclear export signal, causing aberrant accumulation of NPM1 in the cytoplasm, where it dimerizes with and sequesters wild-type NPM1. Although wild-type NPM1 protein is localized to the nucleus, the mutated protein is present in the cytoplasm; this aberrant localization can be identified in NPM1-mutated AML cases by using NPM1 immunohistochemistry (see **Fig. 2B**).

Patients with AML with mutated *NPM1* and wild-type *FLT3* have an overall good prognosis, with an outcome similar to that of patients with favorable-risk cytogenetics; stem cell transplantation is generally not indicated in this AML subgroup.[70] *NPM1* mutations are detected in a small percentage of patients with MDS (approximately 4%), predominantly in cases with excess blasts. When isolated, *NPM1* mutations in MDS do not appear to contribute to progression to AML.[67]

Tumor Protein p53 (TP53)

The tumor protein p53 (TP53) is a transcription factor and prototypical tumor suppressor gene, which can induce cell cycle arrest in G1 or G2 and apoptosis in response to various cellular stresses to allow the activation of the DNA repair system. Somatic *TP53* mutations are detected in 50% of solid tumors, up to 40% of therapy-related myeloid neoplasms, and in 10% to 15% of de novo AML and MDS.[72–74] The mutated TP53 protein is usually overexpressed and the presence of strongly staining cells by TP53 immunohistochemistry is well-correlated with the presence of a TP53 mutation in MDS[74] (see **Fig. 2C**). In AML, *TP53* mutations are almost exclusively seen in the context of a complex karyotype, with more than 50% of such cases showing *TP53* mutations, often consisting of a point mutation together with loss of the other *TP53* locus at chromosome 17p.[75] *TP53* mutations confer poor prognosis in MDS and AML and are associated with chemotherapy resistance and reduced overall and disease-free survival, even in patients undergoing stem cell transplantation.[55,74,76,77] In low-risk MDS with del(5q), detection of a *TP53* mutation even at low frequency is associated with a higher rate of leukemic evolution and a lower likelihood of responding to lenalidomide treatment.[78]

V-kit Hardy-Zuckerman 4 Feline Sarcoma Viral Oncogene Homolog (KIT)

The v-kit Hardy-Zuckerman 4 feline sarcoma viral oncogene homolog (KIT) is a class III transmembrane receptor tyrosine kinase for stem cell factor required for normal hematopoiesis, melanogenesis, and gametogenesis. *KIT* mutations leading to dysregulated receptor activation occur in a variety of solid tumors. In hematological malignancies, they occur predominantly in systemic mastocytosis and in AML with core-binding factor abnormalities: *KIT* mutations are found in approximately 20% to 25% of AML with t(8;21) and 30% of AML with inv(16). The mutations are mostly within exon 17, which encodes the activation loop in the kinase domain, and within exon 8, which encodes the extracellular portion of the KIT receptor.[79,80] In these AML subtypes, both exon 17 and exon 8 mutations are associated with increased risk of relapse. Thus, targeted *KIT* mutational analysis should be considered for core-binding factor AML for prognostic reasons. *KIT* mutations may have therapeutic implications as well, given that potent KIT inhibitors are now available and are active against the imatinib-resistant Asp816 *KIT* hotspot mutation in exon 17.

In myelodysplastic syndromes, *KIT* mutations are uncommon, occurring in less than 1% of cases.[66] They occur mostly in high-grade MDS cases, possibly representing one of the additional genetic events contributing to the progression of MDS to AML.[81]

RNA SPLICING: *SF3B1, SETBP1, SRSF, U2AF1*

Recent NGS efforts have unraveled mutations in the RNA splicing machinery pathway, previously not implicated in cancer.[7,82] Most MDS (35%–85% depending on the subtype), approximately 25% of AML occurring after MDS, and approximately 5% to 10% of de novo AML harbor mutations in one of the components of the spliceosome.[7,83–85] The spliceosome complex, which includes both small nuclear RNAs (snRNA) and proteins (snRNPs), removes introns from genes that encode proteins. Mutations in components of this complex result in altered splicing, altered exon composition, retained introns, unconventional exons, and generation of novel protein isoforms. The biologic mechanisms linking alterations in splicing machinery to cellular transformation and leukemogenesis remain elusive.

More than 50% of MDS cases overall exhibit spliceosome mutations. These include mutations affecting proteins involved in the 3′ splice site recognition: U2 small nuclear ribonucleoprotein auxiliary factor 35 kDa subunit-related protein 2 (ZRSF2), serine/arginine-rich splicing factor 1 (SRSF1), serine/arginine-rich splicing factor 2 (SRSF2), and U2 small nuclear RNA auxiliary factor 1 (U2AF1/U2AF35 and U2AF65/U2AF2). Mutations are also seen that affect the function of the U2 snRNP splicing complex, which includes the Splicing factor 3A subunit 1 (SF3A1) and Splicing factor 3B subunit 1 (SF3B1) proteins.

Mutations of members of the RNA splicing machinery are largely mutually exclusive and occur most frequently in MDS with ring sideroblasts.[7] The genes more commonly mutated, in decreasing order of frequency, are SF3B1, U2AF1, SRSF2, and ZRSR2.[7,86] Mutations are missense and occur in hotspot regions and are therefore likely gain-of-function mutations, except for ZRSR2 in which they occur throughout the entire coding region and are frameshift, splice site, or nonsense mutations, likely causing loss of function. Despite affecting the same complex, different spliceosome mutations are associated with different phenotypes and clinical outcomes. SF3B1 mutations occur in 28% of all MDS, making it the most commonly mutated gene found in MDS to date, are strongly associated with the presence of ring sideroblasts (see Fig. 2D), and are associated with favorable prognosis.[86–88] Conversely, SRSF2 mutations are associated with neutropenia, severe thrombocytopenia, and poor prognosis.[86,89] ZRSR2 mutations are associated with neutropenia, more advanced MDS subtypes and secondary AML.[88] Mutations in U2AF1 are associated with an increased risk of progression to AML.

Spliceosome machinery mutations are also detected in AML, predominantly in cases evolving from MDS or in AML with MDS-related changes, with U2AF1 being the most commonly mutated gene (8%–9%), followed by SRSF2 (4%–6%) and SF3B1 (2%–5%); these mutations appear to have no detectable prognostic impact in this context.[90]

COHESIN COMPLEX

The cohesin complex represents another pathway that, before genome-wide studies, was not known to be altered in myeloid neoplasms.[91] The ring-shaped cohesin complex is composed of 4 subunits (SMC1A, SMC3, RAD21, and either STAG1 or STAG2) that encircle chromatin and are responsible for sister chromatid cohesion and segregation, maintenance of chromatin architecture, gene expression control, DNA replication, and DNA-damage repair. Germline defects in regulators and structural components of the cohesin complex result in cohesinopathies, which are

genetic instability syndromes, such as Cornelia de Lange syndrome, a rare autosomal dominant disorder characterized by craniofacial abnormalities and cognitive deficits. Somatic mutations in the cohesin complex genes are mutually exclusive of one another and mostly result in predicted loss of function. Mutations in genes encoding components of the cohesin complex occur in 8% to 17% of MDS, 6% to 13% of de novo AML, and 8% to 20% of AML following MDS. At least in some large studies, cohesin-mutant patients with AML or MDS showed shorter overall survival compared with cohesin wild-type patients, with those carrying STAG2 mutations having a worse prognosis independently of IPSS score and age.[86,92] Cohesin mutations have been mostly detected as secondary subclonal events, undergoing clonal expansion over time and in some patients achieving clonal dominance at the time of transformation to AML. Despite their involvement in chromatin stability, cohesin mutations have not been associated with aneuploidy or complex cytogenetics in MDS or AML. Therefore, perturbation of other cohesin functions (such as their role in regulating gene expression) could contribute to leukemogenesis.

EPIGENETIC MODIFIERS: GENES THAT METHYLATE DNA AND ALTER CHROMATIN STRUCTURE

Epigenetics refers to heritable processes that regulate gene expression without accompanying changes in the genetic code. It encompasses all modifications of chromatin that determine the transcriptional capacity of a cell. Mutations in genes that regulate DNA methylation and histone modification have been shown to lead to myeloid transformation. This relatively newly discovered class of mutations is now being actively investigated for therapeutic targeting, as epigenetics is theoretically alterable.

DNA methylation, which is the addition of a methyl group at the 5-carbon of cytosine residues, mostly in the CpG-rich regions, results from the activity of the enzyme DNA methyltransferase (DNMT) and affects binding of transcription factors to DNA. Both hypermethylation (resulting in inactivation of tumor suppressor genes) as well as hypomethylation (resulting in transcriptional activation of oncogenes) leads to cancer cell proliferation.[93,94]

Mutations with clinical and potentially relevant consequences have been detected in several genes that affect DNA methylation, including DNA methyl transferases (DNMT)3A, tet methylcytosine dioxygenase 2 (TET2)[95] and isocitrate dehydrogenases 1 (*IDH1*) and 2 (*IDH2*), as well as in genes affecting histone function, like additional sex combslike 1 (*ASXL1*), enhancer of zeste homologue 2 (*EZH2*), and mixed lineage leukemia (*MLL*).

DNA METHYLATION

DNA Methyl Transferase 3A (DNMT3A)

Although both *DNMT3A* and its homologue *DNMT3B* are responsible for initiating de novo DNA methylation, only *DNMT3A* has been found to be recurrently mutated in myeloid neoplasms. *DNMT3A* mutations occur in approximately 22% of AMLs, particularly in those with monocytic features,[5] and in 2% to 8% of MDS.[96] Most (30%–60%) are missense mutations affecting amino acid Arg882 in the methyltransferase domain, whereas the remaining ones are missense, nonsense, indels, and splice site mutations affecting all domains of the protein. Although many mutations result in loss of enzymatic function, the recurrent missense mutation p.Arg882His is a dominant-negative inhibitor of wild-type DNMT3A in that it disrupts the ability of the DNMT3A enzyme to form active homotetramers.[97] *DNMT3A* mutations appear to occur as an early event in the genesis of myeloid neoplasms and they often occur in combination with mutations in *FLT3* (either ITD or TKD), *NPM1*, or *IDH1*, whereas they do not occur in patients with favorable-risk cytogenetics. *DNMT3A* mutations appear to be independently associated with worse overall survival in both MDS and AML,[5,96] but the precise mechanisms through which these mutations act is still unknown.

Ten-Eleven Translocation Gene-2 (TET2)

The ten-eleven translocation gene-2 (*TET2*) gene is homologous to the *TET1* gene involved in t(10;11)(q22;q23) AML, where it is fused to *MLL*. *TET2* encodes a dioxygenase that converts 5-methyl-cytosine (5-mC) to 5-hydroxymethyl-cytosine (5-hmC). Its function is not completely understood, but it may lead to demethylation. Somatic deletions and inactivating mutations in *TET2* are spread across all exons and are predicted to result in loss of function and decreased enzymatic activity. *TET2* mutations have been identified in 10% to 25% of MDS and in 7% to 23% of AML, particularly in MDS-associated AML and in de novo AML with normal cytogenetics. *TET2* mutations are associated with poorer prognosis in patients with cytogenetically normal AML, with lower incidence of complete remission and shorter survival,[98,99] whereas they do not seem to have prognostic relevance in MDS. *TET2* mutations can occur both early in the disease process and

as a late or secondary event during disease evolution. *TET2* mutations predict response to hypomethylating agents,[30] but are associated with shorter overall survival after hematopoietic stem cell transplantation.[55]

Isocitrate Dehydrogenase 1 and 2 (IDH1/IDH2)

The isocitrate dehydrogenase 1 and 2 (*IDH1* and *2*) genes encode for 2 metabolic enzymes, which catalyze the oxidative decarboxylation of isocitrate to α-ketoglutarate (also known as 2-oxoglutarate [2OG]), a tricarboxylic acid cycle intermediate and an essential cofactor for many enzymes. Recurrent somatic mutations in *IDH1* were initially described in glioblastomas. Subsequently, mutations in both *IDH1* and *IDH2*, which are usually, but not always mutually exclusive,[100] were identified in 15% to 25% of AML. *IDH1/2*-mutated AML includes de novo cases as well as AML progressed from MDS or a previous myeloproliferative neoplasm.[87,101–104] *IDH1/2* mutations are less common in MDS, occurring in 5% to 10% cases. The mutations are all located in the active sites of the enzymes affecting codon Arg 132 of IDH1 and Arg140 and Arg172 of IDH2, resulting in a neomorphic catalytic function with conversion of 2OG to (*R*)-2-hydroxyglutarate (2HG), which is thought to function as an oncometabolite, leading to hypermethylation, disruption of TET2 function, and impaired hematopoietic differentiation.[105]

The prognostic relevance of *IDH* mutations in AML and MDS is controversial. Some large studies with uniformly treated patients showed a favorable prognostic role for the *IDH2* Ard140Q mutation in normal karyotype AML[106,107] and no prognostic impact in MDS,[55] while others identified a poor prognostic role for *IDH1* or *IDH2* mutations in AML or found no prognostic significance.[108,109] Clinical trials with specific *IDH1* and *IDH2* inhibitors are ongoing with some promising early results.[110,111]

CHROMATIN MODIFIERS

Additional Sex Combs Like Transcriptional Regulator 1 (ASXL1)

The additional sex combs like transcriptional regulator 1 (*ASXL1*) gene is a member of the polycomb family of chromatin-binding proteins and is involved in the epigenetic regulation of gene expression. Mutations in *ASXL1* are found in all myeloid malignancies, including in about 10% of MDS cases, 6.5% of de novo AML and in up to 30% of AML arising from a prior myeloid neoplasm.[55,112,113] *ASXL1* mutations tend to be heterozygous and cluster in exon 12. They are typically frameshift and nonsense mutations that result in protein truncation just upstream of the

C-terminal plant homeodomain (PHD) motif, which may bind methylated lysines. *ASXL1* mutations are more common in patients with MDS with lower risk disease according to the IPSS, but interestingly have been shown to be associated with shorter overall survival and more rapid to progression to AML.[55,114] In AML, *ASXL1* mutations tend not to occur with *NPM1* or *FLT3* ITD mutations, whereas they frequently co-occur with *RUNX1* mutations. In patients with AML, *ASXL1* mutations are associated with poorer response to chemotherapy and decreased overall survival.[115,116]

Mixed Lineage Leukemia (MLL)

The mixed lineage leukemia (*MLL*) gene, now known as the lysine (K)-specific methyltransferase 2A (*KMT2A*) gene, encodes a histone H3 lysin 4 (H3K4) methyltransferase enzyme that positively regulates expression of target genes, including several homeobox (*HOX*) genes. This transcriptional coactivator plays an essential role in regulating gene expression during early development and hematopoiesis and is deregulated, mainly through translocations with various partners, in B-acute lymphoblastic leukemia and AML. Partial tandem duplications (PTD)[117] in the *MLL* gene also occur in a small proportion patients with AML (3%–8%)[58,118] and MDS (3%).[118] *MLL* PTD abnormalities are more frequently seen in AML with trisomy 11 or in therapy-related AML and MDS with complex karyotype and they often coexist with *TP53* deletion and/or mutation.[119] These cases show distinct clinicopathological features, including cytoplasmic vacuoles and blasts with bilobed nuclei, as well as frequent disseminated intravascular coagulation and an aggressive clinical course.[119,120]

Enhancer of Zeste 2 Polycomb Repressive Complex 2 Subunit (EZH2)

The enhancer of zeste 2 polycomb repressive complex 2 subunit (*EZH2*) gene is a component of the polycomb repressive complex 2 (PRC2), which catalyzes trimethylation of histone H3 lysine 27 (H3K27me3). PRC2 may recruit other polycomb complexes, histone deacetylases, and methyltransferases, targeting transcriptional repressive marks and chromatin compaction at key tumor suppressor gene loci. Overexpression of EZH2 is a marker of advanced disease in many solid tumors, including prostate and breast cancer and *EZH2* mutation has been identified in 10% to 20% of some lymphomas, which may result in enhanced enzymatic activity functionally equivalent to EZH2 overexpression. In myeloid neoplasms, *EZH2* mutations have been identified in

high-risk MDS (occurring in approximately 6% of patients with MDS overall) and appear to convey an unfavorable prognosis.[55,121–123] In contrast to the mutations in lymphomas, *EZH2* mutations in myeloid neoplasms are much more heterogeneous, occurring throughout the gene, and most appear to be inactivating mutations. The mechanisms by which the myeloid *EZH2* mutations participate in leukemogenesis are unknown.

REFERENCES

1. Swerdlow S, Campo E, Harris NL, et al. WHO classification of tumors of hematopoietic and lymphoid tissues. Lyon (France): International Agency for Research on Cancer (IARC); 2008.
2. Greenberg P, Cox C, LeBeau MM, et al. International scoring system for evaluating prognosis in myelodysplastic syndromes. Blood 1997;89:2079–88.
3. Greenberg PL, Tuechler H, Schanz J, et al. Revised international prognostic scoring system for myelodysplastic syndromes. Blood 2012;120:2454–65.
4. Ley TJ, Mardis ER, Ding L, et al. DNA sequencing of a cytogenetically normal acute myeloid leukaemia genome. Nature 2008;456:66–72.
5. Ley TJ, Ding L, Walter MJ, et al. DNMT3A mutations in acute myeloid leukemia. N Engl J Med 2010;363:2424–33.
6. Mardis ER, Ding L, Dooling DJ, et al. Recurring mutations found by sequencing an acute myeloid leukemia genome. N Engl J Med 2009;361:1058–66.
7. Yoshida K, Sanada M, Shiraishi Y, et al. Frequent pathway mutations of splicing machinery in myelodysplasia. Nature 2011;478:64–9.
8. Yan XJ, Xu J, Gu ZH, et al. Exome sequencing identifies somatic mutations of DNA methyltransferase gene DNMT3A in acute monocytic leukemia. Nat Genet 2011;43:309–15.
9. Malcovati L, Hellstrom-Lindberg E, Bowen D, et al. Diagnosis and treatment of primary myelodysplastic syndromes in adults: recommendations from the European LeukemiaNet. Blood 2013;122:2943–64.
10. Seegmiller AC, Wasserman A, Kim AS, et al. Limited utility of fluorescence in situ hybridization for common abnormalities of myelodysplastic syndrome at first presentation and follow-up of myeloid neoplasms. Leuk Lymphoma 2013;55:601–5.
11. Yang W, Stotler B, Sevilla DW, et al. FISH analysis in addition to G-band karyotyping: utility in evaluation of myelodysplastic syndromes? Leuk Res 2010;34:420–5.
12. Vallespi T, Imbert M, Mecucci C, et al. Diagnosis, classification, and cytogenetics of myelodysplastic syndromes. Haematologica 1998;83:258–75.
13. Olney HJ, Le Beau MM. The cytogenetics and molecular biology of myelodysplastic syndromes.

In: Bennett JM, editor. The myelodysplastic syndromes, pathobiology and clinical management. New York: Marcel Dekker, Inc; 2002. p. 89–119.

14. Raimondi SC. Cytogenetics in MDS. In: Lopes LF, Hasle H, editors. Myelodysplastic and myeloproliferative disorders in children. Sao Paulo (Brazil): Le Mar; 2003. p. 119–61.

15. Brunning RD, Orazi A, Germing U, et al. Myelodysplastic syndromes/neoplasms, overview. In: Swerdlow SH, Campo E, Harris NL, et al, editors. WHO classification of tumours of haematopoietic and lymphoid tissues. Lyon (France): International Agency for Research on Cancer; 2008. p. 88–93.

16. Gupta V, Brooker C, Tooze JA, et al. Clinical relevance of cytogenetic abnormalities at diagnosis of acquired aplastic anaemia in adults. Br J Haematol 2006;134:95–9.

17. Jacobs KB, Yeager M, Zhou W, et al. Detectable clonal mosaicism and its relationship to aging and cancer. Nat Genet 2012;44:651–8.

18. Soupir CP, Vergilio JA, Kelly E, et al. Identification of del(20q) in a subset of patients diagnosed with idiopathic thrombocytopenic purpura. Br J Haematol 2009;144:800–2.

19. Hanson CA, Steensma DP, Hodnefield JM, et al. Isolated trisomy 15: a clonal chromosome abnormality in bone marrow with doubtful hematologic significance. Am J Clin Pathol 2008;129:478–85.

20. Woll PS, Kjallquist U, Chowdhury O, et al. Myelodysplastic syndromes are propagated by rare and distinct human cancer stem cells in vivo. Cancer Cell 2014;25:794–808.

21. Barlow JL, Drynan LF, Hewett DR, et al. A p53-dependent mechanism underlies macrocytic anemia in a mouse model of human 5q- syndrome. Nat Med 2010;16:59–66.

22. Starczynowski DT, Kuchenbauer F, Argiropoulos B, et al. Identification of miR-145 and miR-146a as mediators of the 5q- syndrome phenotype. Nat Med 2010;16:49–58.

23. Schneider RK, Adema V, Heckl D, et al. Role of casein kinase 1A1 in the biology and targeted therapy of del(5q) MDS. Cancer Cell 2014;26:509–20.

24. Sanz MA, Grimwade D, Tallman MS, et al. Management of acute promyelocytic leukemia: recommendations from an expert panel on behalf of the European LeukemiaNet. Blood 2009;113:1875–91.

25. Dimov ND, Medeiros LJ, Kantarjian HM, et al. Rapid and reliable confirmation of acute promyelocytic leukemia by immunofluorescence staining with an antipromyelocytic leukemia antibody: the M. D. Anderson Cancer Center experience of 349 patients. Cancer 2010;116:369–76.

26. Falini B, Flenghi L, Fagioli M, et al. Immunocytochemical diagnosis of acute promyelocytic leukemia (M3) with the monoclonal antibody PG-M3 (anti-PML). Blood 1997;90:4046–53.

27. Grimwade D, Hills RK, Moorman AV, et al. Refinement of cytogenetic classification in acute myeloid leukemia: determination of prognostic significance of rare recurring chromosomal abnormalities among 5876 younger adult patients treated in the United Kingdom Medical Research Council trials. Blood 2010;116:354–65.

28. Slovak ML, Kopecky KJ, Cassileth PA, et al. Karyotypic analysis predicts outcome of preremission and postremission therapy in adult acute myeloid leukemia: a Southwest Oncology Group/Eastern Cooperative Oncology Group Study. Blood 2000;96:4075–83.

29. Byrd JC, Mrozek K, Dodge RK, et al. Pretreatment cytogenetic abnormalities are predictive of induction success, cumulative incidence of relapse, and overall survival in adult patients with de novo acute myeloid leukemia: results from Cancer and Leukemia Group B (CALGB 8461). Blood 2002;100:4325–36.

30. Bejar R, Lord A, Stevenson K. TET2 mutations predict response to hypomethylating agents in myelodysplastic syndrome patients. Blood 2014;124:2705–12.

31. Haferlach T, Nagata Y, Grossmann V, et al. Landscape of genetic lesions in 944 patients with myelodysplastic syndromes. Leukemia 2014;28:241–7.

32. Patel JP, Gonen M, Figueroa ME, et al. Prognostic relevance of integrated genetic profiling in acute myeloid leukemia. N Engl J Med 2012;366:1079–89.

33. Kihara R, Nagata Y, Kiyoi H, et al. Comprehensive analysis of genetic alterations and their prognostic impacts in adult acute myeloid leukemia patients. Leukemia 2014;28:1586–95.

34. Zheng Z, Liebers M, Zhelyazkova B, et al. Anchored multiplex PCR for targeted next-generation sequencing. Nat Med 2014;20:1479–84.

35. Tiu RV, Gondek LP, O'Keefe CL, et al. Prognostic impact of SNP array karyotyping in myelodysplastic syndromes and related myeloid malignancies. Blood 2011;117:4552–60.

36. Delhommeau F, Dupont S, Della Valle V, et al. Mutation in TET2 in myeloid cancers. N Engl J Med 2009;360:2289–301.

37. Cancer Genome Atlas Research Network. Genomic and epigenomic landscapes of adult de novo acute myeloid leukemia. N Engl J Med 2013;368:2059–74.

38. Walter MJ, Shen D, Shao J, et al. Clonal diversity of recurrently mutated genes in myelodysplastic syndromes. Leukemia 2013;27:1275–82.

39. Mamanova L, Coffey AJ, Scott CE, et al. Target-enrichment strategies for next-generation sequencing. Nat Methods 2010;7:111–8.

40. Schmitt MW, Kennedy SR, Salk JJ, et al. Detection of ultra-rare mutations by next-generation sequencing. Proc Natl Acad Sci U S A 2012;109:14508–13.

41. Jaiswal S, Fontanillas P, Flannick J, et al. Age-related clonal hematopoiesis associated with adverse outcomes. N Engl J Med 2014;371:2488–98.

42. Steensma DP, Bejar R, Jaiswal S, et al. Clonal hematopoiesis of indeterminate potential and its distinction from myelodysplastic syndromes. Blood 2015;126(1):9–16.

43. Radomska HS, Huettner CS, Zhang P, et al. CCAAT/enhancer binding protein alpha is a regulatory switch sufficient for induction of granulocytic development from bipotential myeloid progenitors. Mol Cell Biol 1998;18:4301–14.

44. Pabst T, Eyholzer M, Haefliger S, et al. Somatic CEBPA mutations are a frequent second event in families with germline CEBPA mutations and familial acute myeloid leukemia. J Clin Oncol 2008;26: 5088–93.

45. Pabst T, Mueller BU. Complexity of CEBPA dysregulation in human acute myeloid leukemia. Clin Cancer Res 2009;15:5303–7.

46. Wen XM, Hu JB, Yang J, et al. CEBPA methylation and mutation in myelodysplastic syndrome. Med Oncol 2015;32:192.

47. Nerlov C. C/EBPalpha mutations in acute myeloid leukaemias. Nat Rev Cancer 2004;4:394–400.

48. Green CL, Koo KK, Hills RK, et al. Prognostic significance of CEBPA mutations in a large cohort of younger adult patients with acute myeloid leukemia: impact of double CEBPA mutations and the interaction with FLT3 and NPM1 mutations. J Clin Oncol 2010;28:2739–47.

49. Renneville A, Boissel N, Gachard N, et al. The favorable impact of CEBPA mutations in patients with acute myeloid leukemia is only observed in the absence of associated cytogenetic abnormalities and FLT3 internal duplication. Blood 2009; 113:5090–3.

50. Pabst T, Eyholzer M, Fos J, et al. Heterogeneity within AML with CEBPA mutations; only CEBPA double mutations, but not single CEBPA mutations are associated with favourable prognosis. Br J Cancer 2009;100:1343–6.

51. Smith ML, Cavenagh JD, Lister TA, et al. Mutation of CEBPA in familial acute myeloid leukemia. N Engl J Med 2004;351:2403–7.

52. De Braekeleer E, Douet-Guilbert N, Morel F, et al. ETV6 fusion genes in hematological malignancies: a review. Leuk Res 2012;36:945–61.

53. Cave H, Cacheux V, Raynaud S, et al. ETV6 is the target of chromosome 12p deletions in t(12;21) childhood acute lymphocytic leukemia. Leukemia 1997;11:1459–64.

54. Barjesteh van Waalwijk van Doorn-Khosrovani SN, Spensberger D, de Knegt Y, et al. Somatic heterozygous mutations in ETV6 (TEL) and frequent absence of ETV6 protein in acute myeloid leukemia. Oncogene 2005;24:4129–37.

55. Bejar R, Stevenson K, Abdel-Wahab O, et al. Clinical effect of point mutations in myelodysplastic syndromes. N Engl J Med 2011;364:2496–506.

56. Okuda T, Nishimura M, Nakao M, et al. RUNX1/ AML1: a central player in hematopoiesis. Int J Hematol 2001;74:252–7.

57. Miyoshi HJ, Shimizu K, Kozu T, et al. t(8;21) breakpoints on chromosome 21 in acute myeloid leukemia are clustered. Proc Natl Acad Sci U S A 1991;88:10431–4.

58. Schnittger S, Dicker F, Kern W, et al. RUNX1 mutations are frequent in de novo AML with noncomplex karyotype and confer an unfavorable prognosis. Blood 2011;117:2348–57.

59. Osato M. Point mutations in the RUNX1/AML1 gene: another actor in RUNX leukemia. Oncogene 2004;23:4284–96.

60. Mangan JK, Speck NA. RUNX1 mutations in clonal myeloid disorders: from conventional cytogenetics to next generation sequencing, a story 40 years in the making. Crit Rev Oncog 2011; 16:77–91.

61. Harada H, Harada Y, Niimi H, et al. High incidence of somatic mutations in the AML1/RUNX1 gene in myelodysplastic syndrome and low blast percentage myeloid leukemia with myelodysplasia. Blood 2004;103:2316–24.

62. Mendler JH, Maharry K, Radmacher MD, et al. RUNX1 mutations are associated with poor outcome in younger and older patients with cytogenetically normal acute myeloid leukemia and with distinct gene and MicroRNA expression signatures. J Clin Oncol 2012;30:3109–18.

63. Gaidzik VI, Bullinger L, Schlenk RF, et al. RUNX1 mutations in acute myeloid leukemia: results from a comprehensive genetic and clinical analysis from the AML study group. J Clin Oncol 2011;29: 1364–72.

64. Song WJ, Sullivan MG, Legare RD, et al. Haploinsufficiency of CBFA2 causes familial thrombocytopenia with propensity to develop acute myelogenous leukaemia. Nat Genet 1999;23:166–75.

65. Nakao MJ, Yokota S, Iwai T, et al. Internal tandem duplication of the flt3 gene found in acute myeloid leukemia. Leukemia 1996;10:1911–8.

66. Bacher UG, Haferlach C, Kern W, et al. Prognostic relevance of FLT3-TKD mutations in AML: the combination matters–an analysis of 3082 patients. Blood 2008;111:2527–37.

67. Bains A, Luthra R, Medeiros LJ, et al. FLT3 and NPM1 mutations in myelodysplastic syndromes: Frequency and potential value for predicting progression to acute myeloid leukemia. Am J Clin Pathol 2011;135:62–9.

68. Kussick SJ, Stirewalt DL, Yi HS, et al. A distinctive nuclear morphology in acute myeloid leukemia is strongly associated with loss of HLA-DR expression and FLT3 internal tandem duplication. Leukemia 2004;18:1591–8.

69. Kayser S, Schlenk RF, Londono MC, et al. Insertion of FLT3 internal tandem duplication in the tyrosine kinase domain-1 is associated with resistance to chemotherapy and inferior outcome. Blood 2009; 114:2386–92.

70. Dohner H, Estey EH, Amadori S, et al. Diagnosis and management of acute myeloid leukemia in adults: recommendations. Blood 2010;115:453–74.

71. Kayser S, Levis MJ. FLT3 tyrosine kinase inhibitors in acute myeloid leukemia: clinical implications and limitations. Leuk Lymphoma 2014;55:243–55.

72. Ok CY, Patel KP, Garcia-Manero G, et al. TP53 mutation characteristics in therapy-related myelodysplastic syndromes and acute myeloid leukemia is similar to de novo diseases. J Hematol Oncol 2015;8:45.

73. Wong TN, Ramsingh G, Young AL, et al. Role of TP53 mutations in the origin and evolution of therapy-related acute myeloid leukaemia. Nature 2015;518:552–5.

74. Cleven AH, Nardi V, Ok CY, et al. High p53 protein expression in therapy-related myeloid neoplasms is associated with adverse karyotype and poor outcome. Mod Pathol 2015;28:552–63.

75. Ohgami RS, Ma L, Merker JD, et al. Next-generation sequencing of acute myeloid leukemia identifies the significance. Mod Pathol 2015;28: 706–14.

76. Bowen D, Groves MJ, Burnett AK, et al. TP53 gene mutation is frequent in patients with acute myeloid leukemia and complex karyotype, and is associated with very poor prognosis. Leukemia 2009;23: 203–6.

77. Bejar R, Levine R, Ebert BL. Unraveling the molecular pathophysiology of myelodysplastic syndromes. J Clin Oncol 2011;29:504–15.

78. Jadersten M, Saft L, Smith A, et al. TP53 mutations in low-risk myelodysplastic syndromes with del(5q) predict disease progression. J Clin Oncol 2011;29: 1971–9.

79. Paschka P, Marcucci G, Ruppert AS, et al. Adverse prognostic significance of KIT mutations in adult acute myeloid leukemia with inv(16) and t(8;21): a Cancer and Leukemia Group B Study. J Clin Oncol 2006;24:3904–11.

80. Park SH, Chi HS, Min SK, et al. Prognostic impact of c-KIT mutations in core binding factor acute myeloid leukemia. Leuk Res 2011;35:1376–83.

81. Lorenzo FJ, Nishii K, Monma F, et al. Mutational analysis of the KIT gene in myelodysplastic syndrome (MDS) and MDS-derived leukemia. Leuk Res 2006;30:1235–9.

82. Papaemmanuil E, Cazzola M, Boultwood J, et al. Somatic SF3B1 mutation in myelodysplasia with ring sideroblasts. N Engl J Med 2011;365: 1384–95.

83. Je EM, Yoo NJ, Kim YJ, et al. Mutational analysis of splicing machinery genes SF3B1, U2AF1 and SRSF2 in myelodysplasia and other common tumors. Int J Cancer 2013;133:260–5.

84. Ogawa S. Splicing factor mutations in AML. Blood 2014;123:3216–7.

85. Ogawa S. Splicing factor mutations in myelodysplasia. Int J Hematol 2012;96:438–42.

86. Thol F, Bollin R, Gehlhaar M, et al. Mutations in the cohesin complex in acute myeloid leukemia: clinical and prognostic implications. Blood 2014;123: 914–20.

87. Patnaik MU, Hanson CA, Hodnefield JM, et al. Differential prognostic effect of IDH1 versus IDH2 mutations in myelodysplastic syndromes: a Mayo Clinic study of 277 patients. Leukemia 2012;26: 101–5.

88. Damm F, Kosmider O, Gelsi-Boyer V, et al. Mutations affecting mRNA splicing define distinct clinical phenotypes and correlate with patient outcome in myelodysplastic syndromes. Blood 2012;119:3211–8.

89. Graubert TA, Shen D, Ding L, et al. Recurrent mutations in the U2AF1 splicing factor in myelodysplastic syndromes. Nat Genet 2012;44:53–7.

90. Cho YU. Preferential occurrence of spliceosome mutations in acute myeloid leukemia with preceding myelodysplastic syndrome and/or myelodysplasia morphology. Leuk Lymphoma 2015;56(8): 2301–8.

91. Rocquain J, Gelsi-Boyer V, Adelaide J, et al. Alteration of cohesin genes in myeloid diseases. Am J Hematol 2010;85:717–9.

92. Thota S, Viny AD. Genetic alterations of the cohesin complex genes in myeloid malignancies. Blood 2014;124:1790–8.

93. Figueroa ME, Skrabanek L, Li Y, et al. MDS and secondary AML display unique patterns and abundance of aberrant DNA methylation. Blood 2009; 114:3448–58.

94. Eden A, Gaudet F, Waghmare A, et al. Chromosomal instability and tumors promoted by DNA hypomethylation. Science 2003;300:455.

95. Jankowska AM, Szpurka H, Tiu RV, et al. Loss of heterozygosity 4q24 and TET2 mutations associated with myelodysplastic/myeloproliferative neoplasms. Blood 2009;113:6403–10.

96. Walter MJ, Ding L, Shen D, et al. Recurrent DNMT3A mutations in patients with myelodysplastic syndromes. Leukemia 2011;25:1153–8.

97. Russler-Germain DA, Spencer DH, Young MA, et al. The R882H DNMT3A mutation associated with AML dominantly inhibits wild-type DNMT3A

by blocking its ability to form active tetramers. Cancer Cell 2014;25:442–54.

98. Metzeler KH, Maharry K, Radmacher MD, et al. TET2 mutations improve the new European LeukemiaNet risk classification of acute myeloid leukemia: a Cancer and Leukemia Group B study. J Clin Oncol 2011;29:1373–81.

99. Weissmann S, Alpermann T, Grossmann V, et al. Landscape of TET2 mutations in acute myeloid leukemia. Leukemia 2012;26:934–42.

100. Platt MY, Fathi AT, Borger DR, et al. Detection of dual IDH1 and IDH2 mutations by targeted next-generation sequencing in acute myeloid leukemia and myelodysplastic syndromes. J Mol Diagn 2015;17(6):661–8.

101. Kosmider O, Gelsi-Boyer V, Slama L, et al. Mutations of IDH1 and IDH2 genes in early and accelerated phases of myelodysplastic syndromes and MDS/myeloproliferative neoplasms. Leukemia 2010;24:1094–6.

102. Pardanani AU, Lasho TL, Finke CM, et al. IDH1 and IDH2 mutation analysis in chronic- and blast-phase myeloproliferative neoplasms. Leukemia 2010;24:1146–51.

103. Tefferi AU, Lasho TL, Abdel-Wahab O, et al. IDH1 and IDH2 mutation studies in 1473 patients with chronic-, fibrotic- or blast-phase essential thrombocythemia, polycythemia vera or myelofibrosis. Leukemia 2010;24:1302–9.

104. Rakheja D, Konoplev S, Medeiros LJ, et al. IDH mutations in acute myeloid leukemia. Hum Pathol 2012;43:1541–51.

105. Figueroa ME, Abdel-Wahab O, Lu C, et al. Leukemic IDH1 and IDH2 mutations result in a hypermethylation phenotype, disrupt TET2 function, and impair hematopoietic differentiation. Cancer Cell 2010;18:553–67.

106. Green CL, Evans CM, Hills RK, et al. The prognostic significance of IDH1 mutations in younger adult patients with acute myeloid leukemia is dependent on FLT3/ITD status. Blood 2010;116:2779–82.

107. Green CL, Evans CM, Zhao L, et al. The prognostic significance of IDH2 mutations in AML depends on the location of the mutation. Blood 2011;118:409–12.

108. Paschka P, Schlenk RF, Gaidzik VI, et al. IDH1 and IDH2 mutations are frequent genetic alterations in acute myeloid leukemia and confer adverse prognosis in cytogenetically normal acute myeloid leukemia with NPM1 mutation without FLT3 internal tandem duplication. J Clin Oncol 2010;28:3636–43.

109. DiNardo CD, Ravandi F, Agresta S, et al. Characteristics, clinical outcome, and prognostic significance of IDH mutations in AML. Am J Hematol 2015;90:732–6.

110. Hansen E, Quivoron C, Straley K, et al. AG-120, an oral, selective, first-in-class, potent inhibitor of mutant IDH1, reduces intracellular 2HG and induces cellular differentiation in TF-1 R132H cells and primary human IDH1 Mutant AML patient samples treated ex vivo. Blood 2014;124:3734.

111. Stein EM, Altman JK, Collins R, et al. AG-221, an oral, selective, first-in-class, potent inhibitor of the IDH2 Mutant metabolic enzyme, induces durable remissions in a phase I study in patients with IDH2 mutation positive advanced hematologic malignancies. Blood 2014;124:115.

112. Gelsi-Boyer V, Trouplin V, Adelaide J, et al. Mutations of polycomb-associated gene ASXL1 in myelodysplastic syndromes and chronic myelomonocytic leukaemia. Br J Haematol 2009;145:788–800.

113. Gelsi-Boyer V, Brecqueville M, Devillier R, et al. Mutations in ASXL1 are associated with poor prognosis across the spectrum of malignant myeloid diseases. J Hematol Oncol 2012;5:12.

114. Thol F, Friesen I, Damm F, et al. Prognostic significance of ASXL1 mutations in patients with myelodysplastic syndromes. J Clin Oncol 2011;29:2499–506.

115. Chou WC, Huang HH, Hou HA, et al. Distinct clinical and biological features of de novo acute myeloid leukemia with additional sex comb-like 1 (ASXL1) mutations. Blood 2010;116:4086–94.

116. Pratcorona M, Abbas S, Sanders MA, et al. Acquired mutations in ASXL1 in acute myeloid leukemia: prevalence and prognostic value. Haematologica 2012;97:388–92.

117. Schichman SA, Caligiuri MA, Gu Y, et al. ALL-1 partial duplication in acute leukemia. Proc Natl Acad Sci U S A 1994;91:6236–9.

118. Bacher U, Haferlach T, Kern W, et al. A comparative study of molecular mutations in 381 patients with myelodysplastic syndrome and in 4130 patients with acute myeloid leukemia. Haematologica 2007;92(6):744–52.

119. Tang G, DiNardo C, Zhang L, et al. MLL gene amplification in acute myeloid leukemia and myelodysplastic syndromes is associated with characteristic clinicopathological findings and TP53 gene mutation. Hum Pathol 2015;46:65–73.

120. Dolan M, McGlennen RC, Hirsch B. MLL amplification in myeloid malignancies: clinical, molecular, and cytogenetic findings. Cancer Genet Cytogenet 2002;134:93–101.

121. Ernst T, Chase AJ, Score J, et al. Inactivating mutations of the histone methyltransferase gene EZH2 in myeloid disorders. Nat Genet 2010;42:722–6.

122. Nikoloski G, Langemeijer SM, Kuiper RP, et al. Somatic mutations of the histone methyltransferase

gene EZH2 in myelodysplastic syndromes. Nat Genet 2010;42:665–7.

123. Makishima H, Jankowska AM, Tiu RV, et al. Novel homo- and hemizygous mutations in EZH2 in myeloid malignancies. Leukemia 2010;24:1799–804.

124. Falini B, Mecucci C, Tiacci E, et al. Cytoplasmic nucleophosmin in acute myelogenous leukemia with a normal karyotype. N Engl J Med 2005;352(3):254–66.

125. Falini B, Gionfriddo I, Cecchetti F, et al. Acute myeloid leukemia with mutated nucleophosmin (NPM1): any hope for a targeted therapy? Blood Rev 2011;25(6):247–54.

126. Marcucci G, Maharry K, Wu YZ, et al. IDH1 and IDH2 gene mutations identify novel molecular subsets within de novo cytogenetically normal acute myeloid leukemia: a Cancer and Leukemia Group B study. J Clin Oncol 2010;28(14):2348–55.

127. Wang X, Dai H, Wang Q, et al. EZH2 mutations are related to low blast percentage in bone marrow and -7/del(7q) in de novo acute myeloid leukemia. PLoS One 2013;8(4):e61341.

Myeloid Neoplasms with Germline Predisposition

A New Provisional Entity Within the World Health Organization Classification

David R. Czuchlewski, MD[a],*, LoAnn C. Peterson, MD[b]

KEYWORDS

- Germline predisposition mutation • Familial cancer • Acute myeloid leukemia
- Myelodysplastic syndrome

ABSTRACT

The forthcoming update of the World Health Organization (WHO) classification of hematopoietic neoplasms will feature "Myeloid Neoplasms with Germline Predisposition" as a new provisional diagnostic entity. This designation will be applied to some cases of acute myeloid leukemia and myelodysplastic syndrome arising in the setting of constitutional mutations that render patients susceptible to the development of myeloid malignancies. For the diagnostic pathologist, recognizing these cases and confirming the diagnosis will demand a sophisticated grasp of clinical genetics and molecular techniques. This article presents a concise review of this new provisional WHO entity, including strategies for clinical practice.

Key Features

- Some cases of myeloid neoplasms are associated with predisposing germline mutations, and the new revision of the World Health Organization (WHO) classification specifically recognizes such cases as a provisional diagnostic entity.

- Some cases of acute myeloid leukemia (AML) and myelodysplastic syndrome (MDS) with germline predisposition mutations are associated with specific clinical phenotypes, whereas others may lack any identifying clues, thus demanding a high index of suspicion.

- Recognizing the true genetic basis of these cases is important for proper clinical management and follow-up.

OVERVIEW

Among all areas of diagnostic pathology, the field of hematopathology has long been a leader in the application of molecular genetic information to the classification of malignancies. Beginning with the identification in 1960 of the Philadelphia chromosome and continuing through the recognition of the *PML-RARA* fusion as pathognomonic for acute promyelocytic leukemia, genetic findings have been closely linked with advances in the understanding and classification of myeloid neoplasms. The importance of genetics was recognized in the original WHO *Classification of Tumours of Haematopoietic and Lymphoid Tissue* released in 2001. These trends continued in the 2008 revision of the WHO classification, which saw the creation of categories of AML defined either by genetic features (for example, the provisional AML with mutated *NPM1*) or by clinical history (for example, therapy-related myeloid neoplasms).

The upcoming revision of the WHO classification continues to highlight the central role of genetic

Disclosure Statement: The authors have nothing to disclose.

[a] Department of Pathology, University of New Mexico, 1001 Woodward Place NE, Albuquerque, NM 87102, USA; [b] Department of Pathology, Northwestern University Feinberg School of Medicine, NMH/Feinberg Room 7-344, 251 East Huron, Chicago, IL 60611, USA

* Corresponding author.

E-mail address: DCzuchlewski@salud.unm.edu

Surgical Pathology 9 (2016) 165–176

http://dx.doi.org/10.1016/j.path.2015.09.010

and clinical data in the diagnosis of myeloid neoplasms, as exemplified by the new provisional diagnostic category "Myeloid Neoplasms with Germline Predisposition." These cases are associated with inherited or de novo mutations within the germline that markedly increase the likelihood that a patient will develop a myeloid neoplasm, especially MDS or AML. As such, they are defined and characterized by specific genetic and clinical phenotypic findings. These mutations and syndromes are rare and, consequently, somewhat outside the current scope of daily pathology practice. This article provides a primer for this new diagnostic area. Because the WHO chapter remains in final revisions at the time of this writing, the authors strongly recommend correlation with the forthcoming published classification for final diagnostic considerations and terminology.

SPECIAL CLINICAL FEATURES OF MYELOID NEOPLASMS ASSOCIATED WITH GERMLINE PREDISPOSITION MUTATIONS

An initial question that might be asked on learning of this new category is, "Why create a special provisional diagnostic category for these cases? Perhaps these should just be considered ordinary cases of MDS or 'AML, not otherwise specified' that happen to occur in genetically predisposed individuals." The committee charged with revising the WHO thought that the genetic and clinical features were sufficiently unique that MDS/AML arising in this setting should be specially recognized. In particular, these patients frequently require specialized approaches to therapy and other aspects of clinical management.

In cases of MDS, for example, patients with germline predisposition mutations often have a poor outcome that is not apparent if traditional diagnostic and risk assessment tools, such as the Revised International Prognostic Scoring System, are applied. (Such prognostic systems exclude cases of MDS with known underlying genetic predisposition.) Patients with MDS and certain types of germline predisposition may benefit from early hematopoietic cell transplantation.[1] Furthermore, patients with MDS in the setting of a classic hereditary bone marrow failure disorder (BMFD) often present at a young age with a hypocellular bone marrow. In patients with non-syndromic MDS, these are features associated with better response to immunosuppressive therapy.[2] In the setting of BMFD, however, immunosuppressive therapy is ineffective and possibly detrimental, increasing the risk of infectious complications.[1]

Cases of MDS/AML with germline predisposition mutations also differ from typical sporadic MDS and AML in that they are frequently associated with unique nonhematopoietic manifestations. Patients with Fanconi anemia, for example, are at greatly increased risk for developing other solid tumors, with up to 75% developing a nonhematologic cancer by age 45.[3] Possible clinical events in the disease course of dyskeratosis congenita include a wide range of nonhematopoietic pathology, from esophageal stenosis to avascular necrosis of the femoral head, pulmonary fibrosis, and retinal detachment.[4] Patients with germline GATA2 mutations may be susceptible to infection by nontuberculous Mycobacteria, such as M avium complex or by other opportunistic pathogens, in addition to developing pulmonary alveolar proteinosis.[5] Patients with RUNX1, ANKRD26, or ETV6 mutations may bleed out of proportion to their platelet counts due to underlying platelet dysfunction. Because a diagnosis of AML or MDS may be the initial presenting sign of these underlying syndromes, classification as uncomplicated MDS or AML, not otherwise specified, would tend to understate the full clinical picture and potentially deprive these patients of necessary follow-up care and surveillance. One important aspect of follow-up care that is common to all cases of myeloid neoplasia with germline predisposition mutations is the necessity of formal genetic counseling with a certified genetic counselor and/or geneticist, including consideration for testing of at-risk relatives.

Finally, special treatment approaches may be called for in some cases of AML/MDS associated with germline predisposition mutations. Patients with BMFD characterized by increased susceptibility to genotoxic stress must follow reduced-intensity conditioning regimens prior to allogeneic bone marrow transplantations.[6] Extra scrutiny of related stem cell donors is also indicated due to the familial nature of the pathogenic mutation. Screening of the potential related donor for the mutation in question is necessary to avoid transplanting cells that harbor the very defect the transplant procedure is intended to correct.[5] Some parents consider and/or undergo preimplantation genetic diagnosis in an effort to provide transplantable stem cells free of the mutation.[7] If a germline susceptibility mutation is present, some clinicians may consider the eradication of cells with the mutation from the hematopoietic compartment as an added advantage of allogeneic transplant.[8] Special considerations in the post-transplant settings include high rates of graft-versus-host disease in Fanconi anemia and cardiac toxicity in Shwachman-Diamond syndrome.[9,10] Because of the unique challenges associated with clinical management of these patients, some experts advocate that they be preferentially treated at national referral centers with experience in patients with germline mutations.[1] It is hoped that the WHO-recognized provisional diagnostic label will facilitate the detection and optimal treatment of these patients.

WHAT ARE THE SPECIFIC MYELOID NEOPLASMS ASSOCIATED WITH GERMLINE PREDISPOSITION MUTATIONS?

There are 3 main types of myeloid neoplasms associated with germline predisposition mutations (Box 1). First, certain mutations tend to be associated with "pure" familial MDS and AML, with no significant nonhematopoietic pathology. Second, a group of MDS/AML-susceptibility mutations cause concomitant platelet abnormalities. And third, cases of MDS/AML may occur in the setting of well-defined clinical genetic syndromes, including those characterized by bone marrow failure. The key genetic and diagnostic features of each of the entities in these groups are briefly described.

MYELOID NEOPLASMS WITH GERMLINE PREDISPOSITION WITHOUT A PREEXISTING DISORDER OR ORGAN DYSFUNCTION

The WHO classification will provisionally recognize 2 types of germline susceptibility to MDS/AML in which the clinical picture is dominated by the myeloid neoplasm, without other significant phenotypic abnormalities.

Acute Myeloid Leukemia with Germline CEBPA Mutation

Familial AML with mutated *CEBPA* is characterized by germline mutation of the CCAAT/enhancer-binding protein (C/EBP), alpha gene, which encodes a myeloid transcription factor essential for granulopoiesis. *CEBPA* is often affected by acquired, somatic mutations in cases of sporadic AML, in which setting the presence of biallelic mutation is specifically associated with favorable prognosis.[11] The biallelic mutations typically affect the N-terminal and the C-terminal regions of the protein, respectively. Familial cases are also characterized by biallelic *CEBPA* mutation, with 1 mutated allele present in the germline, and the mutation in the second allele acquired as a second hit in accordance with the Knudson 2-hit hypothesis. Of the 2, the N-terminal mutation is usually the one found in the germline.

The familial and sporadic *CEPBA*-mutated cases share morphologic and immunophenotypic features in common. Thus, familial AML with *CEBPA* mutation may be indistinguishable from sporadic AML with *CEPBA* mutation, both clinically and based on the results of the initial molecular analysis of the blasts. Because familial AML with *CEBPA* mutation is thought to be inherited in an autosomal dominant fashion with near-complete penetrance, a careful family history may reveal relatives with myeloid neoplasms and raise additional suspicion of an inherited mutation. Consideration of a germline predisposition mutation, however, should be given in any case of AML with double-mutated *CEBPA*. Mutational analysis of a germline specimen (ideally a skin biopsy, as discussed later) is indicated to definitively distinguish germline from somatic *CEBPA* mutation.

Some sense of the incidences involved in these cases is provided by studies that have screened large numbers of AML patients for both somatic and germline *CEPBA* mutations. Although *CEBPA* mutations are detected in 5% to 14% of cytogenetically normal cases of AML, one of the mutations is in the germline in approximately 7% to 11% of the *CEPBA* double-mutated cases,[12,13] for an overall germline *CEBPA* mutation incidence of approximately 0.4% to 1.5% in cytogenetically normal AML. The average age of presentation is 24.5 years (1.75–46 years).[14] There are data to suggest that patients with familial AML with mutated *CEBPA* may be more likely to relapse.[8,14,15] The prognosis seems to remain favorable, however, despite the multiple relapses, reaching 67% overall survival at

---

Box 1
Anticipated World Health Organization–defined provisional myeloid neoplasms with germline predisposition

Myeloid neoplasms with germline predisposition without a preexisting disorder or organ dysfunction
- *CEBPA* mutation

- *DDX41* mutation

Myeloid neoplasms with germline predisposition and preexisting platelet disorders
- *RUNX1* mutation

- *ANKRD26* mutation

- *ETV6* mutation

Myeloid neoplasms with germline predisposition and other organ dysfunction
- *GATA2* mutation

- See Table 1 for further inherited syndromic disorders.

10 years in 1 series.[14] The clones at relapse showed novel second-hit *CEBPA* mutations unrelated to the original clone,[14] indicating a unique pattern of disease recurrence and evolution that underscores the need for proper recognition of this entity.

Myeloid Neoplasms with Germline DDX41 Mutation

The DEAD (Asp-Glu-Ala-Asp) box polypeptide 41 gene (*DDX41*) encodes a protein that seems to function as an RNA helicase with a role in the spliceosome. Thus, *DDX41* joins several other spliceosomal components that have recently been shown to contribute to myeloid neoplasia when mutated.[16] Next-generation sequencing (NGS) studies have identified this gene as infrequently mutated in MDS and AML. Similar to the situation with *CEBPA*, however, there is a significant subset of cases in which the *DDX41* mutation is biallelic, with 1 mutation occurring in the germline. These germline mutations predispose to the development of a high-grade myeloid neoplasm, as evidenced by the strong family history of such malignancies described in several cohorts with germline *DDX41* mutation.[17] These familial cases are associated with a late onset, advanced disease, normal karyotype, and poor prognosis.[17] The penetrance of disease remains to be fully established, although close scrutiny of even apparently unaffected carriers in several families has shown unexplained monocytosis and morphologic abnormalities.[17] Although the most common germline *DDX41* mutation (a frameshift mutation c.419insGATG, p.D140fs) is present in only 0.008% of the population, a screening study identified 0.8% of unselected MDS and AML patients as harboring germline *DDX41* mutations.[17] There are some emerging data to suggest that patients with *DDX41* mutations may respond favorably to lenalidomide therapy,[17] although this remains to be fully established.

MYELOID NEOPLASMS WITH GERMLINE PREDISPOSITION AND PREEXISTING PLATELET DISORDERS

The subcategory, myeloid neoplasms with germline predisposition and preexisting platelet disorders, provisionally defines 3 disease subsets in which the hematologic malignancy arises due to a germline mutation that also causes familial platelet disorders.

Myeloid Neoplasms with Germline RUNX1 Mutation

Germline mutations in *RUNX1* cause "familial platelet disorder with associated myeloid malignancy" (MIM 601399). Runt-related transcription factor 1 (*RUNX1*) encodes a subunit of the core binding factor transcription complex that is frequently affected by somatic mutation in sporadic myeloid neoplasms and is also a partner in the *RUNX1-RUNX1T1* fusion associated with the t(8;21) (q22;q22) in AML. Patients with germline *RUNX1* mutations have variable mild-to-moderate thrombocytopenia from birth, with or without bleeding tendency. Further testing may show decreased platelet aggregation to collagen and epinephrine and dense granule storage pool deficiency. In carriers of the mutation, the likelihood of developing MDS or AML is approximately 35% to 44%,[18,19] although both the severity of the thrombocytopenia and the degree of risk of AML/MDS seem to depend on the specific location of the mutation within *RUNX1*.[5] The average age of onset of MDS/AML is 33 years (range 6–76 years),[15] although this disease seems to show anticipation, in which successive generations show younger age of onset.[19] In some cases, development of MDS or AML is accompanied by somatic mutation of a patient's second *RUNX1* allele and/or the development of trisomy of chromosome 21, which harbors the *RUNX1* gene.[20] Constitutional microdeletions of the *RUNX1* region at chromosome 21q22 are also associated with platelet abnormalities and MDS/AML predisposition as well as congenital abnormalities.[5,19] Thus, additional testing for copy number changes should be considered if sequencing analysis fails to identify a *RUNX1* mutation in a suspected case.[19]

Myeloid Neoplasms with Germline ANKRD26 Mutation

Thrombocytopenia 2 (MIM 188000) is an autosomal dominant thrombocytopenia caused by *ANKRD26* mutations.[21,22] Affected patients have mild thrombocytopenia and bleeding tendency with normal platelet aggregation studies.[5] The *ANKRD26* mutation is characteristically a single nucleotide substitution within a short stretch of the 5'-untranslated region of the gene,[21] which seems to result in increased gene expression[5] by preventing binding of transcriptional repressors.[19] Increased expression of *ANKRD26* leads to increased signaling through the MPL pathway.[19] A significantly increased incidence of AML (approximately 30 times higher than the general population) has been identified in germline mutation carriers, with 4.9% of patients developing acute leukemia and 2.2% of patients developing MDS,[21,23] although this is based on only a few affected families. The spectrum of myeloid malignancies associated with *ANKRD26* mutations may also include CML and CMML,[23,24] and some carriers may also show increased hemoglobin and leukocyte counts. Dysmegakaryopoiesis – consisting of increased megakaryocytes that are small in size with hypolobation and micromegakaryocytes – is observed in carriers of the *ANKRD26* mutation even in the absence of overt MDS,[19,21] a complicating factor discussed later.

Myeloid Neoplasms with Germline ETV6 Mutation

Several kindreds with autosomal dominant thrombocytopenia caused by germline *ETV6* mutations have recently been described[25] and referred to as thrombocytopenia 5 (MIM 616216). Affected individuals have an increased likelihood of developing several types of hematologic malignancies. The mutations seem to affect DNA-binding properties of the encoded protein, which is also a partner in rearrangements in lymphoblastic and myeloid malignancies.[26] Patients have platelets of normal size with variable thrombocytopenia and mild to moderate bleeding tendency. Bone marrow biopsies in affected patients without leukemia have shown small hypolobated megakaryocytes and mild dyserythropoiesis.

MYELOID NEOPLASMS WITH GERMLINE PREDISPOSITION ASSOCIATED WITH OTHER ORGAN DYSFUNCTION

Several otherwise well-characterized inherited syndromes also feature increased risk for myeloid neoplasia. These include *GATA2* mutated cases and cases arising in the setting of inherited bone marrow failure.

Myeloid Neoplasms with Germline GATA2 Mutation

The GATA-binding protein 2 gene (*GATA2*) encodes a protein that assists in gene expression regulation by binding to DNA at the specific sequence G-A-T-A. Germline *GATA2* mutations were originally identified in families with autosomal dominant inheritance of MDS/AML. At the same time, germline *GATA2* mutations were also recognized as causative of other inherited syndromes, including MonoMAC syndrome and Emberger syndrome, both of which also feature increased risk of myeloid neoplasms. *GATA2* mutations are now recognized as causing a small subset of cases with the phenotype of severe congenital neutropenia or bone marrow failure. Because all these manifestations are caused by germline *GATA2* mutations, these are now regarded as a single syndrome with variable expressivity.[27] The historical

Emberger syndrome (MIM 614038) is characterized primarily by lymphedema of the lower limbs and the historical MonoMAC syndrome by monocytopenia; functional defects of B cells, natural killer cells, and macrophages; susceptibility to atypical infections (including mycobacterial and fungal infections); and pulmonary alveolar proteinosis. Generalized warts and autoimmune manifestations are also part of this clinical spectrum. Any of these features in a patient's clinical history could be a tip-off to the presence of a *GATA2* mutation, although it should be emphasized that some *GATA2*-mutated patients present with MDS/AML without these clinical clues (**Figs. 1** and **2**). Furthermore, because up to two-thirds of germline *GATA2* mutations are de novo rather than inherited,[27] probands may lack a suggestive family history. The lifetime risk of MDS in these patients is approximately 70%[19]; the median age of MDS diagnosis is between ages 21 and 33, and the features often include a hypocellular bone marrow, multilineage dysplasia (most prominent in megakaryocytic lineage), increased fibrosis, and monosomy 7 or trisomy 8.[15,27] Good outcomes have been reported with hematopoietic stem cell transplantation in this MDS patient population.[15,27]

Myeloid Neoplasms with Germline Predisposition Associated with Inherited Bone Marrow Failure Syndromes and Telomere Biology Disorders

These clinical syndromes include Fanconi anemia and dyskeratosis congenita as well as severe congenital neutropenia, Shwachman-Diamond syndrome, and Diamond-Blackfan anemia. Key features and references are provided in **Table 1**.

EMERGING SYNDROMES THAT LIKELY PREDISPOSE TO MYELOID MALIGNANCIES

Finally, there are additional mutations that are considered likely to predispose to myeloid malignancy, although the rarity of these cases makes investigation and complete characterization difficult. Familial MDS and congenital nerve deafness associated with germline *SRP72* mutations have been described; this mutation is also associated with aplastic anemia,[28] and thus may ultimately fit best among the other BMFDs described in **Table 1**, although the precise clinical phenotype remains to be fully defined. Four families in the French West Indies show a germline duplication of a 700 kb region of 14q32.3, including *ATG2B* and *GSKIP* genes, that is strongly associated with myeloid neoplasms, in particular essential thrombocythemia. These mutations may emerge

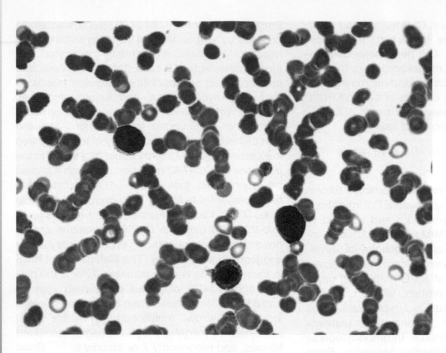

Fig. 1. Peripheral blood smear from a 50-year-old woman with AML with *GATA2* mutation. Note the presence of blasts as well as a dysplastic neutrophil (Wright stain ×60).

as myeloid neoplasm predisposition syndromes as further information becomes available.

GERMLINE ALTERATIONS AND SYNDROMES NOT DESCRIBED UNDER THE PROVISIONAL WORLD HEALTH ORGANIZATION–DEFINED CATEGORY

In addition to the list of germline mutations provisionally recognized by the WHO as meeting

criteria for myeloid neoplasms associated with germline predisposition, there are several scenarios that require additional clarification. First, there are several germline mutations that cause abnormalities of hematopoiesis, which nevertheless are nonclonal. A prime example of this is *GATA1* X-linked cytopenia, which is caused by inherited *GATA1* mutations and associated with significant dyspoiesis and cytopenias. Similarly, *MYH9* mutations cause thrombocytopenia and other peripheral blood abnormalities. Because

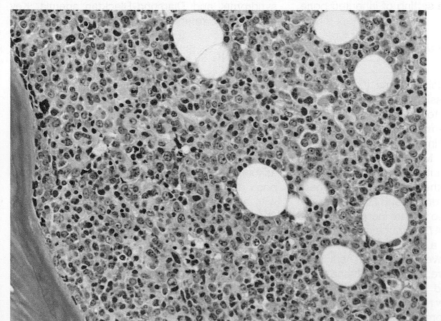

Fig. 2. Bone marrow biopsy from a 50-year-old woman with AML with *GATA2* mutation is hypercellular with many blasts and abnormal megakaryocytes (H&E ×50).

Table 1
Additional selected syndromes with germline predisposition to myeloid neoplasms

Disease	Germline Genes Mutated	Key Clinical Phenotypic Clues (in Addition to Cancer Predisposition)[a]	Inheritance Pattern	Approximate Risk of Myeloid Malignancy	Best Initial Test	Key Reference for Further Details
Fanconi anemia	*FANCA, FANCB, FANCC, BRCA2 (FANCD1), FANCD2, FANCE, FANCF, FANCG (XRCC9), FANCI, BRIP1(FANCJ or BACH1), FANCL, FANCM, PALB2 (FANCN), RAD51C (FANCO), SLX4 (FANCP), FANCQ (ERCC4)*	Bone marrow failure; short stature, radial/thumb abnormalities, abnormal skin pigmentation, other congenital abnormalities	AR, XLR	9%–13% AML, 7% MDS	Chromosomal breakage analysis	4
Dyskeratosis congenita (and telomere biology disorders)	*CTC1, DKC1, TERC, TERT, TINF2, NHP2, NOP10, WRAP53, RTEL1*	Bone marrow failure; dysplastic nails, lacy reticular pigmentation of the upper chest and neck, oral leukoplakia; pulmonary fibrosis	AR, AD, XLR	2%–30%[1]	Flow-FISH for telomere length	4
Severe congenital neutropenia	*ELANE, GFI1, HAX1, G6PC3, WAS, VPS45, USB1, CSF3R*[32]	Preceding persistent isolated neutropenia	AD, AR, XLR	21%–40%, but depends on subtype	Sequencing for relevant mutations	33
Shwachman-Diamond syndrome	*SBDS*	Preceding persistent isolated neutropenia; pancreatic insufficiency; short stature; skeletal abnormalities including metaphyseal dysostosis	AR	5%–24%	Sequencing for *SBDS* mutations	4
Diamond-Blackfan anemia	*RPS19, RPS17, RPS24, RPL35A, RPL5, RPL11, RPS7, RPS26, RPS10, GATA1*	Preceding anemia with reticulocytopenia and selective deficiency of red blood cell precursors; short stature, congenital abnormalities (including craniofacial, cardiac, skeletal, genitourinary)	AD, XLR	5%	Screening: elevated erythrocyte adenosine deaminase and hemoglobin F; sequencing of relevant genes (possibly starting with *RPS19*, which is most commonly mutated)	4

Abbreviations: AD, autosomal dominant; AR, autosomal recessive; XLR, X-linked recessive.

[a] Phenotypes are highly variable, and cases may show additional features or in some instances lack these key findings.

these sorts of mutations mainly impair functional production of peripheral blood elements, however, these non-neoplastic cases are not classified as familial MDS or AML. Second, the presence of a germline predisposition mutation itself – without overt MDS or AML – would not cause a patient to be placed into the category of familial MDS/AML unless or until the appearance of MDS/AML as ordinarily defined. Third, several specific presentations are definitively classified elsewhere in the WHO classification. For example, Down syndrome is certainly caused by a germline genetic abnormality (ie, the presence of an extra copy of chromosome 21). Myeloid neoplasia in patients with Down syndrome is associated with several unique features, including the phenomenon of transient abnormal myelopoiesis and a propensity to develop acute megakaryoblastic leukemia at a young age. Thus, myeloid neoplasia associated with Down syndrome is described elsewhere in the WHO classification. Myeloid proliferations related to Noonan syndrome are also separately described.

WHICH PATIENTS WITH MYELOID NEOPLASMS SHOULD BE TESTED FOR GERMLINE PREDISPOSITION MUTATIONS?

Although the availability of NGS continues to expand, currently it is not suggested that all the genes (discussed previously) be assessed in all patients with MDS or AML. Thus, it is necessary to select a subset of patients for detailed and extensive molecular analysis. During deliberations relating to this provisional entity, the WHO panel discussed guidelines (modified from Churpek and colleagues[29]) that suggest genetic counseling for the following patients:

1. Any patient with acute leukemia or MDS with a first-degree or second-degree relative with AML, acute lymphocytic leukemia, or MDS; abnormal nails or skin pigmentation; oral leukoplakia; idiopathic pulmonary fibrosis; unexplained liver disease; lymphedema; atypical infections; immune deficiencies; congenital limb anomalies; or short stature
2. Any patient with thrombocytopenia, a clinical bleeding propensity, or macrocytosis preceding a diagnosis of MDS/AML by several years
3. Any patient with a hematologic malignancy occurring at a young age (<45 years old) with a first-degree relative with any cancer occurring at a young age (<45 years old) or multiple first-degree and second-degree relatives with cancers (especially sarcoma, early-onset breast cancer [<50 years old], and brain tumors)

4. Any healthy related potential hematopoietic stem cell donor who is found to have any of the conditions listed and is planning to donate for a family member with a hematologic malignancy or who fails to mobilize stem cells well using standard protocols

One key consideration is the age of the patient at diagnosis. Although many of these germline predisposition mutations result in disease at a young age, and, therefore, suspicion may be higher in younger patients, age alone is an unreliable guide. In particular, many of these germline mutations are associated with disease presenting into mid-adulthood or even late adulthood; and even for characteristically pediatric entities, like severe congenital neutropenia, rare later presentations are possible.[1]

In some cases, specific testing may be dictated by further clinical and laboratory clues. A highly simplified schematic overview of key phenotypic clues is provided in **Tables 1** and **2**. For example, a patient with hypoplastic or absent thumbs prompts consideration of Fanconi anemia; however, even in Fanconi anemia, approximately one-third of patients lack such classic physical abnormalities, and several of the germline mutations (discussed previously) are associated with isolated myeloid neoplasia without additional phenotypic findings. Thus, although the history and physical examination are crucial components of this investigation, a normal examination and unremarkable history do not exclude a myeloid neoplasm with a germline predisposition mutation.

Another possible clue to certain specific germline mutations is the presence of previously diagnosed cytopenias or a bleeding diathesis. Thus, for example, a known history of longstanding thrombocytopenia prompts consideration of *RUNX1*, *ANKRD26*, and *ETV6* mutations. Significant bone marrow hypocellularity at diagnosis or delay in bone marrow recovery after chemotherapy suggests the presence of an inherited BMFD.

Finally, because patients with AML in particular are subjected with increasing regularity to extended NGS myeloid panels in an effort to identify somatic mutations, in some cases evidence is found via this route that could point to a germline predisposition mutation. Genes (discussed previously) that are commonly present on such panels include *CEBPA*, *RUNX1*, *ETV6*, and *GATA2*. The identification of mutations involving any of these genes in the appropriate pattern – such as a biallelic *CEBPA* mutation – should prompt additional consideration for germline testing. In the end, it may be necessary for a pathologist to amend a diagnosis to include a germline predisposing

Table 2
Schematic approach to phenotypic correlation in suspected familial myelodysplastic syndrome/acute myeloid leukemia

If the Patient Has...	Think in Particular of...
Evidence of preceding bone marrow failure	• Fanconi anemia • Dyskeratosis congenita
Preceding persistent neutropenia	• Severe congenital neutropenia • Shwachman-Diamond syndrome
Preceding persistent platelet disorder	• RUNX1 mutation • ANKRD26 mutation • ETV6 mutation
Lymphedema, preceding monocytopenia, immunodeficiency with atypical infections, pulmonary alveolar proteinosis	• GATA2 mutation
No specific phenotypic features but general suspicion of germline mutation based on age of presentation or family history	• Fanconi anemia • Dyskeratosis congenita • CEBPA mutation • DDX41 mutation

condition if it is identified by testing performed after the original diagnosis.

HOW SHOULD THE PRESENCE OF A GERMLINE PREDISPOSITION MUTATION BE ESTABLISHED?

Once the decision is made to pursue a diagnosis of a germline predisposition mutation, a laboratory testing strategy must be selected. If there are clues to any specific germline predisposition mutation or syndrome, then testing for that entity first is warranted. In suspicious cases without phenotypic clues to a specific mutation, a general initial screening could include chromosomal breakage analysis for Fanconi anemia, telomere length measurement by flow–fluorescence in situ hybridization (FISH) analysis for dyskeratosis congenita, and mutation analysis for selected genes.

Chromosomal breakage testing for Fanconi anemia is a specialized cytogenetic study in which the cultured patient cells are exposed to clastogenic agents that induce DNA damage. In a normal individual, the resulting DNA breaks are repaired by the cells; in a Fanconi patient, however, the defect in the DNA repair pathway prevents the cells from repairing the damage, and when chromosomal analysis is performed the damaged DNA is visible in the form of broken or abnormal chromosomes.

The flow-FISH assay is the preferred technique for telomere length assessment in diagnosis of dyskeratosis congenita. In this analysis, leukocyte subsets identified via flow cytometry are simultaneously assessed for the length of their telomeres, as indicated by the amount of fluorescently labeled probe targeted to the telomeres.

Current NGS panels for somatic mutations often include RUNX1, GATA2, ETV6, and CEBPA. More recently described or rare familial MDS/AML genes, such as DDX41, are less likely, at this point, to be included on these panels, although DDX41 is targeted on some commercially available myeloid panels. Specific sequencing for the remaining syndromic mutations, if indicated based on clinical and phenotypic clues, is currently available from laboratories that specialize in genetic testing for rare inherited genetic diseases, either as stand-alone tests or grouped into panels relating to phenotype (eg, a panel with genes relevant to bone marrow failure). It is possible that, in the future, NGS panels comprising all the genes known to be mutated in familial myeloid neoplasms will be devised.

It should be apparent that any mutations identified by an NGS panel run on a sample containing leukemic blasts or clonally related hematopoietic cells may well be present in the neoplastic cells only (ie, somatic) rather than in the germline. It is only a small subset of mutations identified in this setting that turn out to be germline in nature. If a relevant mutation is discovered and the clinical situation warrants, the next step is to definitively determine whether the mutation is germline or somatic. The preferred method for making this determination is to obtain a small skin biopsy from the patient, grow fibroblasts from the patient in culture, and then perform the sequencing analysis on the cultured fibroblasts. This procedure yields a pure population of cells that are nonhematopoietic and, therefore, reliably reflective of the germline makeup. Hair and nail samples may also provide germline DNA, although many clinical laboratories do not currently accept these specimen types for established AML assays. Alternative approaches have serious shortcomings. For example, saliva or buccal swabs may be significantly contaminated with leukocytes, opening the possibility of a false-positive result when seeking a germline mutation. Performing sequencing on a postremission specimen might yield evidence for potential germline status of a mutation, in that a somatic mutation is expected to be decreased in frequency or absent relative to the diagnostic specimen. It is difficult, however, to completely exclude a low-level or underlying myelodysplastic component of cells that could persist and cloud the analysis. Testing of a patient's parents could be informative, but a negative result dies not exclude a de novo mutation arising in the proband. NGS yields information about the frequency with which different alleles are detected. Thus, a germline mutation is expected to show a frequency of approximately 50%. In practice, however, it is often difficult to rely on the detected allele frequency, which is altered by the relative concentration of tumor cells; the presence of additional genetic alterations within the tumor cells, such as loss of heterozygosity; and technical factors that may lead to preferential detection of one allele over another.

For all these reasons, sequencing analysis of cultured fibroblasts is the gold standard method for establishing the germline status of an allele in the setting of a myeloid neoplasm. In the authors' experience, however, this remains a challenging endeavor.[5] Although some laboratories certified under the Clinical Laboratory Improvement Amendments of 1988 (in particular those with capabilities for cytogenetic analysis) are capable of the necessary cell culture, many laboratories lack this ability and it remains far from routine. Furthermore, the turn-around time for cell cultures may be rather long, approximately weeks. Finally, clinical colleagues may express some resistance at the prospect of subjecting a patient to a skin biopsy procedure for the sole purpose of this analysis.

WHAT ARE THE REMAINING CHALLENGES RELATED TO THIS NEW PROVISIONAL WORLD HEALTH ORGANIZATION CATEGORY?

Although the addition of this new provisional WHO category is intended to systematize the approach to familial myeloid neoplasms, the emphasis on clinical genetics ties this new diagnostic area to certain inherent challenges. For example, one area of difficulty in the era of NGS is the detection of variants of uncertain significance – that is, rare or unique sequence changes that cannot be reliably linked to pathogenic impact on protein function. The detection of this type of poorly characterized variant within a patient's germline may provide equivocal evidence for inclusion within this disease category. The raw sequencing power of NGS is also a challenge in that more sequencing of more genes tend to lead to the discovery of additional germline mutations that are not accounted for in the static WHO list. In some cases, it will be challenging to link a given novel mutation definitively to the development of a myeloid neoplasm – a process that generally requires a critical aggregation of multiple cohorts to establish an etiologic link. If the mutation in question is rare, aggregating that kind of data may be difficult or, for an isolated individual case, impossible.

The designation of MDS cases as belonging in this category may also gloss over difficulties in diagnosing MDS in the setting of some of these entities. For example, dysmegakaryopoiesis has been observed in carriers of the *ANKRD26* and *ETV6* mutations even in the absence of overt MDS.[21] For this reason the WHO will recommend that these cases not be called neoplastic unless there is additional evidence of neoplasia, such as increased blasts, increasing bone marrow cellularity in the presence of cytopenias, increasing cytopenias, or relevant cytogenetic or additional molecular abnormalities. Similarly, patients with Fanconi anemia may have a clinical course in which fluctuating clonal hematopoiesis precedes the onset of MDS and can be difficult to distinguish from MDS,[30] and somatic clonal *CSF3R* mutations are known to precede by many years the development of overt myeloid neoplasia in patients with severe congenital neutropenia.[31]

In response to many of these challenges, as well as in the general implementation of this new provisional WHO category, close collaboration with clinical geneticists and certified genetic counselors will be essential. These cases are somewhat unusual in the realm of hematopathology, in that proper diagnosis has implications for a patient's entire family.

SUMMARY

With "Myeloid Neoplasms with Germline Predisposition," the WHO classification provisionally extends the scope of relevant genetic information beyond the somatic and into the germline. In the ongoing saga of the convergence between hematopathology and molecular genetics, this is a seminal development. The analysis of these germline mutations in the research and clinical setting has been highly dependent on NGS. As NGS continues to make inroads into standard patient care, it is hoped that this new area of the WHO classification will be a useful rubric for categorizing germline mutations and familial cases of myeloid neoplasms. The added scrutiny brought to bear on these cases may also help to uncover the full extent of familial contribution to the development of myeloid malignancies.

REFERENCES

1. Babushok DV, Bessler M. Genetic predisposition syndromes: when should they be considered in the work-up of MDS? Best Pract Res Clin Haematol 2015;28:55–68.

2. Myelodysplastic syndrome (Version 2.2015). Available at: http://www.nccn.org/professionals/physician_gls/pdf/mds.pdf. Accessed May 15, 2015.

3. Alter BP, Greene MH, Velazquez I, et al. Cancer in Fanconi anemia. Blood 2003;101:2072.

4. Shimamura A, Alter BP. Pathophysiology and management of inherited bone marrow failure syndromes. Blood Rev 2010;24:101–22.

5. Nickels EM, Soodalter J, Churpek JE, et al. Recognizing familial myeloid leukemia in adults. Ther Adv Hematol 2013;4:254–69.

6. Shimada A, Takahashi Y, Muramatsu H, et al. Excellent outcome of allogeneic bone marrow transplantation for Fanconi anemia using fludarabine-based reduced-intensity conditioning regimen. Int J Hematol 2012;95:675–9.

7. Zierhut H, MacMillan ML, Wagner JE, et al. More than 10 years after the first 'savior siblings': parental experiences surrounding preimplantation genetic diagnosis. J Genet Couns 2013;22:594–602.

8. Stelljes M, Corbacioglu A, Schlenk RF, et al. Allogeneic stem cell transplant to eliminate germline mutations in the gene for CCAAT-enhancer-binding protein alpha from hematopoietic cells in a family with AML. Leukemia 2011;25:1209–10.

9. MacMillan ML, Wagner JE. Haematopoeitic cell transplantation for Fanconi anaemia - when and how? Br J Haematol 2010;149:14–21.

10. Bhatla D, Davies SM, Shenoy S, et al. Reduced-intensity conditioning is effective and safe for transplantation of patients with Shwachman-Diamond syndrome. Bone Marrow Transplant 2008;42:159–65.

11. Pabst T, Eyholzer M, Fos J, et al. Heterogeneity within AML with CEBPA mutations; only CEBPA double mutations, but not single CEBPA mutations are associated with favourable prognosis. Br J Cancer 2009;100:1343–6.

12. Pabst T, Eyholzer M, Haefliger S, et al. Somatic CEBPA mutations are a frequent second event in families with germline CEBPA mutations and familial acute myeloid leukemia. J Clin Oncol 2008;26:5088–93.

13. Taskesen E, Bullinger L, Corbacioglu A, et al. Prognostic impact, concurrent genetic mutations, and gene expression features of AML with CEBPA mutations in a cohort of 1182 cytogenetically normal AML patients: further evidence for CEBPA double mutant AML as a distinctive disease entity. Blood 2011;117:2469–75.

14. Tawana K, Wang J, Renneville A, et al. Disease evolution and outcomes in familial AML with germline CEBPA mutations. Blood 2015;126(10):1214–23.

15. West AH, Godley LA, Churpek JE. Familial myelodysplastic syndrome/acute leukemia syndromes: a review and utility for translational investigations. Ann N Y Acad Sci 2014;1310:111–8.

16. Cho YU, Jang S, Seo EJ, et al. Preferential occurrence of spliceosome mutations in acute myeloid leukemia with preceding myelodysplastic syndrome and/or myelodysplasia morphology. Leuk Lymphoma 2015;56:2301–8.

17. Polprasert C, Schulze I, Sekeres MA, et al. Inherited and somatic defects in DDX41 in myeloid neoplasms. Cancer Cell 2015;27:658–70.

18. Owen CJ, Toze CL, Koochin A, et al. Five new pedigrees with inherited RUNX1 mutations causing familial platelet disorder with propensity to myeloid malignancy. Blood 2008;112:4639–45.

19. Godley LA. Inherited predisposition to acute myeloid leukemia. Semin Hematol 2014;51:306–21.

20. Preudhomme C, Renneville A, Bourdon V, et al. High frequency of RUNX1 biallelic alteration in acute myeloid leukemia secondary to familial platelet disorder. Blood 2009;113:5583–7.

21. Noris P, Perrotta S, Seri M, et al. Mutations in ANKRD26 are responsible for a frequent form of inherited thrombocytopenia: analysis of 78 patients from 21 families. Blood 2011;117:6673–80.

22. Pippucci T, Savoia A, Perrotta S, et al. Mutations in the 5' UTR of ANKRD26, the ankirin repeat domain 26 gene, cause an autosomal-dominant form of inherited thrombocytopenia, THC2. Am J Hum Genet 2011;88:115–20.

23. Noris P, Favier R, Alessi MC, et al. ANKRD26-related thrombocytopenia and myeloid malignancies. Blood 2013;122:1987–9.

24. Perez Botero J, Oliveira JL, Chen D, et al. ASXL1 mutated chronic myelomonocytic leukemia in a patient with familial thrombocytopenia secondary to germline mutation in ANKRD26. Blood Cancer J 2015;5:e315.

25. Zhang MY, Churpek JE, Keel SB, et al. Germline ETV6 mutations in familial thrombocytopenia and hematologic malignancy. Nat Genet 2015;47:180–5.

26. Haferlach C, Bacher U, Schnittger S, et al. ETV6 rearrangements are recurrent in myeloid malignancies and are frequently associated with other genetic events. Genes Chromosomes Cancer 2012;51:328–37.

27. Collin M, Dickinson R, Bigley V. Haematopoietic and immune defects associated with GATA2 mutation. Br J Haematol 2015;169:173–87.

28. Kirwan M, Walne AJ, Plagnol V, et al. Exome sequencing identifies autosomal-dominant SRP72 mutations associated with familial aplasia and myelodysplasia. Am J Hum Genet 2012;90: 888–92.

29. Churpek JE, Lorenz R, Nedumgottil S, et al. Proposal for the clinical detection and management of patients and their family members with familial myelodysplastic syndrome/acute leukemia predisposition syndromes. Leuk Lymphoma 2013;54: 28–35.

30. Alter BP, Scalise A, McCombs J, et al. Clonal chromosomal abnormalities in Fanconi's anaemia: what do they really mean? Br J Haematol 1993;85:627–30.

31. Beekman R, Valkhof MG, Sanders MA, et al. Sequential gain of mutations in severe congenital neutropenia progressing to acute myeloid leukemia. Blood 2012;119:5071–7.

32. Triot A, Jarvinen PM, Arostegui JI, et al. Inherited biallelic CSF3R mutations in severe congenital neutropenia. Blood 2014;123:3811–7.

33. Hauck F, Klein C. Pathogenic mechanisms and clinical implications of congenital neutropenia syndromes. Curr Opin Allergy Clin Immunol 2013;13: 596–606.

Therapy Effect
Impact on Bone Marrow Morphology

K. David Li, MD, Mohamed E. Salama, MD*

KEYWORDS

• Bone marrow • Post-therapy and treatment effects • Hematologic malignancies

ABSTRACT

This article highlights the most common morphologic features identified in the bone marrow after chemotherapy for hematologic malignancies, growth-stimulating agents, and specific targeted therapies. The key is to be aware of these changes while reviewing post-therapeutic bone marrow biopsies and to not mistake reactive patterns for neoplastic processes. In addition, given the development and prevalent use of targeted therapy, such as tyrosine kinase inhibitors and immune modulators, knowledge of drug-specific morphologic changes is required for proper bone marrow interpretation and diagnosis.

OVERVIEW

This article highlights the morphologic changes in the bone marrow associated with various treatment modalities for hematologic malignancies. Because some of the morphologic findings can mimic residual disease or malignant neoplasms, pathologists must be aware of the distinguishing features between reactive and residual neoplastic processes. It is common to see a spectrum of morphologic changes in the bone marrow, and they are dependent on the type of therapy and/or the time frame in which a biopsy is performed. After an initial diagnostic bone marrow biopsy, the purpose of the subsequent biopsies is usually to assess residual disease, therapeutic efficacy, and/or marrow regeneration. Occasionally, there might be a change in a patient's clinical status or laboratory results, which also prompts a bone marrow biopsy to evaluate disease relapse. Knowledge of clinical history, including concurrent drug therapy in addition to chemotherapy, is the most important piece of information that can aid in the diagnostic process. This article reviews the most common bone marrow and/or peripheral blood findings associated with traditional therapy for hematologic malignancies and presents additional findings that have become important to recognize given the development and use of newer treatment modalities, including immune modulators and tyrosine kinase inhibitors. Morphologic changes that occur in the bone marrow after hematopoietic stem cell transplant are not included.

BONE MARROW POST MYELOABLATION

The most common traditional treatment modality for hematologic malignancies, especially in the setting of acute leukemias, is myeloablative chemotherapy. The intent of this systemic therapy is to eliminate the neoplastic population; however, it also indiscriminately destroys all proliferating normal hematopoietic elements.[1–3] Depending on the time in which the bone marrow biopsy is performed, a wide spectrum of morphologic changes can be seen. Some of these changes, subdivided into early and late, are presented in **Box 1** and demonstrated in **Figs. 1–6**.

FIBROSIS

Bone marrow fibrosis can be associated with a wide variety of malignant diseases, including leukemia, lymphoma, myeloid neoplasms, and metastatic carcinoma. It can also be seen in a postinduction chemotherapy bone marrow biopsy, most commonly in the form of mild reticulin fibrosis.[4] This fibrosis usually disappears or decreases after the treatment of the primary

Disclosure Statement: The authors have nothing to disclose.
Hematopathology, Department of Pathology, University of Utah/ARUP Laboratories, 500 Chipeta Way, 115-G04, Salt Lake City, UT 84108, USA
* Corresponding author.
E-mail address: mohamed.salama@path.utah.edu

Surgical Pathology 9 (2016) 177–187
http://dx.doi.org/10.1016/j.path.2015.09.006

surgpath.theclinics.com

> **Box 1**
> **Morphologic changes associated with myeloablative therapy**
>
> *Early*
> - Prominent necrosis
> - Edema
> - Dilated sinuses
> - Marrow aplasia
> - Residual histiocytes, stromal cells, and plasma cells
> - Mild reticulin fibrosis
>
> *Late*
> - Increased lobulated fat cells
> - Foci of immature myeloid and erythroid precursors
> - Gradual return of megakaryocytes
> - Resolution of reticulin fibrosis
> - Restoration of marrow cellularity

disorder.[5] It is important to be aware of this finding, especially in a patient with prior history of myeloproliferative neoplasm, and to not characterize the fibrosis as residual disease (**Figs. 7** and **8**).

NECROSIS

Bone marrow necrosis is most commonly associated with marrow involvement by malignancy, such as leukemias, non-Hodgkin and Hodgkin lymphomas, and metastatic carcinoma.[6] It is also common to see marrow necrosis after induction chemotherapy. Post-therapy marrow necrosis is usually characterized by complete replacement by so-called ghost cells with pyknotic nuclei and degenerative cytoplasm. Bone marrow aspirate smear may show an abundance of nonviable stripped nuclei. Depending on the time of the post-therapeutic biopsy, the bone marrow may show areas of normal regeneration or fibrosis. It is also important to exclude or document areas of residual viable tumor (**Fig. 9**).

SEROUS ATROPHY

Also known as gelatinous transformation, serous atrophy is characterized by increased gelatinous

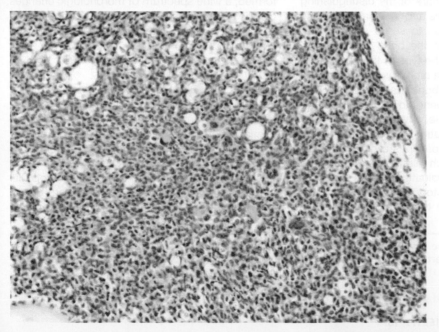

Fig. 1. Diagnostic bone marrow biopsy from a patient with AML demonstrating near 100% cellular marrow composed of mainly myeloid blasts (hematoxylin-eosin ×20).

Fig. 2. Same patient as in Fig. 1. Bone marrow biopsy from postinduction day 14 demonstrating an aplastic marrow with rare residual plasma cells and stromal cells (hematoxylin-eosin ×20).

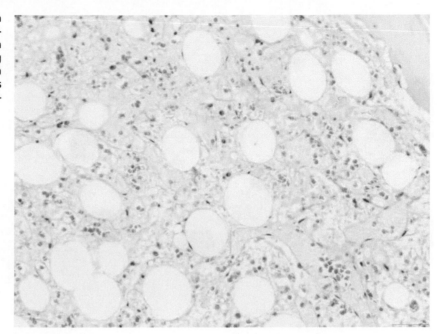

extracellular material with fat atrophy and marrow hypoplasia, which is commonly associated with starvation and cachexia. The morphologic changes seen after myeloablative therapy,[7,8] including edema and deposition of fibrin, may mimic serous atrophy but are an uncommon finding. The edema and fibrin deposition are transient and should resolve over time.

GROWTH FACTORS AND CYTOKINE EFFECTS

Growth factors, such as granulocyte colony-stimulating factor (G-CSF) and granulocyte-macrophage colony-stimulating factor (GM-CSF), are commonly administered for enhancing marrow recovery after chemotherapy and for priming the marrow or peripheral blood before stem cell

Fig. 3. Bone marrow biopsy from postinduction day 21 in a patient with AML. In addition to the aplastic appearing marrow and serous atrophy, there is residual disease with focal areas of residual myeloid blasts (*center*) (hematoxylin-eosin ×20).

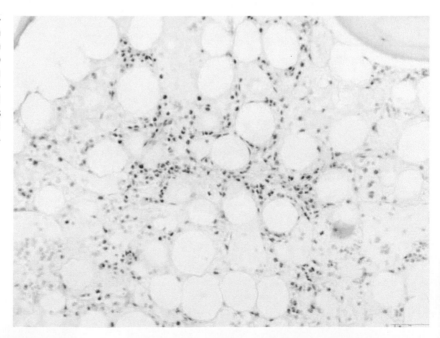

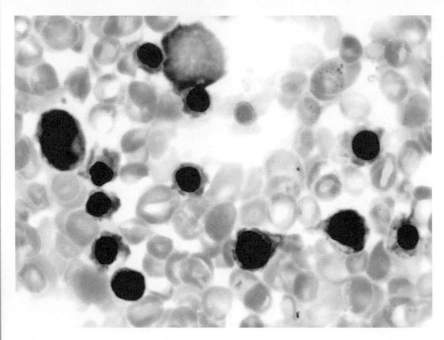

Fig. 4. Aspirate smear from postinduction bone marrow biopsy demonstrating erythroid regeneration with mild dyserythropoiesis (Wright's stain ×100).

collection.[9] Both agents can cause a peripheral blood leukocytosis with a granulocytic left shift and may give the appearance of a reactive proliferation with the presence of toxic granulation and Döhle bodies.[10–12] The granulocytic left shift often includes a transient increase in myeloblasts, rarely exceeding 5%.[13] The excess myeloblasts due to growth factors are usually associated with a high number of promyelocytes; therefore, increased blasts without increased promyelocytes are suspicious for residual disease. It may not always be possible, however, to distinguish residual disease versus growth factor effect; other ancillary results, such as prior immunophenotype and cytogenetics, can be helpful in this setting.[14] The bone marrow typically shows myeloid hyperplasia with

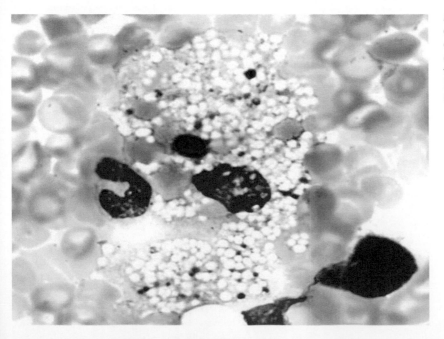

Fig. 5. Vacuolated histiocytes with phagotized cellular debris are commonly seen in patients undergoing myeloablative chemotherapy (Wright's stain ×100).

Fig. 6. Bone marrow biopsy from a patient post consolidation, 5 months after diagnosis, showing regenerated trilineage hematopoiesis (hematoxylin-eosin ×20).

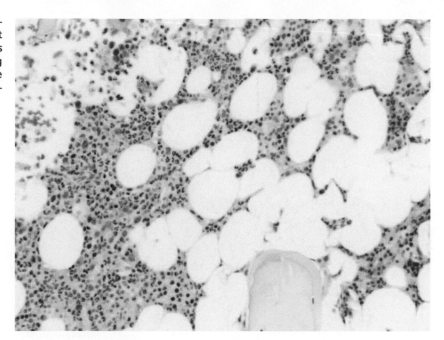

a left shift. Changes in myeloid precursors include increase in size and toxic granulation. Other morphologic findings secondary to growth factors include necrosis and histiocytosis (**Figs. 10** and **11**).

Interleukin (IL)-2 and IL-3 are agents that also stimulate the production of granulocytes.[15] In particular, IL-3 infusion may result in eosinophilia.[16]

Erythropoietin is given to increase marrow red cell precursors usually in patients with various causes of red cell aplasia.[17] The increase results in decreased myeloid:erythroid (M:E) ratio and may show mild dysplastic changes. This should not be confused with myelodysplasia because there are usually dysplastic changes in other lineages as well.

Fig. 7. Bone marrow biopsy with postinduction mild fibrosis. Note the islands of regenerating erythroid precursors (*lower middle*) (hematoxylin-eosin ×20).

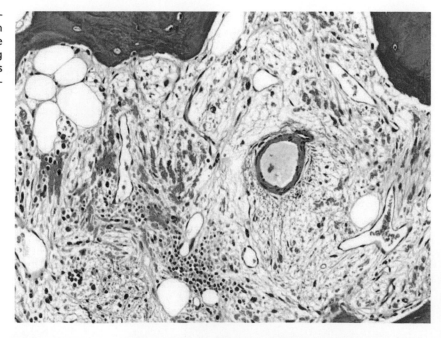

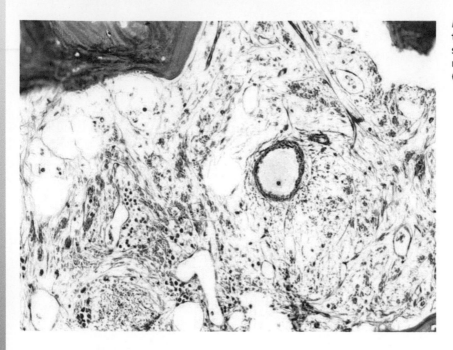

Fig. 8. Reticulin stain of the biopsy from *Fig.* 7 showing very mild to minimal reticulin fibrosis (×20).

Thrombopoietin is usually administered in combination with other growth factors to stimulate platelet production after bone marrow suppression. The peripheral blood typically shows thrombocytosis and the bone marrow is hypercellular with megakaryocytic hyperplasia. Similar to erythroid dysplastic changes associated with erythropoietin therapy, thrombopoietin can also cause dysplastic changes in megakaryocytes, including hypolobate and hyperlobate forms. Dysplastic changes are usually absent, however, in other lineages. The differential diagnosis can include MDS and myeloproliferative neoplasms.[18] Clinical history and other morphologic findings are important for distinguishing these entities (**Table 1**).

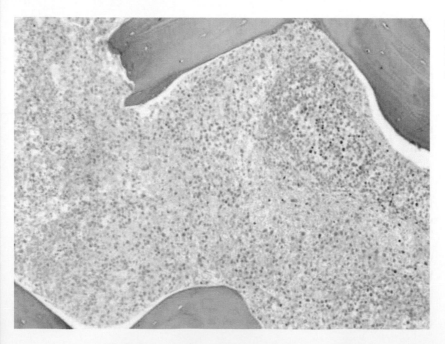

Fig. 9. A mostly necrotic bone marrow core from postinduction day 14 in a patient with AML (hematoxylin-eosin ×20).

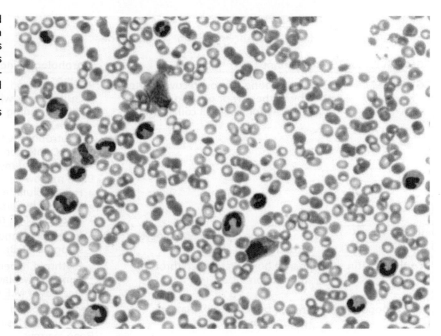

Fig. 10. Peripheral blood smear from a patient on G-CSF therapy 30 days post induction. There is a granulocytic leukocytosis with left shift and occasional toxic granulation and Döhle bodies (Wright's stain ×40).

EFFECT OF SPECIFIC THERAPEUTIC AGENTS

The morphologic changes associated with specific therapeutic agents used in the hematology are discussed. Although the findings associated with all known drugs cannot be elucidated, the most commonly used therapeutic agents are focused on and the most clinically relevant elements highlighted.

IMATINIB

The hallmark of chronic myeloid leukemia (CML) is the Philadelphia chromosome that arises from a reciprocal translocation between chromosomes 9 and 22. The bone marrow cellularity typically is increased in the chronic phase of CML due to granulocytic proliferation with a maturation pattern similar to those often noted in the peripheral blood

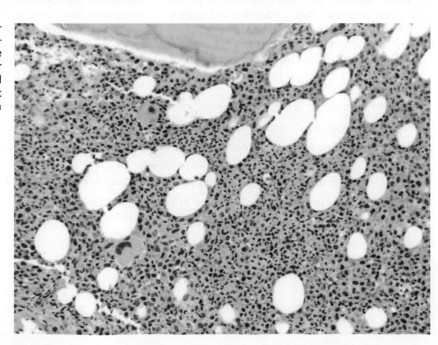

Fig. 11. Bone marrow biopsy from the same patient as in Fig. 10. The marrow is hypercellular with relative myeloid predominance and left shift (hematoxylin-eosin ×20).

Table 1
Common growth factors with associated morphologic changes

Growth Factors	Indications	Morphologic Findings
G-CSF/GM-CSF	Enhance bone marrow recovery after chemotherapy or priming bone marrow for stem cell collection	Peripheral blood • Leukocytosis with neutrophilic left shift including increased myeloblasts (<5%) • Neutrophils with toxic granulation and Döhle bodies • Spectrum of myeloid precursors Bone marrow • Hypercellular marrow • Myeloid hyperplasia with left shift • Increased M:E ratio
IL-2/3	Enhance bone marrow granulocyte production	• Increased granulocytes including eosinophils (IL-3).
Erythropoietin	Enhance bone marrow erythroid production	• Erythroid hyperplasia with mild to minimal dysplasia • Decreased M:E ratio
Thrombopoietin	Enhance bone marrow platelet production	Peripheral blood • Thrombocytosis Bone marrow • Hypercellular marrow with increased megakaryocytes • Mild to minimal dysmegakaryopoiesis

with bulge in the myelocytes and neutrophils. The bone marrow shows characteristically hypolobate and small megakaryocytes. M:E ratio is often increased and ranges from 3.5 to 16,[19] with variable basophils and frequently identified sea-blue histiocytes.[20] Imatinib mesylate (Gleevec, Novartis, East Hanover, NJ) was discovered in the 1990s and is shown highly effective in blocking ABL tyrosine kinase in the leukemic cells in CML.[21] A spectrum of bone marrow histopathologic changes (Box 2) that correlates with a decreased percentage of BCR-ABL–positive cells have been reported in patients with CML treated with imatinib mesylate. Several new tyrosine kinase inhibitors with improved survival in CML are increasingly in use.

A decrease in bone marrow cellularity and decreased myelopoiesis is often observed in patients who show initial favorable response to therapy regardless of the persistence of BCR-ABL fusion signal by fluorescence in situ hybridization (FISH) at 3- to 9-month follow up.[19] The decrease

Box 2
Morphologic changes associated with imatinib therapy

- Reduction in bone marrow cellularity, often first evident in 3 months even in those with no molecular response

- Prominent decreases in myeloid proliferation with M:E ratios of 2 or less at 3 months

- Megakaryocytes appearing normal, often at 18 to 24 months

- Basophilia disappear, often at 18 to 24 months

- Reticulin fibrosis decreased

- Sea-blue histiocytes prominent in patients who retained BCR-ABL

- Osteosclerosis

- Less commonly described changes: gelatinous transformation, bone marrow aplasia, and variable increase in bone marrow lymphocytes in marrow cellularity corresponded, however, to the decrease in FISH fusion signals. It is difficult to predict recurrence based on histopathologic findings alone in the few months after initiation of therapy. Patients who retained evidence of the BCR-ABL fusion by FISH, however, ultimately regained morphologic evidence of CML because cellularity increased after the nadir biopsy.[19]

Sea-blue histiocytes were prominent in many of the patients receiving imatinib mesylate, in particular those who continued to exhibit t(9;22).[19] A reduction in arrow fibrosis in CML cases treated with imatinib mesylate has been reported[22]; however, it was also proposed that imatinib mesylate possibly could contribute to reduction in marrow fibrosis even in cases in which the malignant clone is not eradicated.[19] Imatinib therapy can alter trabecular bone in bone marrow biopsy specimens of CML patients, most often resulting in an increase in trabecular volume.[23]

LENALIDOMIDE

Lenalidomide is an immunomodulatory agent with anti-inflammatory and antiangiogenic effect and have been used to treat myelodysplastic syndrome (MDS) and multiple myeloma. Thalidomide and pomalidomide are also included in the same family of immunomodulatory agents.

Lenalidomide has been used in the management of patients with low-risk MDSs who have no response to conventional therapy.

The morphologic effects of lenalidomide in del (5q) MDS patient bone marrow after 24 weeks of treatment include[24–26]

- Complete resolution of cytologic dysplasia in all hematopoietic lineages noted in approximately one-third of patients
- Myeloblasts in the marrow returned to less than 5% in patients with excess myeloblasts
- Ringed sideroblasts decreased in patients who had refractory anemia with ringed sideroblasts
- Possible progression to a more advanced type of MDS or acute myeloid leukemia.
- Although rare, aplastic anemia developing secondary to treatment of lenalidomide that could be reversible after its discontinuation.[24]
- Neutropenia and thrombocytopenia as common side effects that often result in lenalidomide discontinuation

Lenalidomide maintenance given after autologous stem cell transplant in newly diagnosed multiple myeloma patients resulted in significant prolongation of the progression-free survival; however, concern for the development of MDS/AML

was observed in some trials.[25] Monaghan and colleagues[25] performed longitudinal bone marrow evaluations for myelodysplasia in 40 myeloma patients before and after treatment with lenalidomide and only 1 patient developed MDS. Mild dysplasia (<10%) predominantly affecting megakaryocytes was present predominantly in relapsed/refractory patients. Mild dyserythropoiesis was noted transiently in up to 50% of cases with monotherapy of lenalidomide. Ring sideroblasts were seen in only 1 patient who developed MDS. No significant dysgranulopoiesis was observed; however, a trend of slight shift to more immature granulocytic precursors, including promyelocytes and myelocytes, after 3 to 4 cycles compared with their pretreatment specimens was noted.

Lenalidomide was also used to treat acute myelofibrosis. In a case report of morphologic changes noted after 32 month of continuous lenalidomide treatment, the patient peripheral counts improved with normalization of the white blood cells and her bone marrow biopsy showed a patchy distribution of fibrosis with areas of normal cellularity and morphology; however, clustering of the abnormal megakaryocytes could be observed in the bone marrow. The erythroid precursors showed dysplastic features, whereas, in the myeloid compartment, a marginally elevated number of immature cells were not seen.[27]

RITUXIMAB

Rituximab is a genetically engineered chimeric murine/human monoclonal IgG1 kappa antibody directed against the CD20 antigen and is widely used as immunotherapy often along with conventional chemotherapy in the treatment of various B-cell non-Hodgkin lymphomas.[28] Given the frequent utilization of rituximab, pathologists must be aware of possible bone marrow changes often noted in treated patients.

After rituximab treatment

1. Bone marrow may exhibit lymphoid foci that mimic original lymphoma but are likely composed only of T cells. Immunohistochemistry for T-cell (eg, CD3) and B-cell markers (other than CD20) confirm the impression.
2. Bone marrow or lymph node may show persistent or recurrent disease composed of CD20-negative clone or the result of CD20-blocked epitope (rituximab effect); thus, other B-cell markers, such as CD79a, CD22, and PAX5, should be used to confirm disease.
3. Peripheral blood is depleted from B cells for 2 to 3 months with recovery lasting from 3 to 9 months.

4. Substantial reduction of B-cell compartments occurs in lymph nodes and spleen as soon as 1 month after administration with as few as 3 doses.[29]
5. Neutropenia and thrombocytopenia as well as a picture that could mimic disseminated intravascular coagulation have been reported.

INTERFERON

Interferon therapy has been used in combination with conventional chemotherapy to treat hematologic malignancies, including leukemia and lymphomas. Limited studies reported the morphologic bone marrow changes after the use of interferon-alpha primarily in CML.

The morphologic changes associated with interferon alfa therapy[30]:

- Cellularity decrease
- Regeneration of erythroid precursors for at least 6 months
- Increase in megakaryopoiesis
- Increase in the macrophage population
- Increase in reticulin fibers

REFERENCES

1. Islam A, Catovsky D, Galton DA, et al. Histological study of bone marrow regeneration following chemotherapy for acute myeloid leukaemia and chronic granulocytic leukaemia in blast transformation. Br J Haematol 1980;45:535–40.
2. Wittels B. Bone marrow biopsy changes following chemotherapy for acute leukemia. Am J Surg Pathol 1980;4:135–42.
3. Wilkins BS, Bostanci AG, Ryan MF, et al. Haemopoietic regrowth after chemotherapy for acute leukaemia: an immunohistochemical study of bone marrow trephine biopsy specimens. J Clin Pathol 1993;46:915–21.
4. McCarthy DM. Annotation. Fibrosis of the bone marrow: content and causes. Br J Haematol 1985; 59:1–7.
5. Islam A, Catovsky D, Goldman JM, et al. Bone marrow fibre content in acute myeloid leukaemia before and after treatment. J Clin Pathol 1984;37: 1259–63.
6. Janssens AM, Offner FC, Van Hove WZ, et al. Bone marrow necrosis. Cancer 2000;88:1769–80.
7. Seaman JP, Kjeldsberg CR, Linker A, et al. Gelatinous transformation of the bone marrow. Hum Pathol 1978;9:685–92.
8. Feng CS. A variant of gelatinous transformation of marrow in leukemic patients post-chemotherapy. Pathology 1993;25:294–6.
9. Armitage JO. Emerging applications of recombinant human granulocyte-macrophage colony-stimulating factor. Blood 1998;92:4491–508.
10. Kerrigan DP, Castillo A, Foucar K, et al. Peripheral blood morphologic changes after high-dose antineoplastic chemotherapy and recombinant human granulocyte colony-stimulating factor administration. Am J Clin Pathol 1989;92:280–5.
11. Ryder JW, Lazarus HM, Farhi DC, et al. Bone marrow and blood findings after marrow transplantation and rhGM-CSF therapy. Am J Clin Pathol 1992; 97:631–7.
12. Schmitz LL, McClure JS, Litz CE, et al. Morphologic and quantitative changes in blood and marrow cells following growth factor therapy. Am J Clin Pathol 1994;101:67–75.
13. Meyerson HJ, Farhi DC, Rosenthal NS, et al. Transient increase in blasts mimicking acute leukemia and progressing myelodysplasia in patients receiving growth factor. Am J Clin Pathol 1998;109: 675–81.
14. Harris AC, Todd WM, Hackney MH, et al. Bone marrow changes associated with recombinant granulocyte-macrophage and granulocyte colony-stimulating factors. Discrimination of granulocytic regeneration. Arch Pathol Lab Med 1994;118:624–9.
15. Heslop HE, Duncombe AS, Reittie JE, et al. Interleukin 2 infusion induces haemopoietic growth factors and modifies marrow regeneration after chemotherapy or autologous marrow transplantation. Br J Haematol 1991;77:237–44.
16. Falk S, Seipelt G, Ganser A, et al. Bone marrow findings after treatment with recombinant human interleukin-3. Am J Clin Pathol 1991;95:355–62.
17. Ahn JH, Yoon KS, Lee WI, et al. Bone marrow findings before and after treatment with recombinant human erythropoietin in chronic hemodialyzed patients. Clin Nephrol 1995;43:189–95.
18. Douglas VK, Tallman MS, Cripe LD, et al. Thrombopoietin administered during induction chemotherapy to patients with acute myeloid leukemia induces transient morphologic changes that may resemble chronic myeloproliferative disorders. Am J Clin Pathol 2002;117:844–50.
19. Frater JL, Tallman MS, Variakojis D, et al. Chronic myeloid leukemia following therapy with imatinib mesylate (Gleevec). Bone marrow histopathology and correlation with genetic status. Am J Clin Pathol 2003;119:833–41.
20. Kelsey PR, Geary CG. Sea-blue histiocytes and Gaucher cells in bone marrow of patients with chronic myeloid leukaemia. J Clin Pathol 1988;41: 960–2.
21. Druker BJ, Tamura S, Buchdunger E, et al. Effects of a selective inhibitor of the Abl tyrosine kinase on the growth of Bcr-Abl positive cells. Nat Med 1996;2: 561–6.

22. Beham-Schmid C, Apfelbeck U, Sill H, et al. Treatment of chronic myelogenous leukemia with the tyrosine kinase inhibitor STI571 results in marked regression of bone marrow fibrosis. Blood 2002;99: 381–3.

23. Hoehn D, Medeiros LJ, Kantarjian HM, et al. Digital image analysis as a tool to assess the effects of imatinib on trabecular bone in patients with chronic myelogenous leukemia. Hum Pathol 2012;43: 2354–9.

24. Dasanu CA, Alexandrescu DT. A case of severe aplastic anemia secondary to treatment with lenalidomide for multiple myeloma. Eur J Haematol 2009;82:231–4.

25. Monaghan SA, Dai L, Mapara MY, et al. Longitudinal bone marrow evaluations for myelodysplasia in patients with myeloma before and after treatment with lenalidomide. Leuk Lymphoma 2013;54:1965–74.

26. List A, Dewald G, Bennett J, et al. Myelodysplastic Syndrome-003 Study Investigators. Lenalidomide in the myelodysplastic syndrome with chromosome 5q deletion. N Engl J Med 2006;355(14):1456–65.

27. Vassilopoulos G, Palassopoulou M, Zisaki K, et al. Successful control of acute myelofibrosis with lenalidomide. Case Rep Med 2010;2010:421239.

28. Prichard M, Harris T, Williams ME, et al. Treatment strategies for relapsed and refractory aggressive non-Hodgkin's lymphoma. Expert Opin Pharmacother 2009;10:983–95.

29. Cioc AM, Vanderwerf SM, Peterson BA, et al. Rituximab-induced changes in hematolymphoid tissues found at autopsy. Am J Clin Pathol 2008;130: 604–12.

30. Thiele J, Kvasnicka HM, Schmitt-Graeff A, et al. Effects of chemotherapy (busulfan-hydroxyurea) and interferon-alfa on bone marrow morphologic features in chronic myelogenous leukemia. Histochemical and morphometric study on sequential trephine biopsy specimens with special emphasis on dynamic features. Am J Clin Pathol 2000;114:57–65.

Printed and bound by CPI Group (UK) Ltd, Croydon, CR0 4YY

03/10/2024

01040377-0020